Controversies in Rhinoplasty

Editors

ROXANA COBO
FRED G. FEDOK

FACIAL PLASTIC SURGERY CLINICS OF NORTH AMERICA

www.facialplastic.theclinics.com

Consulting Editor
ANTHONY P. SCLAFANI

November 2024 • Volume 32 • Number 4

ELSEVIER

1600 John F. Kennedy Boulevard • Suite 1800 • Philadelphia, Pennsylvania, 19103-2899

http://www.theclinics.com

FACIAL PLASTIC SURGERY CLINICS OF NORTH AMERICA Volume 32, Number 4
November 2024 ISSN 1064-7406, ISBN-13: 978-0-443-29310-8

Editor: Stacy Eastman
Developmental Editor: Malvika Shah

Facial Plastic Surgery Clinics of North America (ISSN 1064-7406) is published quarterly by Elsevier Inc., 360 Park Avenue South, New York, NY 10010-1710. Months of issue are February, May, August, and November. Business and Editorial Offices: 1600 John F. Kennedy Blvd., Suite 1800, Philadelphia, PA 19103-2899. Periodicals postage paid at New York, NY, and additional mailing offices. Subscription prices are $432.00 per year (US individuals), $487.00 per year (Canadian individuals), $579.00 per year (foreign individuals), $100.00 per year (US students), $100.00 per year (Canadian students), and $255.00 per year (foreign students). For institutional access pricing please contact Customer Service via the contact information below. Foreign air speed delivery is included in all *Clinics* subscription prices. All prices are subject to change without notice. Orders, claims, and journal inquiries: Please visit our Support Hub page https://service.elsevier.com for assistance.

Reprints. For copies of 100 or more of articles in this publication, please contact the Commercial Reprints Department, Elsevier Inc., 360 Park Avenue South, New York, NY 10010-1710. Tel.: 212-633-3874; Fax: 212-633-3820; E-mail: reprints@elsevier.com.

Facial Plastic Surgery Clinics of North America is covered in *MEDLINE/PubMed* (*Index Medicus*).

Contributors

CONSULTING EDITOR

ANTHONY P. SCLAFANI, MD, MBA, FACS
Director of Facial Plastic Surgery
Professor of Otolaryngology - Head & Neck
Surgery, Weill Cornell Medical College New
York, NY

EDITORS

ROXANA COBO, MD
Private Practice, Facial Plastic Surgery,
Service of Otolaryngology, Chief, Department
of Otolaryngology, Clinica Imbanaco, Cali,
Colombia

FRED G. FEDOK, MD, FACS
Adjunct Professor, Department of Surgery,
University of South Alabama, Mobile, Alabama,
USA; Fedok Plastic Surgery, Foley, Alabama,
USA

AUTHORS

SYDNEY C. BUTTS, MD, FACS
Interim Chair and Associate Professor, Chief,
Facial Plastic and Reconstructive Surgery,
SUNY Downstate Health Sciences University
Brooklyn, New York, USA

NAZIM CERKES, MD
Plastic Surgeon, Owner, Cosmed Plastic
Surgery, Istanbul

ROXANA COBO, MD
Private Practice, Facial Plastic Surgery,
Service of Otolaryngology, Chief, Department
of Otolaryngology, Clinica Imbanaco, Cali,
Colombia

FRED G. FEDOK, MD, FACS
Adjunct Professor, Department of Surgery,
University of South Alabama, Mobile, Alabama,
USA; Fedok Plastic Surgery, Foley, Alabama,
USA

GEORGE FERZLI, MD
Facial Plastic and Reconstructive Surgeon,
Ferzli Facial Plastic Surgery, New York, New
York, USA

ANNA FRANTS, MD
Facial Plastic and Reconstructive Surgeon,
NassifMD Plastic Surgery, Beverly Hills,
California, USA; Specialty Aesthetic Surgery,
New York, New York, USA

OREN FRIEDMAN, MD
Director, Facial Plastic Surgery,
Otorhinolaryngology Head and Neck Surgery,
University of Pennsylvania Perelman School of
Medicine, Philadelphia, Pennsylvania, USA

OLIVIER GERBAULT, MD
Director, Policlinique Esthetique Marigny
Vincennes, Vincennes, France

ABDÜLKADIR GÖKSEL, MD
Rino Istanbul Facial Plastic Clinic, Istanbul,
Turkey

ALEXANDER E. GRAF, MD
Resident-Physician, Department of
Otolaryngology–Head and Neck Surgery,
SUNY Downstate Health Sciences University,
Brooklyn, New York, USA

BAHMAN GUYURON, MD, FACS
Plastic Surgeon, Zeeba Clinic, Lyndhurst,
Ohio, USA; Emeritus Professor and Past
Chairman of Plastic Surgery, Case School of
Medicine, University Hospitals Case Medical
Center, Cleveland, Ohio, USA

SEBASTIAN HAACK, MD
Department for Facial Plastic Surgery,
Marienhospital Stuttgart, Stuttgart, Germany

GRANT S. HAMILTON III, MD
Associate Professor, Chair, Division of Facial
Plastic and Reconstructive Surgery, Mayo
Clinic, Rochester, Minnesota, USA

WERNER HEPPT, MD
Professor and Head, Department of
Otorhinolaryngology–Head and Neck Surgery,
Facial Plastic Surgery, Klinikum Karlsruhe,
Karlsruhe, Germany

YONG JU JANG, MD
Professor and Department Chair, Department
of Otolaryngology, Asan Medical Center,
University of Ulsan, Songpa-gu, Seoul, Korea

CHIH-WEN "JEREMY" TWU, MD
Clinical Associate Professor, National Defense
University, Taoyuan City, Taipei; Assistant
Professor, National Yang-Ming University,
Hsinchu City, Taipei; Taichung Veterans
General Hospital, Executive Director, Taiwan
Academy of Facial Plastic and Reconstructive
Surgery, Taichung City, Taiwan

IN-SANG KIM, MD, PhD
Faculty, Be and Young Aesthetic Surgery
Clinic, Representative Surgeon, Department of
Otolaryngology and Fascial Plastic Surgery,
Labom Plastic Surgery Clinic, Seoul, Korea

SUN HONG KIM, MD
Surgeon, Otolaryngologist, Be and Young
Aesthetic Surgery Clinic, Seoul, Korea

RUSSELL W.H. KRIDEL, MD
Clinical Professor, Department of
Otolaryngology, University of Texas Medical
Branch, Galveston Texas and Facial Plastic
Surgery Associates, Houston, Texas, USA

GRACE LEE PENG, MD, FACS
Surgeon, Facial Plastic and Reconstructive
Surgery, Beverly Hills, California, USA

BENJAMIN MARCUS, MD
Director of Facial Plastic Surgery, Department
of Surgery, Division of Otolaryngology–Head
and Neck Surgery, University of Wisconsin
School of Medicine and Public Health,
Madison, Wisconsin, USA

DIRK JAN MENGER, MD, PhD
Department of Otorhinolaryngology, Facial
Plastic Surgery, University Medical Center,
Utrecht, The Netherlands

SAM P. MOST, MD
Chief, Division of Facial Plastic and
Reconstructive Surgery, Professor,
Department of Otolaryngology–Head and Neck
Surgery and Surgery (Plastic Surgery),
Director, Fellowship in Facial Plastic and
Reconstructive Surgery, Stanford University
School of Medicine, Stanford, California,
USA

PAUL NASSIF, MD, FACS
Facial Plastic and Reconstructive Surgeon,
NassifMD Plastic Surgery, Beverly Hills,
California, USA; Assistant Clinical Professor,
Department of Otolaryngology–Head and Neck
Surgery, University of Southern California,
Keck School of Medicine, Los Angeles,
California, USA

JOSE CARLOS NEVES, MD
International and European Board Certified in
Facial Plastic and Reconstructive Surgery
(IBCFPRS - EBCFPRS); Otorhinolaryngology,
Head and Neck Surgery Specialist, Facial
Plastic Surgery, MYFACE, Clinic and
Academy, Lisbon, Portugal

IRA D. PAPEL, MD
Fascial Plastic Surgeon, Aesthetic Center at
Woodholme, Owner, Facial Plastic
Surgicenter, Ltd, Baltimore, Maryland,
USA

PRIYESH N. PATEL, MD
Assistant Professor, Division of Facial Plastic
and Reconstructive Surgery, Department of
Otolaryngology, Vanderbilt University Medical
Center, Nashville, Tennessee, USA

LUCAS G. PATROCINIO, MD, PhD
Private Practice, Otoface, Uberlandia Medical
Center, Uberlandia, Minas Gerais, Brazil

STEVEN J. PEARLMAN, MD, FACS
Director, Pearlman Aesthetic Surgery, Clinical
Professor, Department of Otolaryngology–
Head and Neck Surgery, Columbia University,
New York, New York, USA

EMMANUEL RACY, MD
Maxillofacial Surgeon, Maxillofacial
Department, Clinique saint jean de Dieu, Paris,
France

ENRICO ROBOTTI, MD
Private Practice, Bergamo, Italy; President,
Rhinoplasty Society of Europe; Past President,
Italian Society of Plastic Surgery; Past and
Former Chief of Plastic Surgery, Ospedale
Papa Giovanni XXIII, Bergamo, Italy

THOMAS ROMO III, MD, FACS
Director of Facial Plastic and Reconstructive
Surgery, Lenox Hill Hospital and Manhattan
Eye, Ear & Throat Hospital (MEETH)-Northwell
Health Systems, New York, New York, USA

MONICA K. ROSSI MEYER, MD
Clinical Instructor, Fellow, Division of Facial
Plastic and Reconstructive Surgery,
Department of Otolaryngology–Head and Neck
Surgery, Stanford University School of
Medicine, Stanford, California, USA

PARSA P. SALEHI, MD, MHS
Facial Plastic and Reconstructive Surgeon,
SalehiMD Plastic Surgery, Newport Beach,
California, USA; Facial Plastic and
Reconstructive Surgeon, NassifMD Plastic
Surgery, Beverly Hills, California, USA

MARCO SWANSON, MD
Plastic Aesthetic Surgeon, Plastic Surgery,
Dermatology and Plastic Surgery Institute,
Cleveland Clinic, Cleveland Clinic Foundation,
Cleveland, Ohio, USA

JONATHAN SYKES, MD
Professor Emeritus, Facial Plastic Surgery,
University of California, Davis Medical
Center, Davis, California, USA; Sykes Facial
Plastic Surgery, Beverly Hills, California,
USA

EREN TASTAN, MD
ENT, Private Practice, Ankara, Turkey

DEAN M. TORIUMI, MD
Toriumi Facial Plastics, Professor, Department
of Otolaryngology–Head and Neck Surgery,
Rush University Medical School, Chicago,
Illinois, USA

MATTHEW J. URBAN, MD
Fellow Physician in Facial Plastic and
Reconstructive Surgery, The Williams Center
for Plastic Surgery, Latham, New York,
USA

EDWIN F. WILLIAMS, MD, FACS
Fascial Plastic Surgeon and Chief Executive
Officer, The Williams Center for Plastic
Surgery, Latham, New York, USA

BRIAN WONG, MD, PhD
Professor and Vice-Chairman, Department of
Otolaryngology–Head and Neck Surgery,
University of California Irvine, Irvine, California,
USA

VITALY ZHOLTIKOV, MD
Plastic Surgeon in Private Practice, Saint-
Petersburg, Russia

Contents

> The airway must not be ignored in cosmetic rhinoplasty operations, and it is important to address the 4 areas that restrict airflow namely the septum, the turbinates, the mid-vault, and the external nasal valve. Numerous techniques exist that treat these areas without any compromise in esthetic outcome. Techniques include lateral wall suture suspension methods, specialized sutures of the lateral crus, and articulated alar rim grafts.

> Nasal surgery can be carried out safely in the younger patient. In cases of trauma, it is recommended that corrective surgery be carried out in a short time frame before scar contracture, aberrant remodeling, and malunion of structures occurs. In the less common situation of performing cosmetic surgery on the younger patient there are several principles and guidelines to be considered.

> Rhinoplasty in thick skin patients is challenging because the skin soft tissue envelope (S-STE) is more inelastic, and has a tendency for prolonged postsurgical edema, increased dead space formation, and underlying scar tissue formation. Changes in the S-STE will have an impact on how the final rhinoplasty result will look. When performing surgery, approaches should be targeted to the underlying bony-cartilaginous framework and the S-STE to obtain consistent, improved long term results. In this article, 3 experts will be discussing up to date medical, topical, and surgical management key points, as well as diagnostic options and post-operative treatments.

 Video content accompanies this article at http://www.facialplastic.theclinics.com.

> The reshaping of the nasal pyramid has evolved significantly over the past 20 years. Mechanical instruments have been refined to minimize the bone trauma of

osteotomies. However, these instruments can inadvertently cause radiated fractures and comminuted fractures, which compromise bone stability and can create surface defects. Electric and piezoelectric instruments (PEI) have been developed to address these issues. PEI instruments are selective unlike electric instruments. These instruments allow for precise rhinosculpture and osteotomies under direct visual control. The article reviews the advantages and disadvantages of each method by comparing them for the most frequently performed procedures on the nasal bone pyramid in rhinoplasty.

utilized during a primary rhinoplasty when there is insufficient cartilage from the septum or often in revisional nasal surgeries where the initial septal cartilage has previously been used or removed. Rib cartilage carving can be done on a cutting board prior to the beginning of the rhinoplasty in order to allow time for the cartilage to present any warping while it is soaked in saline. Overall autologous rib cartilage is a good source of copious and often good quality cartilage.

Controversies in Preservation Rhinoplasty" explores the nuanced indications, techniques, and challenges in preservation rhinoplasty (PR), featuring contributions from JC Neves, D Toriumi, and A Göksel. Neves recounts his early career under Wilson Dewes and describes the evolution of PR techniques. Toriumi, having started PR in 2019, discusses his initial cautious approach and subsequent expansion to include patients with more diverse nasal deformities. Göksel highlights the critical role of surgical expertise and individualized patient assessment, advocating for methods like dorsum-plasty osteotomies and the Ballerina maneuver to enhance PR's effectiveness.

Structure rhinoplasty and preservation rhinoplasty are 2 popular philosophies that can be used alone or in combination to provide a hybrid approach. Structure rhinoplasty is the leading option for revision rhinoplasty and utilizes cartilage grafting techniques to support and reconstruct the nose. Preservation rhinoplasty spares bone, cartilage, ligaments, and soft tissues to minimize the need for grafting and preserves the favorable features of the nose. Structural preservation rhinoplasty uses dorsal preservation in the upper two-thirds of the nose and structure rhinoplasty in the lower third. This hybrid approach has great utility in primary, revision, and reconstructive rhinoplasty.

 Video content accompanies this article at http://www.facialplastic.theclinics.com.

Reprojecting the severely damaged nose is a challenging operation fraught with pitfalls. This panel discussion covers 6 fundamental questions answered by 3 surgeons, each with decades of experience. Discussion points include management of the 3 components necessary for successful reconstruction—the soft tissue envelope, the support structure, and the internal lining. The authors also discuss how their practices have changed in the last few years.

Alloplastic materials are well suited for use in rhinoplasty in the right clinical scenarios, specifically in patients with platyrrhine noses and in challenging revision cases. The most commonly used materials today are silicone and high-density porous polyethylene. Both implant materials carry a unique set of properties and offer various advantages and disadvantages for use. Complications can be minimized with appropriate utilization of implants and using proper technique.

Rhinoplasty is one of the most popular operations in the world. Despite its popularity, rhinoplasty complications are common and stem from a myriad of issues both subjective and objective in nature. Complications of rhinoplasty include scar, asymmetries, irregularities, imperfections, nasal airway obstruction, skin ischemia or necrosis, nasal collapse, nasal deformity, and overcorrection or undercorrection of a perceived nasal irregularity. A thorough understanding of these potential complications, along with strategies for avoidance and management, is critical for ensuring patient safety and optimizing surgical outcomes.

FACIAL PLASTIC SURGERY CLINICS OF NORTH AMERICA

FACIAL PLASTIC SURGERY CLINICS
OF NORTH AMERICA

FORTHCOMING ISSUES

February 2025
Updates in Head & Neck Microvascular Surgery
Scott H. Troob, Editor

May 2025
Preservation Rhinoplasty
Sam P. Most and Miguel H. Patel, Editors

August 2025
Face and Neck Trauma

Foreword
Controversies in Rhinoplasty

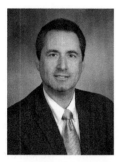

Anthony P. Sclafani, MD, MBA, FACS
Consulting Editor

> *Whenever people agree with me I always feel I must be wrong.*
> —*Oscar Wilde*

"Controversy" is defined as "a discussion marked especially by the expression of opposing views. Synonyms: dispute, quarrel, strife."[1] Drs Fred Fedok and Roxana Cobo have assembled one of the largest groups of contributors to any issue of *Facial Plastic Surgery Clinics of North America* to take on critical topics in rhinoplasty. Each article has been designed to allow experts in rhinoplasty to discuss how they think about specific challenging issues in rhinoplasty, why they use certain techniques and to explain their rationale. While each of these authors strongly believes in their rhinoplasty skills, all discussions were civil, and no surgeons were hurt or injured while preparing these articles. However, the juxtaposition of these experts' opinions can give you, the reader, a deeper understanding of the nuances of rhinoplasty. Whether you fall into one "camp" or another, reading these articles will certainly enhance your understanding and appreciation of the finer points of rhinoplasty.

I am grateful to Drs. Fedok and Cobo, and to the entire Elsevier team in creating this amazing issue, and I am especially grateful to the more than 30 authors who have contributed their time, energy, and expertise to this issue. Enjoy this issue of *Facial Plastic Surgery Clinics of North America*!

> *I think it's counterproductive in many ways to pretend to know things you don't. You surround yourself with people who are the real experts.*
> —*Mario Andretti (referring to race cars, not plastic surgery)*

Anthony P. Sclafani, MD, MBA, FACS
Director of Facial Plastic Surgery
Professor of Otolaryngology-Head & Neck
Surgery
Weill Cornell Medical College
New York, NY

E-mail address:
ans9243@med.cornell.edu

REFERENCE

1. Merriam-Webster. Merriam-Webster.com Dictionary. "Controversy". Available at: https://www.merriam-webster.com/dictionary/controversy. [Accessed 13 July 2024].

Facial Plast Surg Clin N Am 32 (2024) xiii
https://doi.org/10.1016/j.fsc.2024.07.002
1064-7406/24/© 2024 Published by Elsevier Inc.

Preface

Riding the Wave in Rhinoplasty: Changing Paradigms or Embracing Traditional Concepts

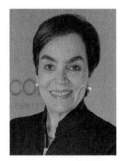 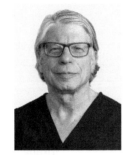

Roxana Cobo, MD   Fred G. Fedok, MD, FACS

Editors

Rhinoplasty has always been a very exciting and prominent part of our practice in the specialty of facial plastic surgery. Its growth and evolution over the years has been achieved through a very creative thought process of many of the leaders in this field.

Techniques have shifted, changed, and evolved. Some have been antagonistic; others have become very popular. We have changed from using endonasal approaches to open or external approaches. From using reductive techniques to structural grafting techniques. Grafting options have shifted from grafting ear conchal cartilage to grafting rib cartilage. Today we are talking about using powered instrumentation like burs, saws, and piezoelectric technology to modify the bony and cartilaginous structures of the nose and septum. Names like Preservation Rhinoplasty, Dorsal Preservation, and Hybrid Structural Preservation Rhinoplasty are becoming increasingly popular.

But despite all these new concepts that have arisen, we have traditional concepts that are still used, are still valid, and have not been changed despite all these developments. And again, like a pendulum, techniques that were being used less, like the endonasal approaches, are becoming popular again. Grafts are being used less by some surgeons and have been replaced by "preservation techniques."

And, of course, we also have all the complications and limitations of these very complex procedures that we still must solve one way or another. The beauty of performing rhinoplasty is that there is not only one solution to the different problems we encounter.

In this very exciting issue, we have grouped some of the very prominent rhinoplasty surgeons from around the world. They are experts, and they do not think alike. This is why this issue is so interesting and engaging. It was designed thinking more of having an open, honest, and

Facial Plast Surg Clin N Am 32 (2024) xv–xvi
https://doi.org/10.1016/j.fsc.2024.07.001
1064-7406/24/© 2024 Published by Elsevier Inc.

updated discussion on varied rhinoplasty topics and the different surgical techniques available today. Questions were designed to promote discussion and offer clear, honest opinions on different techniques being used today. These types of discussions will give readers the chance to immerse themselves in a real panel discussion on the different topics covered.

As editors of this exciting issue, we thank all the authors who participated in this ambitious project. Sharing your expertise and knowledge has been invaluable. We cannot thank you enough for the time spent answering the different questions, explaining your concepts in a precise fashion, and organizing your figures, images, and videos so that the learning experience for readers would be optimal. The Elsevier team did a tremendous job in the compilation of all this information.

We are confident readers will find this an exciting and updated issue that will give everyone a fresh review on many of the important topics in rhinoplasty today. It should be a great learning experience. Enjoy!

Roxana Cobo, MD
International Fellowship in Facial Plastic Surgery -
Face and Nose Institute
Service of Otolaryngology
Clinica Imbanaco
Carrera 38A#5A-100 cons 222A
Cali, Colombia 760044

Fred G. Fedok, MD, FACS
Department of Surgery
University of South Alabama
Mobile, AL, USA

Fedok Plastic Surgery
113 East Fern Avenue
Foley, AL 36535, USA

E-mail addresses:
roxanacobo@gmail.com (R. Cobo)
drfredfedok@me.com (F.G. Fedok)

Cosmetic Rhinoplasty and Nasal Obstruction
What I Look for, How Do I Evaluate the Patient

Brian Wong, MD, PhD[a],*, Werner Heppt, MD[b],
Chih-Wen "Jeremy" Twu, MD[c,d,e]

KEYWORDS

- Functional rhinoplasty • Articulated alar rim grafts • Nasal valve • Nasal obstruction
- Cosmetic rhinoplasty

KEY POINTS

- It is crucial to evaluate patients with cosmetic rhinoplasty for nasal airway obstruction. Cosmetic nasal surgery elements can potentially reduce air space or alter lateral wall mechanical properties.
- A detailed analysis should prioritize the mid-vault and external valve region.
- Turbinate reduction is a critical addition to rhinoplasty surgery, straightforward to perform, and can substantially enhance airflow.
- Grafting and suture techniques play significant roles in establishing nasal airway function and improving cosmetic outcomes.

PANEL DISCUSSION

How do I evaluate the patient?
What surgical techniques do I use to treat the internal nasal valve dysfunction?
What surgical techniques do I use to treat the external nasal valve dysfunction?
In a purely cosmetic rhinoplasty, how do you prevent compromise of nasal function?
How important is the reconstruction of the scroll area in your procedures? Do you do it routinely? What techniques do you use?
How have your cosmetic techniques in this area changed over the last 2 y?

HOW DO I EVALUATE THE PATIENT?
Wong

Each patient completes an intake form, providing a comprehensive medical history and nasal obstruction scoresheet.[1] During examination, I conduct a thorough assessment of the entire head and neck, with particular focus on dynamic valve collapse and nasal endoscopy. The nasal vault is examined both with and without a decongestant, and detailed notes are taken on the geometry of the lower alar cartilages and regions of the septum

[a] Department of Otolaryngology–Head and Neck Surgery, University of California Irvine, 1002 Health Sciences Road East, Irvine, CA 92617, USA; [b] Department of Otorhinolaryngology–Head and Neck Surgery, Facial Plastic Surgery, Klinikum Karlsruhe, Moltkestr. 90, Karlsruhe 76185, Germany; [c] National Defense University, Taipei; [d] National Yang-Ming University, Taipei/; [e] Taichung Veterans General Hospital, Taiwan Academy of Facial Plastic and Reconstructive Surgery
* Corresponding author.
E-mail address: bjwong@uci.edu

Facial Plast Surg Clin N Am 32 (2024) 447–457
https://doi.org/10.1016/j.fsc.2024.06.003

that may restrict airflow. While routine computed tomographic (CT) imaging is not standard practice, it may be selectively ordered for patients undergoing cleft palate rhinoplasty, selected revision procedures, or severe trauma cases. Standardized photography is employed (DSLR, 100 mm macro lens). I photograph a second set of frontal and lateral images with an adhesive specimen marker (millimeter scale) placed on the skin. It provides accurate conversion from pixels to actual distance. In surgery, I utilize a projectometer to ensure precise measurements on photographs displayed in the operating room.[2] Simulation tools are limited to Photoshop (Adobe, San Jose, CA) and PowerPoint (Microsoft, Redmond, WA). Patient consultation is prioritized to identify any factors that may deem them suboptimal candidates for esthetic surgery. For patients with sinonasal disease beyond airflow obstruction, I refer them to 1 of 2 rhinologists for further evaluation. These specialists may recommend additional imaging, such as a CT scan, which I will visualize using Horus (Horosproject.org Nimble Co LLC, Annapolis, MD USA).

Heppt

During the consultation, a structured anamnesis with the aid of a standardized questionnaire such as the Standardized Cosmesis and Health Nasal Outcomes Survey (SCHNOS) is suitable, which allows both esthetic and functional issues to be evaluated.[3] This is followed by endoscopy of the nasal cavity and palpation of the nasal framework, including functional measurement by rhinomanometry and/or acoustic rhinometry. In addition to the assessment of the septum, turbinates, and bony aperture, the detection of constrictions in the isthmus region (so-called inner nasal valve) and of collapse phenomena of the ala (so-called outer nasal valve) is crucial in the evaluation of functional disorders. Cone beam CT combined with the use of computational fluid dynamics (CFD)-based flow simulations is becoming more and more significant as this method can be used to assign functional parameters to morphologic conditions.[4] Finally standard portrait images in lateral, frontal, semi-oblique, inferior, and superior imaging techniques with simulations and morphing are nowadays part of the setting. In addition to the usual rhinological diagnostic procedures, it is also important to assess the skin mantle of the nose and any existing skin diseases in order to obtain the best cosmetic result.

Twu

My evaluation of the patient desiring rhinoplasty includes a comprehensive approach that integrates history-taking, physical examination, laboratory tests, imaging studies, functional measurement, and photography. Initially, recognizing the patient's motivations for seeking rhinoplasty, either esthetic or functional, as well as any prior injury or iatrogenic procedures. This step is crucial in assessing patient expectations and determining the feasibility of achieving desired results. Furthermore, identifying any systemic or psychological diseases through careful history-taking is essential as these may have implications on anesthesia risk and postoperative recovery. Proper history-taking can guide not only clinical decision-making but also establish rapport with the patient by addressing concerns and setting realistic expectations.

Subsequently, a detailed physical examination focuses on both internal and external nasal anatomy to identify structural abnormalities or deviations that might require correction during surgery. Laboratory tests are selectively performed based on the medical history collected; for instance, coagulation profiles can be pivotal in patients with a history suggestive of bleeding disorders. Imaging studies such as sinus plain films or CT scans offer information regarding organic and structural deformities including underlying sinonasal diseases. Objective functional measurements including acoustic rhinometry, rhinomanometry, and olfaction test help detect existing respiratory impediments and can serve as evidence for medicolegal issues.

WHAT SURGICAL TECHNIQUES DO I USE TO TREAT THE INTERNAL NASAL VALVE DYSFUNCTION?
Wong

The internal nasal valve is a region, not a specific area or location within the nose, and is the gateway for airflow to the rest of the airway.[5] Broadly speaking it is where the cross-sectional areas of the airway successively narrow. This tapering leads to increased flow velocity and a pressure drop.[6] Transmural pressure drops result in motion and collapse of lateral wall as the upper lateral cartilage is flexible. During breathing, even a modest inspiratory effort can create a displacement as small as 0.5 mm; this may result in the sensation of obstruction. The perception of nasal obstruction is very sensitive to small changes in geometry in this area. The nose does not have a "flow sensor" per se, sensory nerves detect temperature drops, and shear forces that are produced by the flow of air, and this is more dramatic in turbulent flow.

For internal nasal valve collapse, my workhorse is in the spreader grafts because even the expansion of the mid-vault by 1 to 2 mm results in significant improvement in symptoms. The impact of spreader graft placement between the upper lateral and quadrangular cartilage extends beyond volumetric expansion. Proper suture fixation of the graft results in the creation of tension along the upper lateral cartilage reducing laxity. A substantial amount of improvement from the split hump approach is due to tightening of the upper lateral cartilage.

Heppt

An inner nasal valve stenosis also referred to as isthmus stenosis is often caused by a septal deviation, long upper lateral cartilages, overprojection of tip, and dorsum and last but not least previous rhinoplasty. It is characterized by a reduced isthmus angle and/or a reduced cross-sectional valve area that severely affects breathing, since this anatomic zone is the narrowest in the nose, responsible for airstream regulation. There are several techniques for the correction of an isthmus stenosis generally based on widening of the cross-section area and on opening the angle between the septum and the upper lateral cartilages. Next to septal correction, the most common procedures favored by the author include the Lopez Infante technique and the nasal valve lift. The Lopez Infante technique[7] consists of partial resection of excess cartilage and vestibular skin with refixation in craniolateral direction (**Fig. 1**). It is quick and very effective and indicated when an isthmus stenosis is based on an elongated caudal edge of the upper lateral cartilage.

A very useful and minimal invasive technique is the nasal valve lift (**Fig. 2**). The principle is that a thread is placed in the subcutaneous tissue, elevating the valve area by suspension on bidirectionally orientated cones.[8,9] Further methods for isthmus corrections are upper lateral cartilage splay sutures, spreader flaps, spreader grafts, and titanium implants.

Twu

Techniques for correcting internal nasal valve deformities could be divided into 2 categories: suture techniques and grafting techniques. Suture suspension procedures like transconjunctival approach, Mitek bone anchor, flaring sutures, and lateral pull-up were considered as minimal invasive maneuvers moving the soft tissue away from the stenotic valvular area. On the other hand, grafting and implant methods modified the structure utilizing cartilaginous grafts and artificial implants, for example, the alar batten graft, butterfly graft, spreader graft, spreader flap, and even composite graft.

For Asian noses with internal nasal valve problems, I usually removed the hypertrophic septal cartilage without destructing the L-shape supporting structure first. The removed septal cartilage could be used for further grafting procedures. Then I will correct the caudal septum, cutting off the excessive hypertrophic inferior part, and fix the straightened causal septum to the nasal spine area. Through and through cutting among the dorsal septum was then made if necessary. The cut dorsal septum was then secured by using septal sutures and his maneuver was applied to the middle and posterior part of the septum. Submucosal resection of the inferior turbinates was then performed. Spreader grafts will be placed if necessary. Alar batten graft was seldom used unless there existed a dynamic collapse of the alae while inspiration.

WHAT SURGICAL TECHNIQUES DO I USE TO TREAT THE EXTERNAL NASAL VALVE DYSFUNCTION?
Wong

For external nasal valve dysfunction, it is important to make the diagnosis precisely as this distal airway may collapse as a consequence of restriction of flow in the mid-vault. The external valve is an inlet that

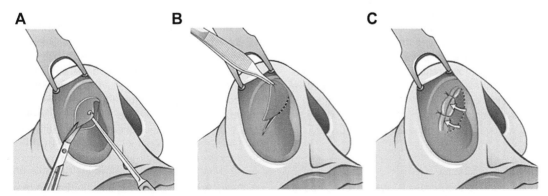

Fig. 1. Lopez Infante technique.

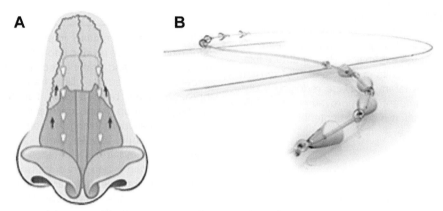

Fig. 2. Nasal valve lift using Silhouette Thread with bidirectional cones.

encompasses what we would call the nostrils/naris and includes the columella, sill, and alar lobule. It extends about 1 cm inwardly and is the inlet for airflow.

There are 2 factors that contribute to airway compromise in this region. First, cross-sectional area of this inlet, as nostril shape varies considerably from a slender and slit-like shape to being circular. Second, pressure drops across this inlet may result in alar lobule collapse. Like the midvault, mechanical stability of the alae depends on the constitutive properties of this composite structure. Hence, improve flow can be accomplished by (1) altering the shape of the aperture and/or (2) mechanically stabilizing the alar lobule. To expand the aperture, a number of maneuvers may be performed such as binding the medial crural footplates together, projecting the nasal tip, and/or introducing a simple rim graft to alter alar margin curvature. Mechanical stability of the alar lobule can be improved by either increasing stiffness with placement of a graft or creating dynamic tension. Both methods will reduce lateral displacement. My personally approach largely relies on the creation of tension (lateral crural tensioning, steps delineated in **Fig. 3**) along with the placement of an articulated alar rim graft (steps delineated in **Fig. 4**), and that usually in combination with some degree of lateral crural tensioning.[10,11] A caveat for lateral crural strut graft placement is that it may reduce airspace in the inlet and thus exacerbate airflow restriction. Narrow, slender noses or narrow nostrils would be a relative contraindication. Use of strut grafts here must be carefully thought out and grafts must be extremely thin, and ideally with convexity facing outward.

Heppt

The surgical concepts of an alar collapse focus mainly on the reinforcement and reconstruction of the ala but on certain widening too. The most effective techniques rely on the strengthening of the alar sidewall and of the lateral crura by placing cartilage grafts on top or under the lateral crus such as the lateral crural splay graft,[12] the articulated alar rim graft,[13] and the lateral crural strut graft.[14] Articulated alar rim grafts (**Fig. 5**) are the most frequently performed procedures I execute. They deliver stable and reliable results from both a functional and esthetic point of view. The grafts best taken from the septum are sewed on the surface of the lateral crura and the edges smoothened using a coarse diamond drill. After fixation of the graft, the lateral portion is inserted into an alar pocket. The use of transcutaneous guiding stitches enables the proper placement and prevents displacement in the early postoperative stage.

Twu

The selection of an appropriate surgical treatment of external nasal valve stenosis relies on a comprehensive assessment of the anatomic structures involved and the degree of functional impairment. I divided the external nasal valve dysfunction into 3 categories: deformities of the soft tissue, deformities of the cartilaginous and bony framework, and deformities of the abnormal tissue like scars and contracture.

Suspension sutures might help the simple soft tissue deformities; however, I usually started from correction of the caudal septum. Resection and reposition of the innate septum, as well as replacement or reinforcement of the deformed structures, are essential techniques. The dysfunction of the external nasal valve may need modification of the lower lateral cartilage and/or the columella. Additional grafting like alar batten graft or alar rim graft might be needed.

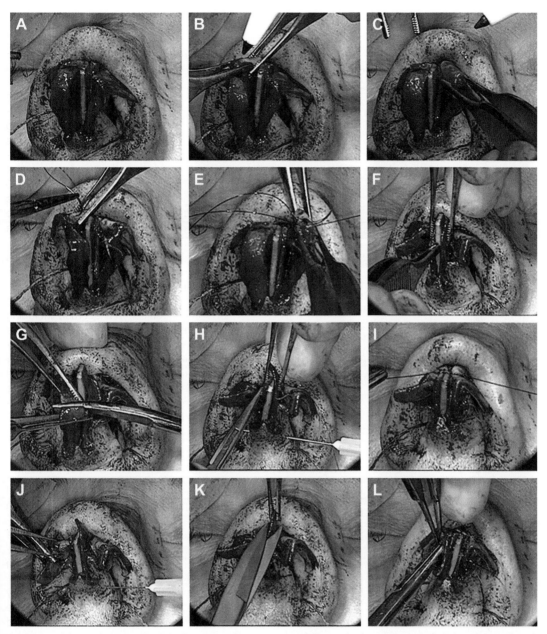

Fig. 3. Lateral crural tensioning (*A*), the native domes are carefully marked to delineate their position within the lower alar cartilages. Subsequently, (*B*) the precise amount of lower lateral cartilage recruited to achieve tension and stability across the alar lobule is identified using a Brown-Adson forceps and marked accordingly. (*C*) Markings are made on the left lower lateral cartilage to guide the surgical procedure. Dome sutures are then meticulously placed on the right side (*D*) and on the left side in (*E*). Upon identification of excess medial crura, as depicted in (*F*), the inferior part of the medial crura is approximated to the septal extension graft with sutures, in anticipation of medical crural division. Subsequent steps, detailed in (*G*), involve the dissection of excess medial crura from the vestibular skin along the lateral columella, followed by division with a scissor. (*H*) Illustrates the secure positioning of the medial crura using a hypodermic needle, with additional sutures utilized to anchor the medial crura to the septal extension graft. Concurrently, interdomal sutures are placed to firmly secure the new domes to the septal extension graft, as depicted in (*I*). A caliper is employed in (*J*) to accurately measure the amount of cartilage recruited for the procedure. Lastly, (*K*) demonstrates the removal of excess medial crura from both sides of the incision, followed by their suture fixation (*L*). Excess medial crural may be overlapped or sectioned.

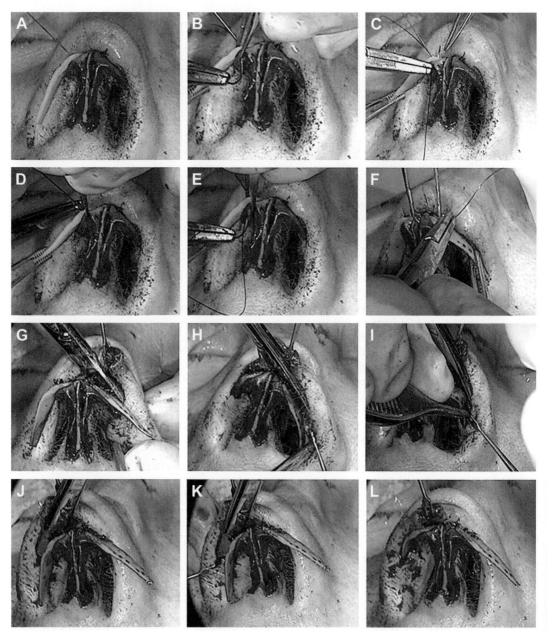

Fig. 4. Articulated alar rim graft placement. (*A*) A triangular-shaped alar rim graft is meticulously secured to the lower alar cartilage just lateral to the dome using a 30 gauge needle. Suture fixation involves passing a needle through the graft and the lower alar cartilage, ensuring it does not penetrate the vestibular skin. Precision is paramount, necessitating the use of a very fine forceps to guide the process. (*B*) The first pass of the needle through the cartilage of the graft and then through the cartilage of the lower alar cartilage. (*C*), The second pass of this suture traverses the margin of the lower alar cartilage and then the graft. It is then tied. The second suture is subsequently placed lateral to the first along the rim graft, traversing both the rim graft and the caudal margin of the lower alar cartilage. It is imperative to avoid piercing the vestibular skin (*D*). The second pass of this suture once again is placed through the margin of the lower alar cartilage and the graft (*E*). This step can pose challenges, particularly if the triangular rim graft is relatively narrow or if there is cephalic malposition of the lower alar cartilage. (*F*) The third suture is placed through the graft, the dome, and, if feasible, the septal extension graft, providing 3 point fixation of the graft in space. With both grafts now secured, (*G*) demonstrates the use of a sharp iris scissor to create a precise pocket parallel to the alar margin, broader and wider medially and narrowing to a point distally toward the alar base. This pocket provides a trajectory path for placement of the rim

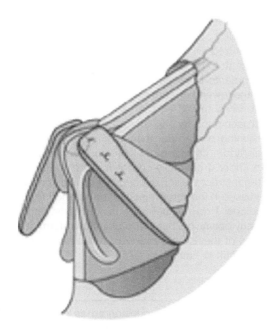

Fig. 5. Articulated alar rim graft.

IN A PURELY COSMETIC RHINOPLASTY, HOW DO YOU PREVENT COMPROMISE OF NASAL FUNCTION?
Wong

I believe every cosmetic rhinoplasty operation is also a functional procedure, especially when part of the operation involves maneuvers that reduce nasal size. This occurs most commonly with dorsal hump reduction. Too often, esthetic rhinoplasty operations are performed without regard for functionality of the airway, and a common reason for performing revision surgery in patients referred to my practice. First and foremost, surgery must create a completely straight septum, and that includes the correction of osseous deformations along the maxillary crest, perpendicular plate, and vomer. Discontinuities in airway topography result in the creation of turbulence. Turbulence leads to pressure drops, and hence reduction in flow velocity. Spurs in particular should not be ignored and must be corrected. I use a piezo

device (Sonopet, Stryker, Kalamazoo, MI) to smooth and contour all bony midline deformities.[15] Second, any maneuver that reduces a dorsal hump could precipitate internal nasal valve collapse, as geometry and by extension pressure and flow change. As I perform a component hump reduction, I consider spreader grafts placement (or auto spreader graft use) in virtually all cases. If there is no hump reduction required, and potential mid-vault issues exist with airflow, I will either split the hump and place spreader grafts or insert a small endonasal–submucosal spreader graft without performing a split.

Tip refinement in cosmetic nasal surgery may also result in a reduction in airflow, particularly esthetic maneuvers cause narrowing at this inlet. Amorphous and boxy-tipped noses may present a challenge, as they are commonly associated with lateral crural recurvature. Many isolated tip suture techniques can exacerbate this recurvature and further compromise nasal airflow. Specific techniques to address recurvature are numerable, and beyond the scope of this study. Finally, turbinate surgery is reasonable in most cases where nasal obstruction is evident preoperatively. I use the NOSE scale as a screening device. There is virtually no downside to performing a conservative turbinate reduction in terms of either a submucous resection of soft tissue and again expands the airway facilitating airflow. My practice is biased in that in an academic center, the vast majority of patients have significant nasal airway obstruction regardless of whether their indication for surgery is primarily cosmetic or functional.

Heppt

With a few exceptions, purely esthetic rhinoplasties such as reduction rhinoplasty or nasal tip corrections run the risk of negatively affecting nasal breathing. One reason for this is that the cross-section of the main nasal cavity is often reduced and dynamic structures such as the nasal valve region are impaired or destroyed. The risk of functional impairment is particularly high if preoperative deviations of the septum,

graft. Prior to this maneuver, it is crucial to inject a small amount of lidocaine and epinephrine at the alar base. Once the pocket has been established, (*H*) a small skin hook gently retracts the skin soft tissue flap, while a second small double-prong hook pulls the apex of the marginal incision infero-laterally to stretch the incision and facilitate placement of the graft into the precise pocket (*H*). (*I*) The index finger on the nondominant hand pushes the entire nasal tip cartilages to the contralateral side, enabling gentle insertion of the tip of the cartilage into the pocket using a Brown-Adson forceps with teeth to grasp the rim graft 3 to 5 mm away from its apex. Similarly, on the right, the pocket is created (*J*), followed by placement of double-prong skin hooks to provide visualization and traction on the apex of the incision before the graft (*K*) is carefully positioned into the pocket, as illustrated in (*L*). The skin flaps are then gently manipulated to facilitate the grafts gliding into the pocket.

turbinates, nasal valve, or chronic diseases of the paranasal sinuses with nasal polyps are overlooked and not addressed. To prevent compromise of nasal function, care must be taken to protect important bony and cartilaginous supporting structures, including muscles and ligaments. Given they are destroyed or no longer present, they should be reconstructed either with sutures or cartilage transplants. Excessive cartilage and bone resections, aggressive mucosal reductions, uncontrolled osteotomies, and dead spaces predisposing to uncontrolled scarring harbor the risk of postoperative functional disorders. Cephalic resections of the lower lateral cartilage edges are particularly critical, as the scroll region is considerably traumatized and nasal valve stenosis can result from scarring.

Twu

In the realm of cosmetic surgery, rhinoplasty stands out as a procedure deeply intertwined with both esthetic desires and functional integrity. The pursuit of enhanced nasal appearance must be carefully balanced against the preservation of nasal functionality, given that any compromise could lead to significant respiratory distress or dysfunction. This balance hinges on a thorough preoperative assessment of the patient's esthetic goals as well as the internal nasal structures.

The surgical technique employed during rhinoplasty plays a pivotal role in ensuring that the functionality of the nose is not jeopardized for cosmetic enhancements. Since contracture and fibrosis might occur after any procedure in rhinoplasty, techniques aimed at preserving or even improving airway flow should be prioritized, such as careful modification rather than aggressive destruction of structural elements not only the cartilages but also the soft tissue and ligaments.

Special care should be taken if we use costal cartilage for septal reconstruction such as septal extension graft or strut. The thickness of the costal cartilage might cause widened septal structure and subsequent airway compromise.

HOW IMPORTANT IS THE RECONSTRUCTION OF THE SCROLL AREA IN YOUR PROCEDURES? DO YOU DO IT ROUTINELY? WHAT TECHNIQUES DO YOU USE?
Wong

The "scroll" is classically described as the region where the upper and lower alar cartilages meet. There are many anatomic relationship anatomic relationships between these 2 cartilages varying from overlapping, end to end, and interdigitation. It is less a contemporary subject of discussion

because of the dominance of the open structure techniques. Scroll anatomy was much more emphasized when endonasal rhinoplasty was dominant. In general, I try not to upset any of the attachments between the upper lateral cartilage and the lower alar cartilage, as I generally do not perform an aggressive cephalic trim. My mainstay approach to correcting lateral crural convexity is a tensioning procedure, though often with a large crura and a convex crura I will do a lateral crural turn under. I generally do not make any attempt to reconstruct the scroll, nor do I reattach connective tissue in the scroll region to the skin soft tissue envelope. I do not believe suture reconstruction has any downside, but at this point, long-term outcomes of these sutures are unknown and results are difficult to gauge.

Heppt

The scroll area can be considered as one of the most important zones of the upper respiratory tract. It is located between the upper and lower lateral cartilages and can be equated with the inner nasal valve (isthmus nasi). As the narrowest part of the upper airway, the inner nasal valve area acts as an accelerator and diffuser of the inhaled air. Due to its location and dynamic construction, the zone is very sensitive to changes. According to Hagen–Poiseuille's law, even small constrictions lead to disproportionately high increases of the resistance.[16] This is the reason why ligaments such as the horizontal and vertical scroll ligament and even fine muscles have to be preserved or reconstructed during every rhinoplasty procedure. The structures can be spared by subperichondrial and pocket-like preparation or rebuilt by suturing or adding cartilage transplants. Spreader grafts[17] and spreader flaps[18] used for reconstruction of the middle vault also have a stabilizing effect on the scroll area, whereas spreader flaps are preferable from the authors point of view due to their better dynamic effect.

Twu

The scroll area plays a significant role in determining the nasal contour and ensuring optimal airflow dynamics. Precise surgical intervention like suture techniques to autologous grafting procedures to restore or enhance its structural integrity and appearance following trauma, congenital defect, or previous surgical modifications is important, because it ensures harmonious integration and reestablishing the delicate balance between maintaining nasal function while improving cosmetic outcomes.

In Asian rhinoplasty, I usually do subperichondrial dissection of the lower lateral cartilage in order to achieve maximal mobilization and then perform extended modification like reposition of the lower lateral cartilages to the neo-causal septum that is reconstructed with septal extension graft. These maneuvers can correct the short nose, underprojected tip, upward rotated tip, and sort of bulbous tip. I will not intend to damage the scroll ligaments, nor reconstruct them.

HOW HAVE YOUR TECHNIQUES IN THIS AREA CHANGED OVER THE LAST 2 YEARS?
Wong

An overwhelming majority of patients with rhinoplasty in my practice have a nasal obstruction score over 75, a fairly morbid degree of nasal airway obstruction. Generally, this indicates that the airway obstruction is multilevel. I have become more aggressive and detailed in terms of correcting the airway in all 4 principal areas—internal nasal valve, external valve, septum, and turbinates. In patients who have very narrow nose is that tend to be thin and steeple-like with very narrow nostrils, I believe performing any maneuver to improve airflow would be justified. A key point lost upon most clinician relates to an understanding of basic fluid mechanics, namely upstream changes alter downstream flow, and vice versa downstream changes alter upstream flow. Study flow when turbulent is complex, and turbulent flow exists in the nose under physiologic conditions. Understanding flow is sublime, but in short, the take-home lesson is that eliminating obstruction anywhere in the nasal airway will create overall better flow. This is particularly crucial in patients with narrow nasal passages, where addressing inferior turbinate issues can be highly beneficial. I am fortunate to collaborate with a skilled rhinologist proficient in medial flap inferior turbinoplasty technique.[19,20] This procedure involves an aggressive resection of the inferior turbinate, creating a soft tissue flap to cover the raw edges, and removal of the inferior aspect of the turbinate bone. Initially, I had concerns about potential complications such as empty nose syndrome. With several hundred procedures performed, we have not observed any cases of empty nose syndrome. While this is a significant turbinate resection, I believe it is best performed under endoscopic guidance. The outcomes have been exceptionally positive, particularly in patients with narrow nasal passages, and we intend to publish our findings soon.

Another cause of iatrogenic obstruction that is largely preventable is the side-to-side placement of the septal extension graft. I make every effort to perform and end-to-end graft whenever possible. Straightening the caudal septum should be an objective of every rhinoplasty. Side-to-side grafts would be indicated in airways with an expansive external valve geometry, and a modest deviation of the anterior septal angle to one side. Imprudent design of a side-to-side septal extension graft may block the airway. Our recent publication compared the side-to-side to end-to-end, and so we saw no difference in obstruction, in over 200 patients, but it is important to recognize the indications for each is entirely different.[21]

Finally, what I am doing differently now compared to the previous decade is become increasingly aggressive with achieving stability in the alar lobule. I am aggressive with placing alar rim grafts if I feel at the end of the operation, there is instability or lack of support. It does not take much time or skill to place a classic free-floating fusiform graft along the alar margin, and the benefits are massive.

Heppt

As a rhinoplasty surgeon with a background in otorhinolaryngology, the nasal valve is always of particular importance not only in purely functional but also primarily esthetic procedures. The focus on this region has certainly become even greater in recent years due to the groundbreaking findings of airstream simulations, detailed anatomic studies, and innovative concepts of preservation rhinoplasty.[22] Personally, my surgical approach has changed in such a way that in recent years, I have again increasingly favored endonasal techniques, specifically sparing ligamentous structures In the scroll region. In part, this Is achieved by pocket-like dissection, in part by completely bypassing the central nasal valve region through a strict medial and lateral approach toward the nasal bridge or lateral nasal flank. If the ligaments of the scroll region have to be severed or are no longer present, I try to either readapt them with sutures or stabilize them by inserting cartilage grafts. In recent years, I have paid particular attention—and this is the most important change in my approach over the last 2 years—to preventing dead space not only in the supratip but also in the scroll region by using sutures.[23] I try to avoid the classic intercartilaginous incision that often destroys the scroll region as well as cephalic trimming of lower lateral cartilages in favor of incisions on the caudal rim of the lower lateral cartilage and suturing techniques for reorientation of the nasal tip and the lateral crura.

Twu

My changes of techniques in rhinoplasty could be divided into 3 categories: the approach, the surgical design, and the material. Rhinoplasty has been approached through either open or closed methods, each with distinct advantages and limitations. The open technique provides surgeons with a better view of nasal structures, facilitating more accurate modifications, whereas the closed technique offers reduced scarring and recovery times. I did more and more endonasal operations in recent years and left open approach only to those suffered from severe damages, multiple revisions, and those without clear preoperative diagnoses. For those who came to me for cosmetic nasal problems, I usually set the surgical goal as correcting the appearance and function at 1 time, since most of the patients had both cosmetic and functional insufficiency. My belief in surgical design is that "less is more." I tried my best to conduct procedure with minimal invasive ways and also tried to preserve the innate tissue as much as I could. Although preservation rhinoplasty was much promoted in recent years, the Asian noses need much augmentation then destruction, and thus, I seldom follow those popular preservation ways. As for the material, I use only autologous cartilage in the past 2 decades. But complete fixation of the cartilage with sutures was not always easy if I do endonasal approach, for example, fixation of the autologous costal cartilage to the glabella through endonasal incisions like intercartilaginous and marginal incisions. Therefore, I use tissue glue (sealer protein with human fibrinogen) for fixation of the upper most of the inserted costal cartilage.

REFERENCES

1. Stewart MG, Witsell DL, Smith TL, et al. Development and validation of the Nasal Obstruction Symptom Evaluation (NOSE) scale. Otolaryngol Head Neck Surg 2004;130(2):157–63.
2. Webster RC, Davidson TM, Rubin FF, et al. Recording projection of nasal landmarks in rhinoplasty. Laryngoscope 1977;87(7):1207–11.
3. Moubayed SP, Ioannidis JPA, Saltychev M, et al. The 10-Item Standardized Cosmesis and Health Nasal Outcomes Survey (SCHNOS) for Functional and Cosmetic Rhinoplasty. JAMA Facial Plast Surg 2018;20(1):37–42.
4. Hildebrandt T, Heppt WJ. Nasal breathing assessment using computational fluid dynamics: an update from the rhinologic perspective. Facial Plast Surg FPS 2024;40(3):331–3.
5. Tripathi PB, Elghobashi S, Wong BJF. The myth of the internal nasal valve. JAMA Facial Plast Surg 2017;19(4):253–4.
6. Hakimi AA, Sharma GK, Ngo T, et al. Coupling pressure sensing with optical coherence tomography to evaluate the internal nasal valve. Ann Otol Rhinol Laryngol 2021;130(2):167–72.
7. Kasperbauer JL, Kern EB. Nasal valve physiology. Implications in nasal surgery. Otolaryngol Clin North Am 1987;20(4):699–719.
8. Saban Y, Javier DB, Massa M. Nasal lift-nasal valve lift and nasal tip lift-preliminary results of a new technique using noninvasive self-retaining unidirectional nasal suspension with threads. Facial Plast Surg FPS 2014;30(6):661–9.
9. Heppt H, Vent J, Alali M, et al. Nasal valve lift in nasal valve stenosis-a 2 years clinical trial. Facial Plast Surg FPS 2019;35(1):14–22.
10. Calloway HE, Heilbronn CM, Gu JT, et al. Functional outcomes, quantitative morphometry, and aesthetic analysis of articulated alar rim grafts in septorhinoplasty. JAMA Facial Plast Surg 2019; 21(6):558–65.
11. Goodrich JL, Wong BJF. Optimizing the soft tissue triangle, alar margin furrow, and alar ridge aesthetics: analysis and use of the articulate alar rim graft. Facial Plast Surg FPS 2016;32(6):646–55.
12. Timmer FCA, Roth JA, Börjesson PKE, et al. The lateral crural underlay spring graft. Facial Plast Surg FPS 2013;29(2):140–5.
13. Ballin AC, Kim H, Chance E, et al. The articulated alar rim graft: reengineering the conventional alar rim graft for improved contour and support. Facial Plast Surg FPS 2016;32(4):384–97.
14. Gunter JP, Friedman RM. Lateral crural strut graft: technique and clinical applications in rhinoplasty. Plast Reconstr Surg 1997;99(4):943–52. discussion 953-955.
15. Hjelm N, Goldfarb J, Krein H, et al. Sonic Rhinoplasty: Review and Updated Uses. Facial Plast Surg FPS 2021;37(1):107–9.
16. Pape HC, Kurtz A, Silbernagl S. Georg Thieme Verlag KG. Physiologie [Internet]. Thieme. 2019. Available at: https://books.google.com/books?id=W-22DwAAQBAJ.
17. Sheen JH. Spreader graft: a method of reconstructing the roof of the middle nasal vault following rhinoplasty. Plast Reconstr Surg 1984; 73(2):230–9.
18. Gruber RP, Park E, Newman J, et al. The spreader flap in primary rhinoplasty. Plast Reconstr Surg 2007;119(6):1903–10.
19. Barham HP, Knisely A, Harvey RJ, et al. How i do it: medial flap inferior turbinoplasty. Am J Rhinol Allergy 2015;29(4):314–5.
20. Barham HP, Thornton MA, Knisely A, et al. Long-term outcomes in medial flap inferior turbinoplasty

are superior to submucosal electrocautery and submucosal powered turbinate reduction. Int Forum Allergy Rhinol 2016;6(2):143–7.

21. Peters RD, Vasudev M, Hakimi AA, et al. Boomerang modification of the septal extension graft: graft design and functional outcomes. Facial Plast Surg Aesthetic Med 2024. https://doi.org/10.1089/fpsam.2023.0152.

22. Çakır B, Öreroğlu AR, Daniel RK. Surface aesthetics in tip rhinoplasty: a step-by-step guide. Aesthet Surg J 2014;34(6):941–55.

23. Robotti E, Leone F, Malfussi VA, et al. The "3 points compartmentalization" technique in subperichondrial-subperiosteal dissection in primary rhinoplasty to reduce edema and define contour. Aesthetic Plast Surg 2022;46(4):1923–31.

Nasal Surgery in the Younger Patient

Dirk Jan Menger, MD, PhD[a], Fred G. Fedok, MD[b,c], Sydney C. Butts, MD[d],*

KEYWORDS

- Nasal fracture • Pediatric septoplasty • Pediatric rhinoplasty • Nasal growth

KEY POINTS

- Nasal surgery can be carried out safely in the younger patient. In cases of trauma, it is recommended that corrective surgery be carried out in a short time frame before scar contracture, aberrant remodeling, and malunion of structures occurs.
- In the less common situation of performing cosmetic surgery on the younger patient there are several principles and guidelines to be considered.
- Chronic nasal obstruction can have impacts on the growing face which should be considered when making decisions about timing of rhinoplasty.

PANEL DISCUSSION

What is too young for cosmetic rhinoplasty?
What is too young for corrective nasal surgery?
What areas should I preserve in the young patient?
If cartilage grafting is needed, what are your preferred donor sites in the younger patient? Do you ever use alloplasts or cadaver sources?
When will you utilize an endonasal rhinoplasty approach in the younger patients? When will you utilize an open rhinoplasty approach in the younger patients?
How have your techniques in this area changed over the last 2 years?

WHAT IS TOO YOUNG FOR COSMETIC RHINOPLASTY?
Menger

In the Netherlands, where I reside, a legal age limit of 18 years is imposed in private clinics for all forms of aesthetic surgery, encompassing cosmetic rhinoplasty. Conversely, general and academic hospitals do not impose such age restrictions, theoretically allowing aesthetic surgery, including rhinoplasty, in younger patients. Psychologically, the age of 6 is deemed opportune for conducting aesthetic corrections for congenital or acquired facial anomalies, such as protruding ears. This is rooted in the observation that before this age, children are less likely to taunt each other, and often the child remains oblivious to cosmetic concerns.

However, for nasal deformities, a challenge arises as the nasal skeleton is not fully developed at the age of 6. Consequently, performing cosmetic rhinoplasty at this age holds the potential to impede normal nasal development, leading to unpredictable and distorted long-term postoperative results.[1–4]

[a] Department of Otorhinolaryngology, Facial Plastic Surgery, University Medical Center Utrecht, Heidelberglaan 100, 3584 CX, Utrecht, The Netherlands; [b] Department of Surgery, University of South Alabama, Mobile, AL, USA; [c] Fedok Plastic Surgery, 113 East Fern Avenue, Foley, AL 36535, USA; [d] Facial Plastic and Reconstructive Surgery, State University of New York-Downstate Health Sciences University, 450 Clarkson Avenue, Box 126, Brooklyn, NY 11203, USA
* Corresponding author.
E-mail address: Sydney.butts@downstate.edu

Facial Plast Surg Clin N Am 32 (2024) 459–471
https://doi.org/10.1016/j.fsc.2024.06.012
1064-7406/24/© 2024 Elsevier Inc. All rights are reserved, including those for text and data mining, AI training, and similar technologies.

From a nasal development perspective, the ideal age for surgery aligns with the post-puberty growth spurt when the nose attains full development. This age range varies between 16 years and 18 years in females and 18 years and 20 years in males.[5] Exceptions to this norm, where surgery may be conducted at an earlier age, are limited to cases involving severe psychological issues linked to nasal aesthetics or severe nasal breathing issues. Should cosmetic surgery be contemplated in such instances, the surgeon must apprise both the patient and parents of the associated risks, as outlined above. Cosmetic nasal issues stemming from causes other than the nasal framework, such as nasal fistulas with dermoid cysts, tumors, and so forth, can be addressed at any age but necessitate treatment with minimal trauma to the nasal skeleton. For any indication, the potential benefits of intervention must be carefully balanced against the conceivable adverse effects on nasal and midfacial growth.

Fedok

First, before addressing this question, I think one must delineate the definition of several terms. The term rhinoplasty refers to a procedure to change a nose—(from The 5th Edition of the American Heritage Dictionary) the noun Rhinoplasty: (1) Plastic surgery of the nose. (2) Plastic surgery of the nose to correct deformity or to replace lost tissue. Tissue may be transplanted from the patient's cheek, forehead, arm, and so forth, or even from another person. (3) A type of plastic surgery that is used to improve the function (reconstructive surgery) or appearance (cosmetic surgery) of a person's nose. (4) Cosmetic surgery to improve the appearance of your nose.[6]

In the application of these terms in my practice, I have used the terms cosmetic versus reconstructive in a manner that was derived from my interactions with the insurance industry. The term cosmetic refers to a procedure aimed at enhancing one's appearance beyond the expected "normal"; while the term reconstructive (or functional) denotes that the procedure is aimed at restoring the anatomy (or function) to normal from deformity or malfunction. The deformity can be the result of genetics, injury, tumor, or other entities. I am belaboring these points because I frequently have witnessed surgeons applying the terms cosmetic and reconstructive in variable situations that in my perspective may not apply.

So…What is too young for cosmetic rhinoplasty? For myself, if I see a young patient who truly has a well-proportioned "normal" looking nose without functional impairment and my engagement is to elevate it to something that "looks" exceptionally or pleasingly different, without the need to change function, I consider that a true cosmetic endeavor. If, on the other hand, I am consulted for the care of a patient whose nasal appearance has been impaired by a developmental problem, by trauma or by other deleterious situation, and/or the patient has functional breathing problems, than I consider that a different situation and not cosmetic, but a reconstructive situation or functional situation.

I believe in the case of true cosmetic procedures the surgeon should try to think beyond the immediate possible structural changes one can possibly make in the younger patient's nose. One should consider the motivations of the younger patient and their parents desiring cosmetic rhinoplasty. One should also try to estimate where the patient is in their personal growth curve so one might synchronize the timing of the rhinoplasty with where they are in achieving their adult facial and height proportions. Finally, I believe the surgeon should evaluate the patient to try to predict how the patient's nose might develop as they grow older. It is a goal to avoid removing crucial structural tissues from the younger patient's nose and potentially inhibiting growth. For instance, one should diligently work toward preventing the patient's nose from being too small when they are 25 years of age and older. Surgery should be planned to not adversely affect the future nasal growth. Any alteration in the shape of the nose should be planned to be in harmony for the patient when they are several years older. There are several publications cautioning this.[2,7–9] In general, given the different growth patterns of young males and young females, younger female patients should not undergo cosmetic rhinoplasty until at least the age of 14[10,11] and only if they have growth characteristics of a young adolescent and not that of a child. In the case of the male patient, because of the relative lag in growth compared to females it has generally been advised for young males to not undergo cosmetic rhinoplasty until they are at least the age 16. Therefore, the general guidelines I now apply in my practice: 14–16 years of age for female patients and 16–18 years of age in male patients. There is variation in how I apply these rules of thumb depending on the individual characteristics of the patient as these general guidelines and trends change over time.[12,13]

Butts

Among cosmetic surgical procedures in the adolescent population(<18), rhinoplasty is performed most often.[12] Unlike the patient with nasal airway obstruction, the motivation for cosmetic rhinoplasty can be more challenging to define. Both the patient and parent's wishes must be clearly understood. Articulation of a realistic set of expectations is paramount. The surgeon must ascertain whether any psychological problems exist that should be addressed prior to moving forward with surgery. The patient's overall maturity level and possession of coping skills needed to handle the postoperative recovery should be frankly discussed. Adamson recommends that eligible patients are at least 1 year past menarche or have shown 1 year of stable facial growth, have parental support and show psychological readiness for the procedure.[7] Other guidelines suggest that for male patients, the earliest age cosmetic rhinoplasty should be performed is between 16 and 18 and for female patient between the ages of 15 and 17 years of age.[12]

WHAT IS TOO YOUNG FOR CORRECTIVE NASAL SURGERY?
Menger

Corrective or secondary nasal surgery encompasses any procedure necessary in the future following an initial rhinoplasty. This surgical intervention is distinct from a planned follow-up. In younger patients, corrective nasal surgery may be prompted by the unpredictable postoperative outcomes, stemming from the incomplete development of the nasal skeleton during the initial procedure. As elucidated previously, the optimal timing for rhinoplasty is post the puberty growth spurt, typically between the ages of 16 years and 20 years. Nevertheless, certain indications may warrant (corrective) rhinoplasty at an earlier stage, such as in children experiencing severe psychological distress associated with nasal aesthetics or substantial functional impairment leading to dental issues, sleep disturbances, or hindrances in daily activities. In cases like cleft lip patients, both aesthetic and functional issues often coexist. It is noteworthy to inform both the patient and their parents about the advantages and disadvantages of performing rhinoplasty before the full development of the nasal skeleton is achieved. This communication is of paramount importance to ensure informed decision-making regarding the timing and necessity of the procedure.

Fedok

I consider patients for "corrective" nasal surgery in many situations and in age ranges different than those I would consider for a cosmetic procedure. I consider corrective indications to include a spectrum of issues, including trauma, reconstructive situations after current or past tumor treatment, congenital and developmental abnormalities, and significant nasal obstruction caused by anatomic stenosis, collapse, or severe anatomic deviations. Many of these younger patients have been referred to me from primary care doctors, pediatricians, and pediatric otolaryngologists. Thus, in the case of corrective rhinoplasty and functional nasal surgery my considerations and goals are quite different than in cosmetic cases.

In corrective and functional situations, as engaged by me, there exists a clear deformity or functional problem. Hence the consideration of "too young" rarely comes into question, unless there are other non-nasal complicating factors, such as anesthesia risks, poor health, among others. We rarely find a "too young limit" when the patient has suffered extensive craniofacial trauma where plates and screws and absorbable devices might be used to aid in the reconstructive process. I have described to many colleagues over the years that the issues are quite similar in other disciplines. I pose the question, "if one was a pediatric orthopedist and was presented with 2-year old patient with a severely crooked forearm from a recent both bone fracture of the forearm would one hesitate to treat the child and correct the deformity?" Obviously again, this is with the caveat that there are no other mitigating factors or health issue that would prevent the medical treatment of the patient. I look at the nasal area in the facial anatomy with similar considerations and goals.

Situations in which I have been asked to intervene with corrective nasal surgery in younger patients have included: following the removal of tumors such as a dermoid where there appears to have been an arrest of growth of the nasal anatomy, following trauma with resultant saddle nose deformity, severe septal deviation, and nasal stenosis. Some of the young patients referred to me with severe nasal and septal deviations have had at least one side of the nose completely obstructed.[13]

In the cases of acute craniofacial trauma such as a nasoethmoid orbital fracture or a badly comminuted nasal fracture resulting in a crooked and collapsed nose, I believe, corrective rhinoplasty after the initial repair should be performed early. In the younger patient with a severely deviated septum corrective rhinoplasty may be in order to improve breathing, which may only be done optimally if the whole nose is straightened. **Fig. 1**A–C. My pediatric otolaryngology colleagues have worried that these younger patients with severe nasal obstruction have long-term midfacial growth complications similar to what occurs with patients with enlarged adenoids. Chronic nasal

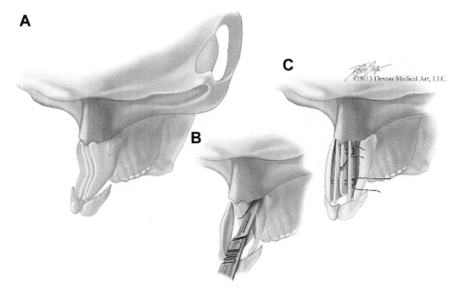

Fig. 1. Surgical Management of Severely Deviated Septum Secondary to Horizontal Fracture or Deviation of Septal Cartilage at the Level of the Maxillary Crest. The technique incorporates the use of spreader grafts to "brace" the septum in correct position. (*A*) Superior view of deviated middle vault and septum. (*B*) Upper lateral cartilages (ULC) have been divided from septum in order to be able to divide septum vertically at the apex of the angulated region. Although it is not always necessary to completely divide septum through its most superior portion, in this depiction, it is divided to allow maximal mobilization. (*C*) Bilateral spreader grafts are sutured in place between ULC and septum. The spreader grafts will hold the septal segments in correct position and reconstitute the middle vault. Image credits: © 2013 Devon Medical Art, LLC.

obstruction will have a definite and profound effect on midfacial growth[14,15] (**Fig. 2**A–F).

Thus, many of the clinical situations where one considers corrective nasal surgery and rhinoplasty in young patients have both anatomic issues causing appearance problems, as well as functional issues. Both of these issues should be addressed.

Butts

Severe nasal obstruction that results from a disturbance of the anatomy of the nasal septum or osseocartilaginous nasal skeleton can occur at any age. Active growth of the nose and the midface are primary factors that determine the extent and timing of nasal surgery in the pediatric patient which is defined as 14 years of age in female patients and 16 years of age in male patients.[13,16–18]

The timing of surgery prior to completion of nasal growth weighs the risks of delays in treating the obstruction with those of performing the surgery. Only the most severe obstructions should be considered for surgery in the pediatric age group, including patients with mouth breathing, snoring, recurrent sinusitis, feeding difficulties (neonates), epistaxis, or a severe deformity causing a negative impact on the quality of life. A graduated approach can be adopted exhausting other treatment options

to include medical therapy (steroid nasal sprays, antihistamines) or surgical procedures that can improve the airway without disturbing the septum (turbinate reduction, adenoidectomy) and buy time that will allow for additional nasal growth.

The quadrangular cartilage attains near complete growth between 2 years and 3 years of age and the remaining growth of the nose develops from increases in height and length of the bony septum.[19,20] 2 main nasal growth spurts have been identified: between the neonatal period and age 2 years to 3 years and the pubertal growth spurt.[16,21] Factors that may alter the growth potential of the nose include trauma or diminished nasal airflow.[22–25] Paties and their families may report that the patient had a straight nose in early childhood but upon entering puberty, the nose became deviated. Some of these patients have a history of a traumatic injury of the nose during elementary school or pre-teen years which was thought to be minor or which was not treated acutely. It is for this reason that I counsel all parents of children diagnosed with nasal fractures (whether operative or non-operative) of the possibility of delayed nasal deformity and/or nasal obstructive symptoms and advise them to come in for regular follow ups to assess the patient upon entering puberty.

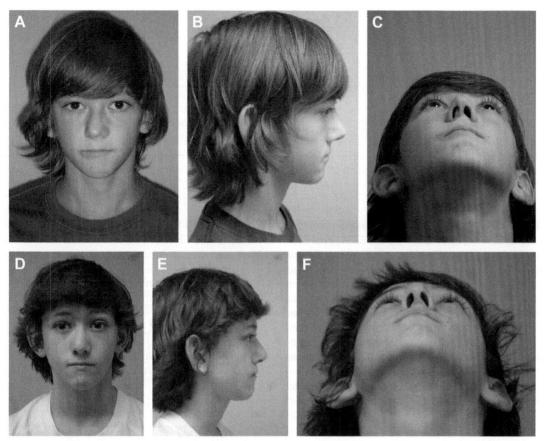

Fig. 2. (*A–C*) Preoperative clinical photographs depicting severe nasal deviation to the right and airway obstruction secondary to underlying septal deformity. (*D–F*) 8-month postoperative clinical photographs after surgical repair involving septoplasty, placement of bilateral spreader grafts, and lateral osteotomies. (*A* and *D*, Frontal view; *B* and *E*, side view; *C* and *F*, base view.) (*From* Adil E, Goyal N, Fedok FG. Corrective nasal surgery in the younger patient. JAMA Facial Plast Surg. 2014 May-Jun;16(3):176-82).

Nasal airway obstruction from a deviated septum can have several downstream negative impacts on growth of the nose and midface. Chronic nasal obstruction often leads to mouth breathing which has been shown to be associated with elongation of the lower face, lip incompetence, and class II malocclusion.[14,26] Additional nasal deformities may develop from chronic septal deviation. Caudal septal deviation can result in presentation of the septum into one nostril causing narrowing and asymmetry (**Fig. 3**A). Displacement of the caudal septum can cause inferior displacement of the ipsilateral nasal sill and in more severe instances, lateralization of the ala Position of the columella and midline support of the nasal tip are linked to the caudal septum. Once displaced from the midline, the growth of these structures is no longer in concert and the columella may be retracted and the tip deviated. Severe nasal obstruction may present in the neonatal period secondary to intra-uterine or birth trauma. Corrective surgery in infants may be

required given their status as obligate nasal breathers. Closed septal reduction can be performed to restore adequate nasal airflow.[19] Cephalometric has shown nasal, dental and midfacial deformities in children who are chronic mouth breathers from septal deviation as early as 7 years old.[26] In severe cases, where conservative therapy is ineffective, patients as young as 6 years old may benefit from septoplasty to avoid secondary deformities and years of quality of life disturbance.[16]

The determination of the severity of the obstruction and/or nasal deformity requires a detailed conversation with the patient and the parents to understand how the patient's quality of life is impacted. The ability to participate in sports, any psychosocial impact (feeling self-conscious, anxious or bullied because of the appearance of the nose) and how poor breathing quality, sleep disturbance or recurrent illnesses impact academic performance should be discussed. Patient reported outcomes (PROs) measures can also be

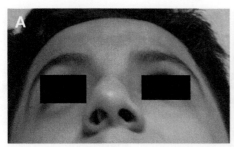 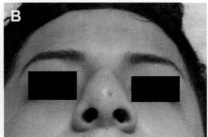

Fig. 3. 13 and a half year old patient with marked caudal septal deviation to the right with narrowing of the nostril and inferior displacement of the nostril sill (*A*). After open septorhinoplasty with caudal septal reconstruction and left internal valve reconstruction (*B*).

utilized in the pediatric patient to assess symptom severity and measure quality of life (QOL) improvement after surgery. The Nasal Obstruction Symptom Evaluation scale is one of the most frequently used PROs in the assessment of nasal obstruction severity.[27] Recently, the scale was validated for use in pediatric patients.[28–30] Other PROs have been used in published studies of outcomes of septoplasty or septorhinoplasty in children to include the SN-5 the Glasgow Benefit Inventory and the EQ5D.[7,17,31,32]

A survey of members of the American Academy of Facial Plastic and Reconstructive Surgery in 2021 assessed practice trends regarding pediatric rhinoplasty. One-third of respondents would perform rhinoplasty in children as young as 14 years of age, 1/3 of respondents choose 16 years old as the recommended age minimum and 10% of surgeons would perform rhinoplasty in children 12 years of age or older.[21]

In summary, septoplasty or septorhinoplasty in children should be performed in patients with severe nasal obstruction or deformity that are caused by deviated septum or abnormality of the osseocartilaginous skeleton. Other causes of obstruction must first be addressed if present. Circumstances that would require a young child (prior to the beginning of puberty and the associated growth spurt) to need a septorhinoplasty are most likely severe trauma, septal hematoma or abscess resulting in septal perforation and nasal reconstruction which may necessitate surgery in school age children in these situations. The beginning of puberty may mark the transition to a course of abnormal nasal growth resulting in symptoms of obstruction and external deformity. The recommendation to families in this circumstance would be to plan surgery at a point after other treatment options have been exhausted, ideally at least 1 year after the onset of puberty, when the patient is more mature and able to best cope with surgery and the recovery phase.

WHAT AREAS SHOULD I PRESERVE IN THE YOUNG PATIENT?
Menger

In the young patient, preservation of the growth centers of the nasal septum is crucial prior to the complete development and outgrowth of the nose. Nasal growth is characterized by 2 distinct spurts, occurring in the first 2 postnatal years and during puberty. The cartilaginous segment of the nasal septum exhibits a 3 dimensional organization during this development, featuring 2 thicker areas with disparate mitotic activity and histologic maturation.[33] These thicker areas, identified as growth zones, possess an approximate thickness of 3 mm, while the intervening thinner region boasts a transverse diameter of approximately 0.4 mm. Both zones extend from the sphenoid.

The "sphenodorsal" zone, situated between the sphenoid and the nasal dorsum, plays a pivotal role in the normal increase in length and height of the nasal dorsum.[34] Meanwhile, the "sphenospinal" zone, positioned between the sphenoid and the anterior nasal spine, serves as the driving force behind the forward outgrowth of the maxilla. Both clinical observations[1,2] and experimental studies[3,4] have demonstrated that the destruction of these growth zones during childhood leads to underdevelopment of both the nose and the maxilla. The impact on midfacial growth is age-related, with more severe outcomes observed in younger children compared to their older counterparts.[1]

A young child experiencing complete destruction of the nasal septum, whether due to surgery, trauma, or infection, will manifest with an underdeveloped nose exhibiting saddle deformity, retraction of the columella, over-rotation of the nasal tip, and retro-positioning of the maxilla. Conversely, complete reconstruction of the septum using autogenous cartilage grafts from the auricle or rib results in a normal development of the nose.[35,36] In summary, preservation of the 2 growth centers of the nasal septum is imperative in the young patient. In cases of severe nasal impairment, such as septum deviations or fracture lines, conservative dissection and mobilization of the septum can be undertaken without resection or removal of septal cartilage in the area of the growth zones.

Fedok

There has been considerable research into nasal growth. Nasal growth has been studied both in the normal patient as well as the effect on growth after various kind of traumas and surgery. The results of studies of children who have undergone extensive septal surgery for transseptal sphenoid surgery demonstrate that nasal growth can be quite resilient.[37,38] The results of research suggest that the center of growth of the nose appears to be at the bony-cartilaginous junction of the septum.[39] The relationship of the septum with the keystone area and the nasal floor appears to be of primary importance.

Surgical changes in the area of the rhinion and in that anatomic vicinity of the septal bony-cartilaginous junction appear to have a profound negative effect on nasal growth such as I have seen in younger patients who have undergone nasal dermoid removal.

In general principles, the surgical management of nasal deformity and malfunction in the younger patient should be performed with conservatism, be minimally invasive but effective. My approach to corrective surgery in the younger patient has been to repair what needs to be repaired, straighten that which needs to be straightened and replace missing tissue. One should utilize the most minimally invasive method of harvesting grafting material and, as much as possible, harvest the cartilage in a way that lessens donor site morbidity.

When presented with a saddle nose deformity that has occurred after trauma or surgery, I will attempt to restore central nasal support[4,40] eliminate the 4, reposition the nasal bones and replace missing structure with cartilage grafts, derived from the auricle or from rib. I will use only a cartilage graft from the septum if the small amount of cartilage from the septum has had to be removed as part of a primary intervention. (Like the minimum amount of cartilage that may be removed along the maxillary or palatine crest to perform a swinging door maneuver).

When presented with the patient with a severely deviated nose I will perform a septal "swinging door" maneuver, removing only a millimeter or 2 of cartilage to allow the repositioning of the septal cartilage. If a large septal spur is present posterior in the nose, almost as mimicking a nasal choanal atresia I will remove that spur and restore the airway. I will retain as much of the septal cartilage and bone in position or fracture it into position. I categorically keep as much septal cartilage and bone between the lining flaps as possible.

In case of the extremely crooked nose with deviation of the nasal bones I will carry out micro-osteotomies using a 1 mm to 2 mm osteotome and reposition the bones into an anatomic position. In the case of severe deformity of the nasal tip I will not carry out "tip refinement surgery" except to reposition and suture the upper lateral and lower lateral cartilages into more beneficial positions.

Finally, in my practice, corrective surgery does not include hump reduction or tip narrowing but instead, as mentioned above, I will manage a saddle nose deformity, and if necessary, I will place a cartilage graft in order to provide tip support.

The overall philosophy is to be surgically minimalistic, repair what needs to be repaired, preserve structure, and do not go beyond that.

Butts

An important decision point in septal surgery in children is whether or not the posterior bony-cartilaginous junction should be separated. Preservation of the bony-cartilaginous junction is advocated to prevent possible interference with growth which would result in diminished dorsal height or length.[13,24] Several reports of septoplasty in children describe open approaches and extracorporeal septoplasty to correct the most severe deviations.[18,20,24] Impacts of this approach varied from no effect on nasal growth[18,20,22] to the development of nasal tip ptosis or diminished dorsal height.[11] In general, leaving the bony-cartilaginous junction intact is attempted unless reconstitution of the airway is not possible otherwise.

Consensus does exist that only small segments of cartilage should be removed and attempts to reshape and replace cartilage and bone that is excised should be made. Techniques that can modify the septal cartilage are prioritized over resection. Cartilage scoring or mattress suture techniques that can correct bends in the septum are preferred. Other suturing techniques can be employed to correct middle vault asymmetries and may minimize the need for osteotomies or grafts to camouflage contour irregularities. Upper lateral cartilage (ULC) suspension to the nasal bone periosteum can correct avulsion of the ULC resulting from nasal trauma and the clocking suture between the ULC and septum can correct twisting of the middle vault.[23,42,43]

IF CARTILAGE GRAFTING IS NEEDED, WHAT ARE YOUR PREFERRED DONOR SITES IN THE YOUNGER PATIENT? DO YOU EVER USE ALLOPLASTS OR CADAVER SOURCES?

Menger

The preferred donor sites for younger patients are auricular and costal cartilage, particularly in the reconstruction of the nasal septum following cartilage destruction due to a septal hematoma, abscess, or severe trauma. In younger children (0–8 years), the use of auricular cartilage from 1 or 2 auricles proves sufficient for septal rebuilding, while rib cartilage becomes more suitable for older children.

The use of alloplasts, such as silicone, Teflon, or mersilene, is discouraged due to their relatively high incidence of postoperative chronic infections and implant extrusion.

Soluble implants, exemplified by the polydioxanone (PDS) plate with a thickness of 0.15 mm and perforations, offer valuable assistance in younger patients. For instance, they can aid in realigning nasal septal cartilage fragments into a straight septum after severe trauma. Additionally, PDS can be employed to reconstruct the nasal septum using auricular or rib grafts in cases of complete destruction, such as after a nasal septal abscess. In these instances, the PDS plate serves as a carrier or template to secure individual cartilage grafts, absorbing within 12 weeks.

Cadaver materials, including homologous implants like irradiated rib grafts derived from human donors, are deemed safe and effective for reconstructing the nasal skeleton in adult patients but are not recommended for younger individuals. This recommendation stems from 2 primary reasons: firstly, homologous materials lack growth potential, whereas autologous cartilage grafts exhibit evidence of growth in the developing nasal septum. Secondly, homologous implants exhibit a higher rate of resorption, often replaced by fibrous material, leading to a diminished support function compared to autologous cartilage.[44] Therefore, the use of homologous materials in children is not advised.

Fedok

This was somewhat addressed in the answer to question number 3. In general, I do not harvest septal cartilage or bone to use as a structural material in the younger patient. I believe the growth of the septum is crucial to the normal growth and maturation of the patient's nose. Where I have removed a millimeter or 2 of septal cartilage to allow mobilization of the septum, I will either put it back within the lining flaps of the septum or use as available for a structural change elsewhere in the nose. I will not remove septal cartilage primarily to be used as grafting material.

The auricular cartilage is my first choice in the pediatric patient as a source of cartilage material for grafting. Here again, the amount of cartilage that I remove will be quite minimal, and being careful not to remove cartilage that will affect the shape of the ear. At times portions of the cymba concha and the concha cavum can be removed while preserving all the native perichondrium.

Where a larger amount of donor cartilage is necessary to repair a more extensive injury such as a saddle nose deformity, I will go to the chest wall. In the younger patient, this is much easier than with the older patient. Because of the ease of dissection, there is less trauma to the soft tissues than might occur with an adult patient. The rib cartilages are quite soft and pliable, so the cartilage is relatively easy to harvest. I leave the perichondrium down at the donor site to allow some of the cartilage to regenerate. I do not advocate the use of cadaver material or the long-term use of an alloplast in any rhinoplasty patients.

Butts

My preference in the younger patient is to use autogenous sources of grafting. Studies have shown that nasal grafts can grow with the patient.[18,20,41] The threshold for using extra-nasal sources of cartilage grafting is lower to preserve the native septal cartilage. In addition, septal cartilage that needs to be removed may be fractured or fibrosed and not of adequate grafting quality to provide needed structural support. The auricles have reached near adult size by the time children are 6 years old and provide a good donor sitebut may not offer the needed structural support that rib cartilage provides. Graft harvesting procedures need to be discussed with families in the context of healing complications (graft resorption, warping) and the possible fate of grafts placed in the growing nose. If future revision surgery is needed and additional grafts must be placed, the patient and the family need to be prepared for this and understand which sites are available to harvest from.

I avoid alloplasts in the growing nose given increased risks of migration and extrusion and a possible future deformity that could occur with continued nasal growth. Cadaveric irradiated rib grafts avoid the donor site morbidity of autogenous rib but there are few reports of their use in pediatric rhinoplasty.There have been studies in cleft rhinoplasty showning some good outcomes.[45,46]

WHEN WILL YOU UTILIZE AN ENDONASAL RHINOPLASTY APPROACH IN THE YOUNGER PATIENTS? WHEN WILL YOU UTILIZE AN OPEN RHINOPLASTY APPROACH IN THE YOUNGER PATIENTS?
Menger

In general, rhinoplasty is discouraged in younger patients due to the potential risk of harm to the nasal skeleton, leading to disruptions in the normal development and outgrowth of the nose and maxilla. Indications for nasal surgery typically arise from conditions such as severely impaired nasal breathing resulting from trauma, infection, fistulas, dermoid cysts, among others. The choice of approach and technique should prioritize causing minimal trauma while achieving optimal results. In the majority of cases, the endonasal approach emerges as the preferred choice, allowing access to all compartments of the nose and facilitating the execution of most surgical techniques.

Conversely, the external approach does not impede nasal development. The open approach provides the advantage of visualizing nasal deformities with both eyes and allows for the use of 2 hands, often enhancing the precision of the reconstruction compared to the endonasal approach. Additionally, osteotomies performed during the procedure do not have a negative impact on nasal development. It is crucial to exercise caution and avoid the resection of cartilage from the nasal septum, especially in regions containing growth centers, to prevent the underdevelopment of the nasal skeleton.

Fedok

As with all of my rhinoplasty cases I decide on what approach to use, endonasal or open, by considering the patients anatomy and the goals I wish to accomplish. In general, the simpler the task, and the more normal the anatomy, the more likely, I am to do an endonasal approach. In doing so I avoid making an external incision, lessen the duration of postoperative edema and the other possible issues that may cause. Therefore, where possible I will perform endonasal approaches and minimize incisions as much as possible.

With the above in mind, however, I will not hesitate to do an open approach if the necessary tasks or the anatomy suggest a complexity that is beyond my ability to execute endonasally. The open approach allows easier access to all of the nasal structures. It allows easier execution of grafting challenges. The open approach, for me, allows better visualization of the existing anatomy and what is being accomplished as you carry out the surgery.

Butts

Open rhinoplasty has an excellent safety profile in young patients and has been used for approaches to the nasal dorsum for excision of benign lesions. Elevation of the soft tissue envelope for exposure to the nasal skeleton offers the same benefits in the pediatric age group as adults with no evidence of increased risks or interference with growth. Many patients require middle vault reconstruction and wide exposures to assess and correct post-traumatic or other complex deformities. The smaller nostril size in younger patients can make the endonasal approach more challenging.

Endoscopic assistance has an important role in septal surgery in the pediatric patients I operate on and can be an excellent adjunct for open or closed septal surgery. The magnified visualization facilitates elevation of the septal mucoperichondrium to avoid tears in the delicate flaps and aids in precise cartilage excision that may prevent over-resection of cartilage and weakening of the caudal and dorsal struts.[47]

HOW HAVE YOUR TECHNIQUES IN THIS AREA CHANGED OVER THE LAST 2 YEARS?
Menger

A critical consideration in performing rhinoplasties at a young age is the recognition that the organ is still undergoing growth and maturation. My general approach to nasal surgery in children remains unchanged. However, new insights into the growth and development of the nasal skeleton have led to adjustments in the timing of reconstruction. Over the last 15 years, I have encountered children who were referred to me with a history of a nasal septal abscess, resulting In complete destruction of septal cartilage. In some cases, no reconstruction was performed, while in others, only an incomplete reconstruction (specifically the L-strut) was carried out. In most instances, the interval between the nasal abscess and referral was 6 months to 12 months.

In an attempt to facilitate optimal conditions for the outgrowth of the nose, I reconstructed these nasal septa completely using autogenous cartilage from the auricle or rib. Unfortunately, during follow-up, the results were better than expected without intervention but not as good as those in children who had undergone a complete and direct reconstruction. These outcomes necessitated a second or third rhinoplasty with considerable reconstruction after the puberty growth spurt. This experience prompted a change in my policy. It is now preferable to allow for natural growth to complete before undertaking a comprehensive reconstruction of the nasal skeleton. In other words, the growth of the nose, both aesthetically and functionally, does not improve when the septum is fully reconstructed in the interim. Only a direct and complete reconstruction of the septum with autogenous cartilage from the rib or auricle allows for the normal development of the nose in children who have experienced complete destruction of septal cartilage due to a nasal septal abscess (**Figs. 4** and **5**).

Fedok

Fortunately, or unfortunately since my move to private practice, I have been seeing fewer of these younger patients except as those after relatively uncomplicated nasal trauma. Although I formerly performed a considerable number of craniofacial trauma procedures when I was working at Level I trauma center, I have not recently performed any significant pediatric craniofacial trauma procedures. I have had some ongoing experience with these younger patients suffering nasal and septal fractures. For those patients I have retained my philosophy for conservative but effective intervention and retention of normal anatomy. I remain, however, firmly a believer that deformity or functional problems after trauma should be treated rather promptly. I continue to consider the need to retore damaged anatomy to normal as paramount.[48] By freeing up these anatomic structures from the more fixed areas of the face, I am able to reposition their septum and improve the crookedness of their nose back to the midline.

I am adamantly not of the philosophy to wait for the younger patient to achieve a certain age (In my career I have heard age 18 is the magic age) for them to undergo correction after trauma. I feel relatively strongly that deformity should be repaired as soon as possible. I do not try to compensate for deformity with things such as the use of fillers. I seek a surgical correction, in that matter nothing has really changed for me in the last few years. In a small number of these patients I have employed a dorsal preservation technique to straighten a crooked nose.

Butts

With the availability of nasal QOL instruments designed for children or existing instruments now validated for pediatric patients, pre and post operative use of PROs in younger patients has been incorporated into my standard patient assessment process.

Patients with severe caudal septal deviation and nostril sill deformities are 1 example of the secondary soft tissue changes that can develop in patients with severe septal deviation during facial growth. With longer-term patient follow ups has come the ability to determine which patients with nostril sill deformities associated with

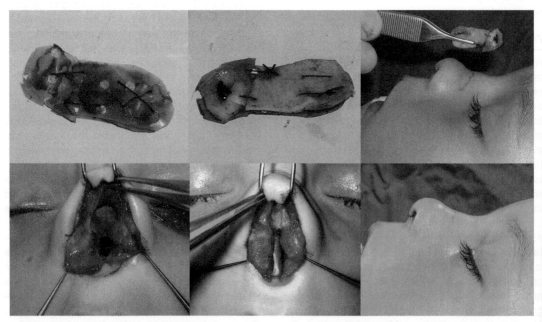

Fig. 4. Perioperative pictures of a direct and complete septal reconstruction with the use of auricular cartilage. The cartilage grafts were fixed to PDS plate to create a perfectly fitting implant in between the ULC and the premaxilla.

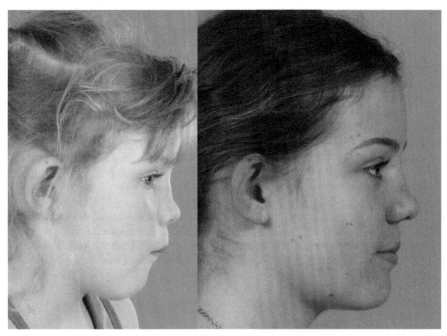

Fig. 5. Pre and postoperative lateral view. On the left side the pre-operative view of a 5-year-old girl with a nasal septal abscess. Notice the early signs of dorsal insufficiency. On the right side the same individual at the age of 16. The outgrowth of the nose and maxilla is within the normal range of standard deviations.

severe caudal septal deviation will correct after septoplasty and relocation of the septum to the midline and which patients will not (**Fig. 3**B). Attention to this asymmetry at the nasal base can be addressed with augmentation of the deficient side using cartilage grafting placed in a subcutaneous pocket.[49] Augmentation of the sill at the time of primary nasal surgery should be considered when the discrepancy between the sides is so significant that adequate improvement after correction of the caudal septal deflection alone is not expected to result in improvement of the asymmetry.

ACKNOWLEDGMENTS

Dr F.G. Fedok would like to recognize 2 co-authors for their roles in the publication: Adil E, Goyal N, Fedok FG. Corrective nasal surgery in the younger patient. JAMA Facial Plast Surg. 2014 May-Jun;16(3):176-82.

REFERENCES

1. Pirsig W. the influence of trauma on the growing nose. In: Mladina R, passali D, editors. Pediatric rhinology. Siena, Italy: Siena Tipografia Sense; 2000. p. 145–59.
2. Verwoerd CD, Urbanus MA, Nijdam DC. The effect of septal surgery on the growth of nose and maxilla. Rhinology 1979;XVII:53–63.
3. Norgaard JO, Kvinnsland S. Influence of submucous septal resection on facial growth in the rat. Plast Reconstr Surg 1979;64:84–8.
4. Nolst Trenite GJ, Verwoerd CDA, Verwoerd – Verhoef HL. Reimplantation of autologous septal cartilage in the growing nasal septum I. The influence of resection and reimplantation of septal cartilage upon nasal growth : an experimental study in growing rabbits. Rhinology 1987;25:225–36.
5. Graber TM. Postnatal development of cranial, facial and oral structures: the dynamics of facial growth. In: Graber TM, editor. Orthodontics: principals and practice. Philadelphia: WB Saunders; 1966. p. 69–78.
6. American Heritage Dictionary. The American heritage dictionary: fifth edition. Boston, MA: Houghton Mifflin Company; 2012.
7. Chauhan N, Warner J, Adamson PA. Adolescent rhinoplasty: challenges and psychosocial and clinical outcomes. Aesthetic Plast Surg 2010;34(4): 510–6.
8. Neuhann-Lorenz C. Adolescent rhinoplasty: challenges and psychosocial and clinical outcomes. Aesthetic Plast Surg 2010;34(4):517–8.
9. Bendre DV, Ofodile FA. Rhinoplasty in adolescent cleft patients. Oral Maxillofac Surg Clin North Am 2002;14(4):453–61.
10. McGrath MH, Mukerji S. Plastic surgery and the teenage patient. J Pediatr Adolesc Gynecol 2000; 13(3):105–18.

11. American Society of Plastic Surgeons Weighs inOn Growing Popularity of Teen Plastic Surgery. Newly-Published Recommendations Explain When Plastic Surgery Is and Isn't Okay for Teens. Connect by Americxan Society of Plastic Surgeons 2018;22.

12. Rohrich RJ, Cho MJ. When Is Teenage Plastic Surgery versus Cosmetic Surgery Okay? Reality versus Hype: A Systematic Review. Plast Reconstr Surg 2018;142(3):293e–302e.

13. Adil E, Goyal N, Fedok FG. Corrective nasal surgery in the younger patient. JAMA Facial Plast Surg 2014; 16(3):176–82.

14. Harari D, Redlich M, Miri S, et al. The effect of mouth breathing versus nasal breathing on dentofacial and craniofacial development in orthodontic patients. Laryngoscope 2010;120(10):2089–93.

15. Principato JJ. Upper airway obstruction and craniofacial morphology. Otolaryngol Head Neck Surg 1991;104(6):881–90.

16. Johnson MD. Management of Pediatric Nasal Surgery (Rhinoplasty). Facial Plast Surg Clin North Am 2017;25(2):211–21.

17. Lee VS, Gold RM, Parikh SR. Short-term quality of life outcomes following pediatric septoplasty. Acta Otolaryngol 2017;137(3):293–6.

18. Walker PJ, Crysdale WS, Farkas LG. External septorhinoplasty in children: Outcome and effect on growth of septal excision and reimplantation. Arch Otolaryngol Head Neck Surg 1993;119(9):984–9.

19. Christophel JJ, Gross CW. Pediatric septoplasty. Otolaryngol Clin North Am 2009;42(2):287–94.

20. El-Hakim H, Crysdale WS, Abdollel M, et al. A study of anthropometric measures before and after external septoplasty in children: a preliminary study. Arch Otolaryngol Head Neck Surg 2001;127(11): 1362–6.

21. Shehan JN, Liu J, LeClair J, et al. Pediatric septorhinoplasty: Current attitudes and practices by facial plastic and reconstructive surgeons. Am J Otolaryngol 2023;44(1):103684.

22. Jugo SB. Total septal reconstruction through decortication (external) approach in children. Arch Otolaryngol Head Neck Surg 1987;113(2):173–8.

23. Cottle MH. Nasal surgery in children. Eye Ear Nose Throat Mon 1951;30(1):32–8.

24. Justicz N, Choi S. When Should Pediatric Septoplasty Be Performed for Nasal Airway Obstruction? Laryngoscope 2019;129(7):1489–90.

25. Derkay CS. A conservative role for septoplasty in young children. Arch Otolaryngol Head Neck Surg 1999;125(6):702–3.

26. D'Ascanio L, Lancione C, Pompa G, et al. Craniofacial growth in children with nasal septum deviation: a cephalometric comparative study. Int J Pediatr Otorhinolaryngol 2010;74(10):1180–3.

27. Stewart MG, Witsell DL, Smith TL, et al. Development and validation of the Nasal Obstruction Symptom Evaluation (NOSE) scale. Otolaryngol Head Neck Surg 2004;130(2):157–63.

28. Yilmaz MS, Guven M, Akidil O, et al. Does septoplasty improve the quality of life in children? Int J Pediatr Otorhinolaryngol 2014;78(8):1274–6.

29. Din H, Bundogji N, Leuin SC. Psychometric Evaluation of the Nasal Obstruction Symptom Evaluation Scale for Pediatric Patients. Otolaryngol Head Neck Surg 2020;162(2):248–54.

30. Kawai K, Dombrowski N, AuYeung T, et al. Validation of the Nasal Obstruction Symptom Evaluation Scale in Pediatric Patients. Laryngoscope 2021;131(9): E2594–8.

31. Fuller JC, Levesque PA, Lindsay RW. Functional septorhinoplasty in the pediatric and adolescent patient. Int J Pediatr Otorhinolaryngol 2018;111:97–102.

32. Saniasiaya J, Abdullah B. Quality of life in children following nasal septal surgery: A review of its outcome. Pediatr Investig 2019;3(3):180–4.

33. Meeuwis J, Verwoerd – Verhoef HL, Verwoerd CDA. Norma land abnormal nasal growth after partial submucous resection of the cartilaginous septum. Acta Otolaryngol 1993;113:379–82.

34. Verwoerd CDA, Verwoerd – Verhoef HL. Rhinosurgery in children: Basic Concepts. Facial Plast Surg 2007;23:219–30.

35. Menger DJ, Tabink I, Nolst Trenite GJ. Treatment of septal hematomas and abscess in children. Facial Plastic Surg 2007;23(4):23–243.

36. Menger DJ, Tabink I, Nolst Trenite GJ. Nasal septal abscess in children: reconstruction with autologous cartilage grafts on polydioxanone plate. Arch Otolaryngol Head Neck Surg 2008;134(8):842–7.

37. Kassam AB, Thomas AJ, Zimmer LA, et al. Expanded endonasal approach: a fully endoscopic completely transnasal resection of a skull base arteriovenous malformation. Childs Nerv Syst 2007;23(5):491–8.

38. Rigante M, Massimi L, Parrilla C, et al. Endoscopic transsphenoidal approach versus microscopic approach in children. Int J Pediatr Otorhinolaryngol 2011;75(9):1132–6.

39. Van Loosen J, Van Zanten GA, Howard CV, et al. Growth characteristics of the human nasal septum. Rhinology 1996;34(2):78–82.

40. Vora NM, Fedok FG. Management of the central nasal support complex in naso-orbital ethmoid fractures. Facial Plast Surg 2000;16(2):181–91.

41. Lawrence R. Pediatric septoplasy: a review of the literature. Int J Pediatr Otorhinolaryngol 2012;76(8): 1078–81.

42. Pontius AT, Leach JL Jr. New techniques for management of the crooked nose. Arch Facial Plast Surg 2004;6(4):263–6.

43. Keeler JA, Moubayed SP, Most SP. Straightening the Crooked Middle Vault With the Clocking Stitch: An Anatomic Study. JAMA Facial Plast Surg 2017; 19(3):240–1.

44. Menger DJ, Nolst Trenite GJ. Irradiated homologous rib grafts in nasal reconstruction. Arch Facial Plast Surg 2010;12(2):114–8.

45. Insalaco LF, Karp E, Zavala H, et al. Comparing autologous versus allogenic rib grafting in pediatric cleft rhinoplasty. Int J Pediatr Otorhinolaryngol 2020; 138:110264.

46. Jenny HE, Siegel N, Yang R, et al. Safety of Irradiated Homologous Costal Cartilage Graft in Cleft Rhinoplasty. Plast Reconstr Surg 2021;147(1):76e–81e.

47. Tasca I, Compadretti GC. Nasal growth after pediatric septoplasty at long- term follow-up. Am J Rhinol Allergy 2011;25(1):e7–12.

48. Ondik MP, Lipinski L, Dezfoli S, et al. The treatment of nasal fractures: a changing paradigm. Arch Facial Plast Surg 2009;11(5):296–302.

49. Adham G, Keyhan SO, Fallahi HR, et al. Nasal sill augmentation: an overlooked concept in rhinoplasty- a technical note and review of the literatures. Maxillofac Plast Reconstr Surg 2021;43(1):14.

Management of Thick Skin in Rhinoplasty

Roxana Cobo, MD[a],*, Lucas G. Patrocinio, MD, PhD[b], Bahman Guyuron, MD[c,d],
Marco Swanson, MD[e]

KEYWORDS

- Rhinoplasty • Thick skin • Thick skin soft tissue envelope • Sebaceous skin • Undefined tip
- Dead space

KEY POINTS

- Thick skin in rhinoplasty can result in noses with poor definition and undesirable results if not managed properly.
- The skin rhinoplasty patients should be pre-conditioned for surgery with a skin care routine, diet and when needed, oral isotretinoin.
- Hemostasis is crucial as blood collections can turn to fibrosis, leading to poor definition.
- Special surgical maneuvers should be utilized to improve definition and decrease dead space.

PANEL DISCUSSION

1. What surgical approaches do you use to treat thick skin?
2. What medical treatments or minimally invasive treatments do you use to treat thick skin?
3. Are skin routines useful to manage the thick skin in rhinoplasty?
4. Can thick skin be evaluated adequately before surgery? What can be used?
5. How do you avoid dead space formation in the thick-skinned patient?
6. How have your techniques in this area changed over the last 2 years?

WHAT SURGICAL APPROACHES DO YOU USE TO TREAT THICK SKIN?

Patrocinio

I have 8 surgical steps which I consider my key points when I perform a rhinoplasty in a thick skin patient.

Costal Cartilage Graft

In thick skin patients, specially from African, Asian, and/or Native Indian descent, there is usually very weak, thin, and cephalic oriented lower lateral cartilages (LLC) associated to a more cephalic, retro-positioned, and flimsy caudal septum.[1] These characteristics make rib graft mandatory because of the amount of grafts that are necessary to accomplish a stable tip work and the inherent weakness and the limited amount of the quadrangular cartilage available as a donor graft.[2]

A piece with 5.0 cm to 7.0 cm can be obtained with a 1.5 cm to 2.0 cm incision. Rectus abdominis fascia can also be harvested through the same

[a] Facial Plastic Surgery, Department of Otolaryngology, Clinica Imbanaco, Carrera 38A #5A-100 cons 222A, Cali 760045, Colombia; [b] Private Practice, Otoface, Uberlandia Medical Center, Rua Rafael Marino Neto, 600 - Jardim Karaiba, Uberlandia, Minas Gerais 38411-186, Brazil; [c] Zeeba Clinic, 29017 Cedar Road, Lyndhurst, OH 44124, USA; [d] Case School of Medicine, University Hospitals Case Medical Center, Cleveland, OH, USA; [e] Dermatology and Plastic Surgery Institute, Cleveland Clinic, Cleveland Clinic Foundation, 2049 East 100th Street, Crile Building, A60 Plastic Surgery, Cleveland, OH 44106, USA
* Corresponding author.
E-mail addresses: Roxana.cobo@quironsalud.com; roxanacobo@gmail.com

Facial Plast Surg Clin N Am 32 (2024) 473–493
https://doi.org/10.1016/j.fsc.2024.06.004

incision. Using the oblique split technique to carve the grafts avoids cartilage wrapping.

Open Approach

Open rhinoplasty is my preferred approach because it allows a better placement and fixation of the grafts (which are very important in tip stabilization and long term outcomes in thick skin patients).[3] Also, the open approach gives the opportunity to better evaluate the subcutaneous tissue and treat it accordingly.

Despite the skin being thick and oily, the transcolumellar scar is inconspicuous.[3] Bilateral marginal incisions are joined with an inverted V incision in the middle of the columella.

Supraperichondral Tip Dissection

Dissection of the LLC is performed in the supraperichondrial plane. The subperichondrial plane may be tricky, because the weakness of the LLC may jeopardize tip sutures. Care should be taken exposing the Pitanguy ligament in the midline and the scroll ligaments (horizontal and vertical). They should be transected carefully and preserved for reconstruction as the final steps of the surgery.

Selective Defatting

The defatting is an important step to help control skin thickness. Selective debulking allows one to maintain the highlights in the center of the tip and to help keep the shadows in the supra tip and scroll areas, giving a better refined tip.[4]

Septal Extension Graft

The septal extension graft (SEG) is the most important graft for thick skin rhinoplasty. Initially described to lengthen a short nose, nowadays its application has expanded and it is particular important in my practice to control tip projection, rotation, and definition.

I routinely use double side-by-side SEG to have the maximum support possible to counteract skin thickness and scar contracture (**Fig. 1**). The graft is carved to span the whole height of the caudal septum and to set the tip position 10 mm to 12 mm above the final dorsum height. The 2 SEGs are fixated to the caudal septum with 5-0 polydioxanone mattress sutures. After the desired projection and rotation are achieved, the tip of the SEG should be trimmed to achieve better tip refinement and projection.[2]

I also use bilateral spreader grafts that are placed in submucosal tunnels and are trimmed to fit exactly end-to-end to each SEG. The combination of the double SEG with the bilateral

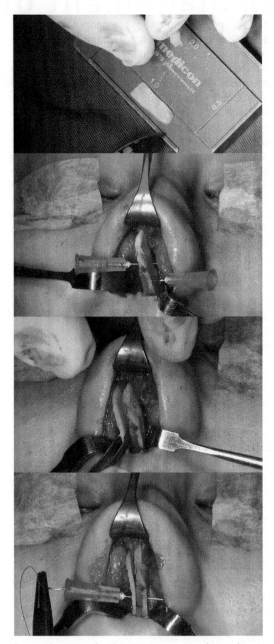

Fig. 1. Photographs showing suturing of costal cartilage side-to-side bilateral septal extension grafts (SEGs).

spreader grafts creates a stronger L-strut, which decreases the possibility of caudal and dorsal septum deviation and subsequent loss of projection and rotation (**Fig. 2**).

Lateral Crural Tensioning

The lateral crural tensioning (LCT)[5] is the workhorse in thick skin with a wide and amorphous

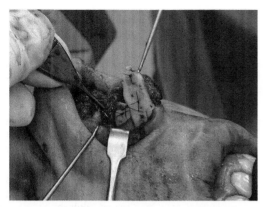

Fig. 2. Photograph showing costal cartilage side-to-side bilateral SEGs connected to end-to-end bilateral spreader grafts.

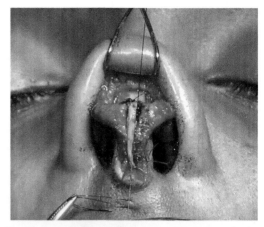

Fig. 3. Photograph showing lateral crural tensioning (LCT) and tongue-in-groove of the lower lateral cartilages (LLC).

nasal tip. The LCT is a modification of the lateral crural steal.[6] LCT stretches and flattens the lateral crura with a noticeable reduction in crural convexity and bulbosity, increasing tension and strength, thus achieving tip definition and better support of nasal valve and preventing alar retraction. Transdomal oblique 5-0 polydioxanone mattress sutures are used to set the new domes in a position that creates a flat lateral crus. Paradomal trimming is used to adjust the domes to 4 mm to 5 mm width.

The tongue in groove is initiated with the interdomal suture to the SEG. A 5-0 polydioxanone mattress suture is used, starting from the right side, transfixing the SEG 2 mm below the margin, then transfixing the center of the dome 1 mm below the margin, returning 2 mm cephalic to this point; then, transfixing again the SEG, 2 mm posterior and cephalic to the first point, and then transfixing the right dome the same way as the other one. The knot is tied carefully so the 2 domes are positioned symmetrically and the lateral crus everted, with the caudal margin higher than the cephalic one. The next suture is an intercrural 6-0 polydioxanone mattress suture, 6 mm to 8 mm below the domes, with the knot medially (**Fig. 3**). If further increase in columella projection is needed, a small strut can be interpolated to this suture to avoid or correct retractions and set better infratip angle.

Control of the Short Axis of the Lateral Crus

First of all, complete separation of the scroll ligament is necessary for adjustment of the lateral crura in the correct resting angle. Second, alar margins are weak in thick skin patients, and usually there is an important concavity around the alar ridge. Thus, lateral crus stabilization sutures and alar rim or lateral crural grafts should be added to achieve better aesthetic and function to the tip.

My first step is to apply a suture to reconnect the lateral crus to the upper lateral. And my second step is a suture to set the best resting angle possible and remove any fullness at the supra-alar and supra tip area. I prefer the pulley suture rather than the conventional spanning suture, which may cause further rotation of the tip, some degree of lateral crus cephalization, and eventually pinching of the tip. In the pulley technique, the suture is passed in the shape of a loop that embraces the lateral crus from the contralateral side of the nasal septum or the SEG.[2] The needle transfixes the SEG or the dorsal septum and upper laterals (2 mm–3 mm from the anterior border) contralateral to the crus that will be rotated. Then, the needle transfixes the lateral crus, from outside in, creating a loop that will act as a pulley to rotate the short axis. The entry point is in the upper face of the lateral crus, approximately 3 mm from the cephalic margin and 3 mm lateral to the dome. Next, the needle transfixes back the SEG or the dorsal septum and upper laterals back to the contralateral side, 2 mm below the first entry. The antero-posterior and cephalocaudal position of the suture may be modified, depending on each case. Finally, the knot is tightened on the same side as the first entry, observing the rotation of the short axis of the lateral crus, until it reaches the desired position (**Fig. 4**). Each crus is sutured separately, because the desired tension of the suture may differ for each side.

If further reinforcement of the caudal margin of the lateral crus is needed, alar rim grafts (articulate or floating) or lateral crus strut grafts can also be added. I prefer lateral crus strut grafts, because they strengthen and further flatten the lateral crus, creating a smooth lobule-all transition, and, usually, no flaring of the nostrils or alar base widening occurs.

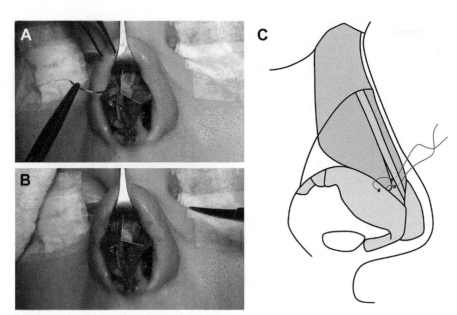

Fig. 4. Photographs and drawing showing the pulley suture and its effect in enhancing the resting angle. (*A*) Suture being passed between cephalic edge of lateral crus to cross the SEG. (*B*) Suture fixed in place. (*C*) Schematic drawing of suture where the "pulley effect" can be visualized.

Reduction of the Dead Space

Repositioning and resuturing the Pitanguy ligament and the vertical scroll ligament are helpful to avoid dead space and redraping of the skin, leading to better outcomes in tip definition. I will comment with more details on question number 5.

Guyuron/Swanson

To address patients with thick dermis there are specific surgical maneuvers focused on the following: (1) removal of interdomal tissue, (2) creation of a sufficiently firm nasal framework, (3) elimination of dead space, and (4) removal of redundant skin envelope.

Patients with thick skin tend to have more fibrofatty tissue both overlying and in between the nasal domes. This can be excised to decrease the bulkiness of the nasal tip. Through a transcolumellar approach, the nasal skin elevation is performed at the supra-superficial muscular aponeurotic system (SMAS) plane while leaving the excess fibrofatty tissue on the LLC. The subcutaneous fat is retained on the dermis to ensure good vascularity, especially in previously heavy smokers. The remaining fibrofatty tissue overlying the domes and between them can then be excised, skeletonizing the cartilaginous frame (**Fig. 5**).

In addition to fibrofatty tissue excision around the domes, it is essential to have a firm underlying cartilaginous frame. A strong frame will be able to withstand the weight of a thick skin envelope. Overtime the gradual and constant gentle pressure applied

by the rigid frame on the thick dermis will cause it to become thinner and more revealing, ultimately improving the definition. The creation of such a frame is achieved by using rigid cartilaginous grafts for tip support. The medial crura is strengthened with a columella strut graft. The lateral crura are frequently supported using lateral crura strut grafts. The domes are further stabilized with a subdomal graft.[7] Tip sutures also contribute significantly to creating a firm bed for the tip, including transdomal and interdomal sutures.[8] Furthermore, to prevent long term derotation of the tip from the weight of the skin, the medial crura are fixed to the caudal septum with 5-0 nylon, if needed. In patients with a long nose, this is performed after excision of a triangular portion of the caudal septum and a proportional amount of membranous septum. The tip should be set at least 8 mm and sometimes 10 mm anterior to the dorsum. The tip width should also not exceed 8 mm on patients with thick skin and 9 mm to 10 mm on those with average skin thickness at the nasal tip.

To mechanically eliminate dead space, a supratip stitch and/or simple splints can be placed as indicated. At the end of the procedure, to place the supratip stitch, the nasal envelope is draped over the nose and the transcolumellar incision is temporarily closed with a single suture. A 25-gauge needle is then dipped into methylene blue and the desired supratip break site is temporarily tattooed, while ensuring that the tip of the needle is deep enough and directed to mark the anterocaudal septal angle with methylene blue. The temporary transcolumellar stitch is then removed and

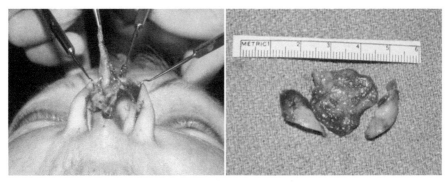

Fig. 5. Fibroadipose tissue over and between the domes being elevated. (*Left*). Tissue removed from between and overlying the domes along with excised cephalic portion of lateral crura (*Right*).

the skin envelope re-elevated. Using the tattoo as a guide, a 6-0 plain gut suture is placed through the deep subcutaneous tissue, through the antero-caudal septal angle and tied VERY GENTLY to the desired amount of supratip break. Caution should be taken as to not tighten the suture excessively, which can lead to overlying skin necrosis (**Fig. 6**). This technique also approximates the skin to the underlying lateral crura, helping eliminate dead space in this area as well.

If extensive dissection around the lateral crura is performed, such as with lateral crural struts or repositioning caudally, external simple splints should be placed.[9] Trapezoidally shaped pieces are cut from silicone sheets to encompass the supra-alar zone of dissection. 2 pieces are cut per side. One is placed internally and the other externally and sutured in place with a 4-0 Prolene suture, taking care to not overtighten and cause skin ischemia and necrosis (**Fig. 7**).

Similarly, if there is any redundant skin envelope after final re-draping, this should be trimmed to allow for an even wrapping of the skin over the created framework. This allows the rigid cartilaginous framework to exert gentle and constant pressure on the dermis and thus lead to good definition over time. The trimming is performed following the incision pattern and tapered laterally along the alar incision. Caution should be taken to not over excise and only trim the redundant tissue. The incision closure at the columella and the alar rims should remain tensionless (**Fig. 8**). At the end of the procedure the newly designed vestibular stents which will be described more elaborately below are placed to enforce elimination of any lateral dead space. Altogether, these surgical maneuvers can minimize the detrimental effects of thick skin on the outcome (**Fig. 9**).

Cobo

The surgical management of the thick skin patient can be divided into 2 big groups: intra-operative management and specific surgical approaches.

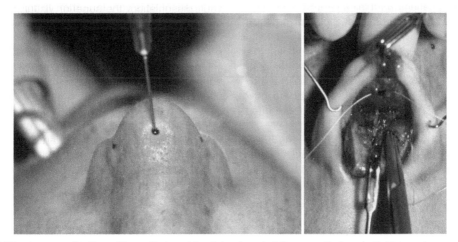

Fig. 6. A 25 gauge needle dipped in methylene blue introduced at the supratip break site transcutaneously down to the anterocaudal septal angle. A supratip suture is placed at the tattooed sites to appose the skin flap to the underlying frame as needed.

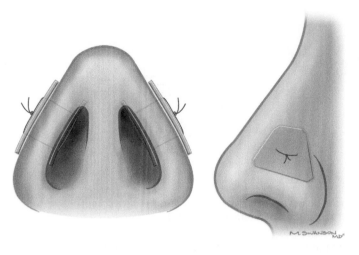

Fig. 7. An illustration of the simple splint design and placement for dead space elimination after extensive lateral dissection.

Intra-operative management is oriented toward controlling bleeding and swelling. The patients head should be slightly elevated above the rest of the body. Blood pressure should be controlled during the procedure and ideally the patient should be under controlled hypotension during the surgery. Intravenous tranexamic acid is routinely used to control bleeding and postsurgical chemosis.[10–12] In cases of severe bleeding desmopressin can also be used.[13] Tissue handling must be done carefully and cautery if used should ideally be done using bipolar cautery.

Surgical techniques in the thick skin patient will vary depending on how thick the skin soft tissue envelope (S-STE) is and on how big or small the underlying nasal skeleton is. They can be divided into 3 big groups: (1) Thinning of the S-STE/resection of the SMAS and fibrofatty layer, (2) Building up the underlying bony and cartilaginous framework, (3) Eliminating dead space formation.

Resection of the underlying fibrofatty layer is performed in patients with thick skin. SMAS resection is reserved for those patients that have an extremely thick inelastic skin (type III thick skin classification-see answer to question 4). In these cases, flap elevation is performed in the subdermal layer leaving all the SMAS and deep fibrofatty tissue attached to the underlying alar cartilages. The flap is elevated in the subdermal plane up to the supratip area and extended laterally to the cephalic edge of the lateral crus of the alar cartilages. The SMAS and deep fibrofatty tissue is then resected off the alar cartilages. This tissue is resected en-bloc and can be used later in surgery as a graft if necessary (**Fig. 10**A, B). Complications with SMAS debulking are uncommon if care is taken not to resect into the subdermal plexus and use of cautery is avoided as much as possible.

Building up the underlying bony and cartilaginous framework is especially important when the idea is to create definition. If necessary the dorsum is augmented and work is done to try and define the dorsal tip aesthetic lines. The nasal tip area can be problematic and difficult to treat in the thick skin patient. It is very important to try and create definition of nasal tip structures. Usually this

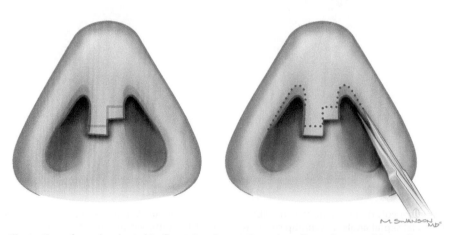

Fig. 8. An illustration of a redundant skin flap trimming at the columella and tapered laterally.

means increasing projection to try and push out the S-STE to create more definition over the nasal tip area. Many times, patients want small defined looking noses and it becomes very important to define how much projection is going to be achieved and to try and reach an agreement with the patient before surgery. If the patient does not want a big nose and has thick skin they must understand that it will not be possible to obtain great definition of the nasal tip after surgery. The objective of the surgery is to create a strong pedestal. This is done with a reinforced overlapping SEG (ROSEG graft) that is placed overlapping the patients existing caudal septum that has been previously aligned in the midline (**Fig. 11**). In addition to this, the lateral crura are tensioned over this pedestal creating a more defined looking tip.[5] If additional definition is needed in the nasal tip area a shield graft can be sutured in place in front of the medial crura or a bar graft can be placed over the dome area (**Figs. 12** and **13**).

Eliminating dead space is a must in all thick skin patients and is done routinely before closing the flap. This is done with sutures and using silicone splints over the lateral crura area. When a full open approach has been performed and wide dissection was done to be able to use powered instrumentation, drains are routinely left in place along the basal lateral osteotomy lines. All of this will be explained more extensively in question 5.

WHAT MEDICAL TREATMENTS OR MINIMALLY INVASIVE TREATMENTS DO YOU USE TO TREAT THICK SKIN?
Patrocinio

The first medical treatment is a detailed conversation with the patient about the extended postoperative care due to the thickness of the skin and the prolonged edema. Patients should be aware that final results can be reached only after 2 years to 3 years.

My main medication for the skin-soft tissue envelope is isotretinoin.[14] Despite few studies on that, I see in my patients the same evidences that are already published in the literature. Oral isotretinoin in patients with thick skin accelerates improvement in cosmetic results during the early months after surgery[15] and the patients were more satisfied with their operation outcomes and experienced fewer skin problems.[16] On the other hand, it seems that isotretinoin does not significantly affect the final cosmetic result in 1 year.[15]

Patients usually receive a drug regimen a dose ranging from 0.25 mg/kg to 0.5 mg/kg for a period of 4 months to 6 months. My routine is to prescribe 20 mg daily, starting 30 days to 60 days before

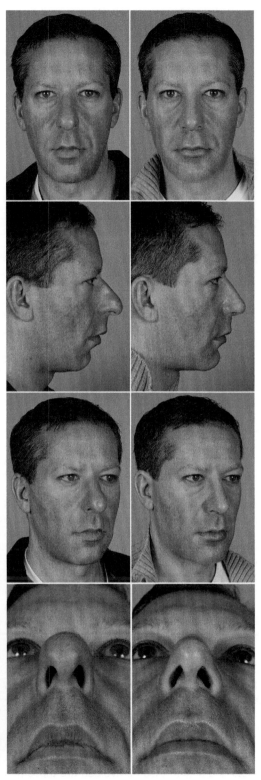

Fig. 9. Before and after photographs of a 48-year-old male patient with thick skin, over-projected nose and cephalically oriented LLC, 12 months after rhinoplasty and a sliding genioplasty.

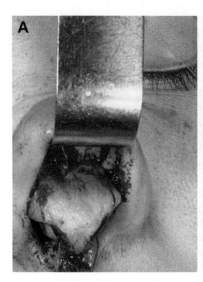 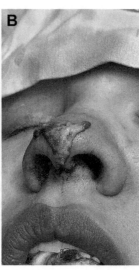

Fig. 10. (*A*) Skin flap elevated in subdermal plane leaving SMAS and deep fibrofatty tissue attached to underlying alar cartilages (*B*). SMAS and deep fibrofatty tissue resected en-bloc.

surgery and suspend it 7 days before surgery. Then, 7 days after surgery it is resumed and kept for 6 months minimum (**Fig. 14**). If the patient complaint of any side effects, I reduce the dose to 3 times a week (mondays, wednesdays, and fridays). All patients are monitored with hepatic function tests, however, I have never had any problem with that using this regimen and I have seen the same outcomes with these doses as recent papers.[17]

External splinting remains for 7 days to 10 days. Taping is used for 1 week more all day and another month during the night. I consider the taping very important and I educate the patient to use it adequately and explain that are evidence that suggest that it is useful.[18] In selected cases, I also use subcutaneous injections of corticosteroids (triamcinolone) postoperatively to help reduce the edema in the supratip area.[19,20] The dose of 0.2 mL to 0.4 mL of 10 mg/mL is used 2 weeks after surgery and repeated subsequently every 4 weeks depending on the response obtained (**Fig. 15**).

In thick skin, is also common to have complications related to incisions, such as hyper or hypopigmentation, hypertrophic scars, and keloids. Dermabrasion, laser, and triamcinolone injections might be applied to help reduce these effects.[21] I am also careful watching the recent advances on the use of other chemical agents to enhance skin adhesion.[22,23]

Guyuron/Swanson

Non-surgical interventions prior to surgery to target sebaceous overactivity and decrease the chances of poor definition after rhinoplasty, include dietary changes, a strict skin care regimen, and oral retinoids if needed.[9,14,24] Foods that have been shown to disrupt sebaceous gland homeostasis and should thus be avoided are those rich in hyperglycemic carbohydrates, milk and dairy products, saturated fats and trans fats. These types of food promote insulin growth factor signaling, leading to a downstream cascade of

Fig. 11. ROSEG Graft. Reinforced Overlapping SEG placed to strengthen the nasal pedestal.

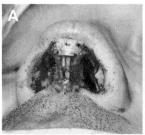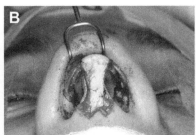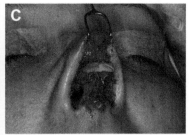

Fig. 12. (*A*) Image of a small shield graft placed in front of domes to help define nasal tip area (*B*). Long shield graft placed caudal to feet of intermediate and medial crura trying to improve nasal tip projection and definition (*C*). Bar graft placed over dome area to increase tip projection and improve definition of nasal tip area.

events that interferes with normal androgen receptor activity.[25,26] This is especially applicable in adolescent patients who are prone to having acne flare-ups.

If the patient does not respond to topical retinoids or presents with severe acne or sebaceous overactivity, oral isotretinoin is recommended.[7,14,27] Ideally these patient should be co-managed with a dermatologist and be closely followed with routine laboratory tests including pregnancy tests, serum lipid profiles, and liver function tests. Isotretinoin is a teratogen, and is thus contraindicated in women able to have children unless there is a strict contraceptive regimen prior to commencing and during therapy. The conventional dosing is 0.5 mg/kg/day to 1 mg/kg/day, but studies have shown that a low dose of 0.25 mg/kg/day to 0.5 mg/kg/day is equally effective in treating acne and associated with fewer side effects and lesser relapse rates.[28] The majority of patients should be acne free about 4 months after starting treatment. Due to its potential to delay healing, isotretinoin should be stopped pre-operatively.[25] We usually stop isotretinoin 6 months prior to rhinoplasty[7] (**Fig. 16**).

Post-operatively, edema and blood accumulation in areas of potential dead space turns into scar tissue, which is severely detrimental to the aesthetic outcome. It leads to loss of tip definition and supratip deformity. In rhinoplasty, especially if the skin is thick, having good hemostasis is crucial. In addition to pre-operative local infiltration of anesthesia with epinephrine and tranexamic acid (TXA) as well as meticulous dissection and precise electrocautery hemostasis, the use of intravenous TXA for cases with persistent bleeding at a dose of 10 mg/kg (including the amount infiltrated with local anesthesia) can be useful. In cases with further persistent bleeding, intravenous desmopressin (DDAVP) (0.3 μg/kg)[13,29] can be used, administered in a period of 30 minutes to 45 minutes. Patients who require TXA and DDAVP intra-operatively are thoroughly counseled and closely followed for deep venous thrombosis prophylaxis post-operatively. Patients who require DDAVP should also be advised about the extremely rare complication of syndrome of inappropriate anti-diuretic hormone with DDAVP, which manifests as excessive thirst and can lead to fatal volumes of water consumption. It is a common occurrence that patients with intra-operative clotting issues have negative routine coagulation screening.[30] Additionally, patients with thick or oily skin, or those with a history of keloid scarring have an increased risk of forming post-operative edema and subsequent fibrosis, especially in the supratip area. In these patients, a prophylactic intra-operative injection of triamcinolone acetonide (0.1 cc–0.2 cc of 40 mg/mL) is recommended in the supratip area before final closure.

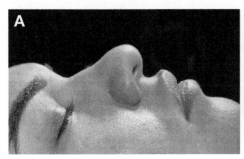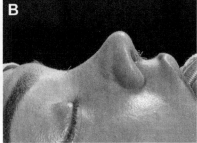

Fig. 13. (*A*) On the table presurgical lateral view of patient with thick skin (*B*). On the table postsurgical lateral view of same patient after SMAS resection, placement of ROSEG graft and small shield graft to improve projection and definition of nasal tip area.

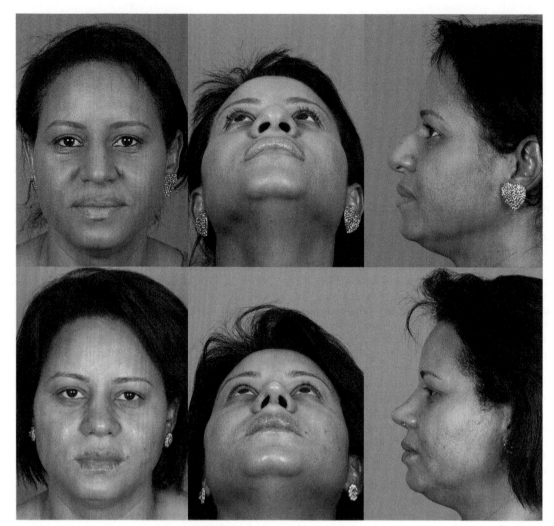

Fig. 14. Pre and post-operative photographs of a patient submitted to rhinoplasty and oral isotretinoin for 6 months after surgery.

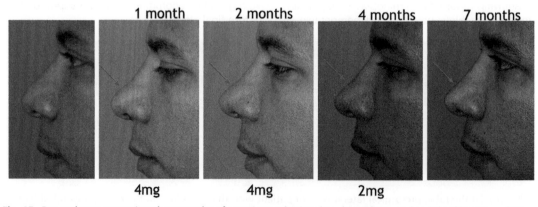

Fig. 15. Pre and post-operative photographs of a patient submitted to rhinoplasty and serial infiltration of triamcinolone showing improvement of the supratip break 7 months after surgery.

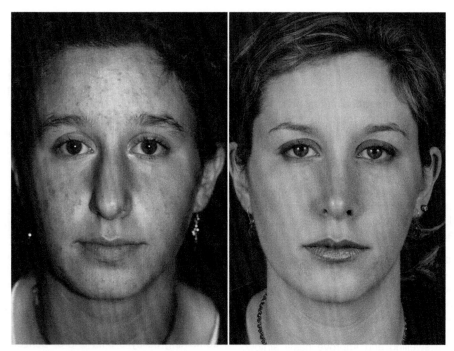

Fig. 16. Patient photograph demonstrating improvement in both nasal skin thickness and overall facial skin quality after skin care and Retin A, followed by rhinoplasty.

Cobo

All thick skin patients are treated not only surgically but also medically. This is called an "integrated management" to the thick skin rhinoplasty patient and several steps must be followed.[24]

1. The thick skin patient's skin is classified into categories I-III depending on the degree of thickness and the findings on the skin (see answer to question 4). Depending on this classification different decisions are made medically and surgically.[24]
2. All patients are prescribed a skin routine that targets sebum formation, controls oil production and exfoliates skin (see answer to question 3).
3. Patients are recommended an anti-inflammatory diet where patients are asked to avoid hyperglycemic carbohydrates, sugary drinks, saturated fats and transfats, milk and milk derivatives. This helps control postsurgical inflammation and helps prevent acne breakouts which are very common in young adults and adolescents.[26,31]
4. In type III thick skin patients (ultra thick skin patients) and patients that have acne prone skin can benefit from taking oral isotretinoin and this has been an important adjuvant when treating thick skin rhinoplasty patients.[14,24]

The dosing has become very important in the treatment of these patients because it has increased patient compliance and reduced side effects. Multiple studies have shown that low dose schemes (0.25 mg/kg/day–0.40 mg/kg/day) are just as efficient as standard dosing regimes (0.5 mg/kg/day–1.0 mg/kg/day), have less side effects and are better tolerated.[32–34]

Today, intermittent dosing (10 mg–20 mg/2–3 times a week) is being used regularly by dermatologists and has better patient compliance of their therapy.[28]

This has become an excellent therapeutic alternative for those patients with sebaceous hyperplasia and oily skin. It is also used frequently in patients with mild acne. It is important though, that patients adhere to treatment to prevent relapse of acne flare-ups.

The improvement of the skin quality and acne can be usually seen after 16 weeks to 20 weeks of treatment. Treatment will shrink oil glands and control sebum production. This effect can be permanent after 6 months of treatment with oral isotretinoin. Today, there is no reason to postpone surgery for patients on oral isotretinoin. Studies show that there is no reason to delay skin surgery, dermabrasion or chemical peels.[27]

For the past 8 years, the author has been using oral isotretinoin without any type of complications and without having to postpone surgery. The medication is stopped right before surgery and re-started 2 weeks after surgery when tapes come off.

On patients who were not able to receive treatment before surgery, oral isotretinoin can also be started right after surgery with good results. With these patients, the author starts them on medication 2 weeks after surgery when the tapes are taken off.

All patients on oral isotretinoin must be followed periodically. Before starting treatment, routine laboratory tests including pregnancy tests, serum lipid profiles, and liver function tests must be performed and repeated during the treatment as needed. Pregnancy is an absolute contraindication while on this medication due to the teratogenic side-effects of the medication. All patients (and their legal guardians) must be counseled properly before starting treatment.[14,27,28,32–34]

5. Late post-operative treatments include the use of intranasal topical steroid sprays (fluticasone, mometasone). These are routinely used to improve intranasal swelling. They are started 3 weeks after surgery and continued for 3 months after surgery. They will help reduce intranasal swelling and improve nasal airflow. In specific cases where there is localized fibrosis or scar tissue formation, subdermal steroid injections using triamcinolone acetonide (10 mg/cc) can be used. These injections can be repeated every 4 weeks to 6 weeks if necessary. The use of these injections in my practice has reduced dramatically after using the isotretinoin protocol with our thick skin patients.

ARE SKIN ROUTINES USEFUL TO MANAGE THE THICK SKIN IN RHINOPLASTY?
Patrocinio

The thick skin is also oily, sebaceous, and inelastic, thus, skin treatment usually helps in some point and a treatment regimen is performed on an individual basis to reduce skin inflammation.[24,35]

First of all, sunblock should be used pre and postoperatively. Pre-operative skin cleansing and exfoliation is recommended for all the patients to control oil production and remove dead skin cells while also opening clogged pores. Most commonly I use salicylic acid or benzoyl peroxide, but alternatives such as topical antioxidants, alpha-hydroxy, and retinoids can be used. I use the same regimen as for the oral medications (starting 30 days–60 days before surgery and suspend it 7 days before surgery; then, 7 days after surgery it is resumed and kept for 6 months minimum).

Guyuron/Swanson

Strict adherence to an individualized skin care routine is also crucial and involving a dermatologist can be essential. Skin regimens usually include a combination of a skin cleansing, exfoliation, whether mechanical or chemical, and sebum controlling agents to decrease inflammation. Common skin cleansing and exfoliating agents contain salicylic acid or benzoyl peroxide, which help control sebum production, promote exfoliation, clear pores, and decrease trapped debris and sebum. Additionally, topical antioxidants, retinoids (ie, tretinoin), and the generous application of sunblock aid with stabilization of the epidermis.

Cobo

For the past 8 years, the author is using skin routines in all rhinoplasty patients. If possible a skin protocol is started before surgery at the time of the initial consultation and is continued at least for 6 months post surgery. Treatment is aimed at treating the epidermis and dermis with exfoliation, pore unclogging, and control of sebum production. This is achieved through the use of cleansing agents containing salicylic acid and/or benzoil peroxide and when needed topical treatments with retinoic acid and benzoil peroxide. The final objective of treatment is to diminish the inflammatory response of the skin and control edema.[24,36,37]

Before surgery all patients receive a facial where blackheads and comedones are removed. Additionally, after surgery, patients are treated with manual lymphatic drainage of the perinasal area and face. This will help reduce swelling and will control edema.

CAN THICK SKIN BE EVALUATED ADEQUATELY BEFORE SURGERY? WHAT CAN BE USED?
Patrocinio

The difficulty in evaluating the skin in rhinoplasty patients occurs because it is not only a matter of thickness of the skin, but also color, elasticity, oiliness, vascularity, sebaceous glands alterations, subcutaneous characteristics, and many others. In my practice, we have a big mixture of a bit of everything. Brazil is a mixing pot of different cultures and an interracial reproduction for the last 500 years.

I have been using ultrasonography to evaluate the skin and soft tissue envelope of the nose for the last 13 years.[38] During these periods, we have tried to standardize the method of evaluation and to compare pre and post-operative thickness and other characteristics of the skin and subcutaneous tissue. Nowadays, we use high-frequency (22 MHz) ultrasound evaluation of the epidermis and dermis. We have found that the original findings by Jack Sheen that the more you stretch the soft tissue envelope, the more you can achieve better tip definition. Unfortunately, a great part of the patients do not want their tips (over)projected. So, I had to direct my efforts toward better control of the lateral crus position, the suturing of the dead space, and the medical treatment of the soft tissue envelope.

Anyway, clinical evaluation and skin pinch is still my preferred method to evaluate and to educate the patient on the difficulties of achieving tip definition on thick skin patient, specially in the inelastic skin.[39]

Guyuron/Swanson

The pre-operative assessment before rhinoplasty should include an evaluation of the skin for pigmentation, consistency, elasticity, porosity, as well as sebaceous gland activity. Skin quality is different between individuals, but can also vary within the same individual depending on the stage of life. Studies on nasal skin thickness have demonstrated that it is thickest at the radix (1.25 mm–3.96 mm) and nasal tip (2.3 mm–3.32 mm) and thinnest at the rhinion (0.6 mm–1.86 mm) and columella (0.73 mm–2.3 mm).[40–42] Skin thickness is influenced mainly by genetics and ethnicity, however, certain medications, trauma, prior surgery, anatomic region, as well as age and gender also play a determining role.

Sebaceous glands are integral to the structure and function of skin, contributing to the majority of skin lipids secreted in the form of sebum. They are directly involved in hormone formation and regulation and thus are highly influenced by systemic hormonal changes, including androgens, estrogens, glucocorticoids, and prolactin.[43] Furthermore, diets high in fatty and hyperglycemic contents can increase their activity. Despite their skin protective role, certain conditions are associated with dysregulation or hyperactivity of these glands, such as acne vulgaris as well as rosacea and rhinophyma. Sebaceous glands are present in highest density around the nasal supratip and tip areas.[44] Highly sebaceous skin appears oily and highly porous on examination. In contrast, skin with thick dermis tends to have less density in sebaceous glands, is less porous and is often described as somewhat red and shiny (**Fig. 17**). Dermal thickness is mainly influenced by ethnicity, age, anatomic region, and certain chronic medication use, namely steroids. Certainly, ultrasound measurements are possible and provide accurate information. However, not every office possesses this device and its value is debateable. The skin thickness can readily be assessed by both the experienced and beginners alike.

Cobo

The thickness of the S-STE varies in patients. Patients can have a thick deep fatty areolar tissue and SMAS or both. Authors have constantly been trying to measure the S-STE to try and plan surgery accordingly.[36,40,45–47]

For this they have used ultrasound, computed tomography scans, cone bean tomography, and MRI. All of these tools can be helpful if they are available but many times increase the cost of consultation. What is done by most surgeons though is a clinical diagnosis to try and define skin quality and thickness.

For over 8 years, the author has been using a skin evaluation sheet where thickness, oiliness, pore description, changes in coloration, and skin elasticity are documented.[24] A pinch test is routinely done over the rhinion and supratip area to define skin elasticity and define how easily the S-STE can be detached from the underlying skeleton at the supratip and rhinion of the nose. Depending on the result and on the description of skin findings like pore size, presence of acne, oiliness, and so forth the skin is classified into 3 categories (**Fig. 18**).

Type I is the thick skin patient with good skin quality that has a "positive" pinch test over rhinion and supratip.

Type II is the thick skin patient that has less elasticity especially when the pinch test is done over the supratip area. They can have slight to moderate acne, oiliness, and open pores.

Type III patients have thick inelastic skin and a negative pinch test over rhinion and supratip area. There is a clear tendency for acne formation, skin will be oily with high sebum production.

Type II and Type III patients are patients that can additionally benefit from oral isotretinoin schemes. All thick skin patients need an integrated approach to their surgery where topical, medical, and surgical approaches are combined to obtain the best result possible.

HOW DO YOU AVOID DEAD SPACE FORMATION IN THE THICK SKINNED PATIENT?
Patrocinio

Control of dead space is one of the main points in thick skin and revision rhinoplasty. There are medical and surgical approaches to it. In my routine, the medical approach is the use of isotretinoin and triamcinolone associated to prolonged external splinting and taping as detailed on question number 2. The surgical approach is the reconstruction of the deep Pitanguy ligament and the vertical scroll ligament. The transection of these 2 ligaments (along with the horizontal scroll

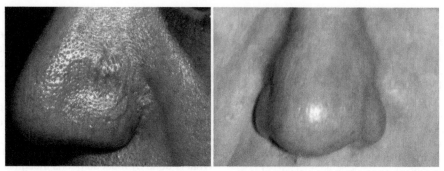

Fig. 17. A patient example with sebaceous overactivity (*left*) and a patient with thicker dermis (*right*).

ligament) are mandatory in thick skin patients, otherwise one can not correct the position of the tip and the resting angle.

The deep Pitanguy ligament is reinserted using 4-0 polydiaxonone sutures between the medial crura and the vestibule mucosa reaching the preserved ligament and them returning to the contralateral side.[48] This suture increases supratip break and prevents pollybeak deformity (**Fig. 19**). The vertical scroll ligaments are resutured in the same fashion, but the suture is passed through the inner lining of the scroll region. A second option is to use external splint to avoid dead space and redirect the reconnection of the scroll region. Alternatively, externals sutures can be used to achieve the same goals (**Fig. 20**). Care should be taken with the knot pressure not to damage the vascularization to the skin.[49]

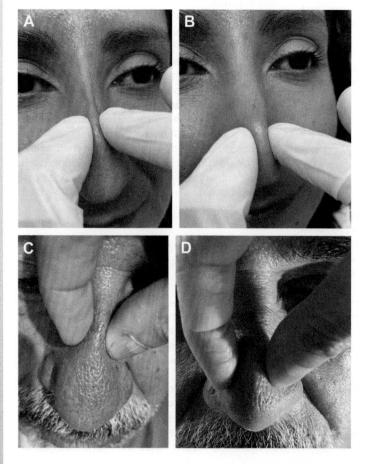

Fig. 18. Pinch Test Supratip and Rhinion. The pinch test measures elasticity and how easily skin can be detached from underlying skeleton. (*A, B*) Positive pinch tests at rhinion and supratip area in a type I thick skin patient. (*C, D*) Negative pinch test ar rhinion and supratip area in a type III thick skin patient.

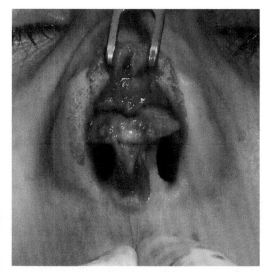

Fig. 19. Photograph showing re-suture of the Pitanguy ligament.

Guyuron/Swanson

In addition to medical adjunct measures, dead space must be mechanically eliminated by means of a supratip stitch and/or simple splints as indicated. As mentioned above, a supratip stitch can be placed by means of a 25-gauge needle dipped in methylene blue or brilliant green to tattoo the supratip break over the skin and the underlying anterocaudal septum.[50] Care must be taken so as not to tighten the stitch excessively and lead to skin dimpling with potential necrosis. If extensive lateral dissection is performed to reposition the lateral crura or place lateral crura strut grafts, external simple splints are recommended. As indicated earlier, these are cut pieces of silicone sheet

placed intranasally and externally, and sutured in place using a 4-0 Prolene. As described below, the newly designed internal nasal splint helps further eliminate dead space by means of gentle outward pressure from intranasally.

Cobo

Dead space formation should always be managed in rhinoplasty but especially in the thick skin patient. This will help decrease blood accumulation in the supra tip area and will help control swelling and secondary scar tissue formation in these regions.

A supratip suture that approximates the S-STE in the supratip area to the most anterior portion of the dorsal septum (behind the anterior septal angle and behind the dome area) is placed using an absorbable suture. The supratip break point is marked with a needle in the area where this suture is going to be placed. Care must be taken not to overtighten the suture as this could produce skin necrosis. When extended lateral dissection has been performed over the lateral crura, additional sutures are placed between the subcutaneous tissue and the scroll area. These sutures can also be placed as full thickness sutures tying them over the skin in the supratip and scroll area[37,49] (**Fig. 21**).

Another option to control dead space formation is the placement of silastic splints over the lateral crura area intranasally and externally suturing them in place to reduce swelling and dead space formation. The author routinely places gelfoam inside the vestibule area of the nose to reduce edema in this region.

In the cases where a full open approach was used, additional drains are placed following lateral osteotomy sites and secured inside the nasal

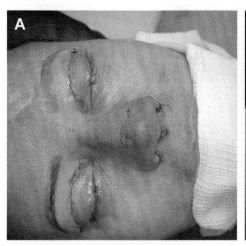
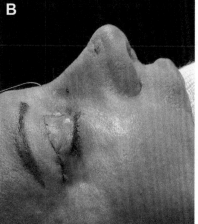

Fig. 20. Photograph showing external suturing to avoid dead space at the supra tip (*A*) and scroll area (*B*).

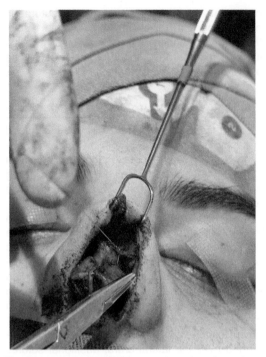

Fig. 21. Internal Scroll Sutures. Are placed to close dead space area in scroll area.

vestibule to facilitate blood drainage from this area and prevent chemosis formation. Drains are removed after 72 hours.

HOW HAVE YOUR TECHNIQUES IN THIS AREA CHANGED OVER THE LAST 2 YEARS?
Patrocinio

We usually change our technique if either one of the 2 situations occur: complications or patient dissatisfaction. In thick skin patient, it is usually the latter.

The usual unsatisfied thick skin patient returns after 2 years to 3 years of rhinoplasty and complaints about loss of tip projection, loss of tip rotation, and/or underachievement of tip definition. In the last 2 years (and also in the last 20 years), I have focused on improving my techniques for tip definition and long term stability.

Nowadays, I use costal cartilage in 100% of my thick skin patients. If the patient does not accept costal cartilage harvesting, he/she is not suitable to my practice. It used to be very uncomfortable to me when a patient of mine returned to my office after 2 years to 3 years and complained about the loss of rotation or projection. It was difficult to me

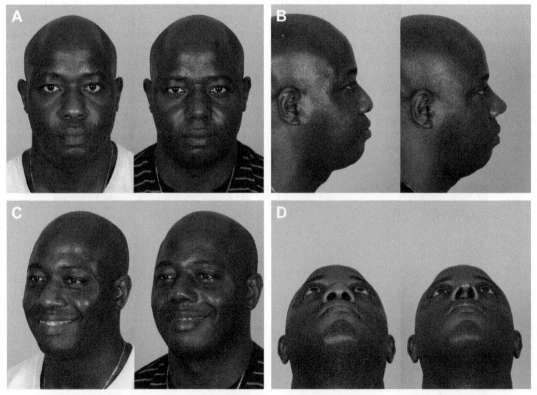

Fig. 22. Pre and 1-year postoperative photographs of a 35-year-old male that underwent open rhinoplasty with bilateral side-to-side SEGs connected to en-to-end bilateral spreaders grafts to achieve better support of the nasal tip. (*A-D*) Preoperative views, left image, Postoperative views, right image.

to admit that there was another donor site for grafts (the rib), that could have had more stability and that we could have used it at the first surgery. We now have more control of complications related to rib grafting and it is not an issue that should make surgeons avoid it.

At the same page, that is why I use bilateral side-by-side SEG connected to end-to-end to bilateral spreader grafts. These grafts span the whole L-strut and provide, in my hands, the best structural tip support for suturing of the LLC (**Fig. 22**).

A second point that I changed was the control of the lateral crus. I now spend much more time during the surgery trying to suture the lateral crus in the correct resting angle and reinforcing it with grafts (usually underlay grafts). I really think the surgeon have to spend all his/her efforts on setting the lateral crus on the correct position (short and long axis), otherwise all the other maneuvers will not be of much help (**Fig. 23**).

A third point is the focus on avoiding dead space. I have tried external splints, internal suturing, and external suturing. In my opinion, internal suturing for the supratip is technically easy to perform and provides excellent outcomes. On the other hand, internal suturing for the vertical scroll ligament is technically difficult and provides the same outcomes as the other option. So, I changed to external suturing for the vertical scroll ligament (**Fig. 24**).

Finally, I keep studying and incorporating medical skin treatment. Probably, it is the new frontier that we, as surgeons, still lack the ability to control.

Guyuron/Swanson

We have designed the BG Splint™, a new nasal internal splint that combines a paired set of modified nostril stents and modified septal splints into one single piece of flexible silicone (**Fig. 25**). The stent and septal splint for each side are connected anteriorly by an isthmus, which prevents inadvertent migration of the construct into the nasal cavity. The BG Splint™ serves the function of nostril

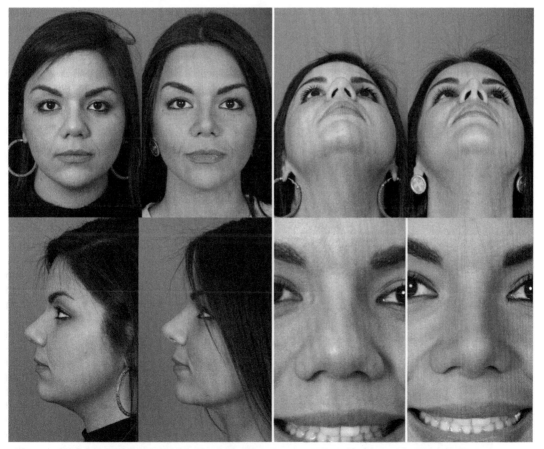

Fig. 23. Pre and 1-year postoperative photographs of a 25-year-old female that underwent open rhinoplasty with bilateral side-to-side SEGs connected to en-to-end bilateral spreaders grafts, associated LCT and lateral crus repositioning sutures (pulley suture) to achieve better definition of the nasal tip.

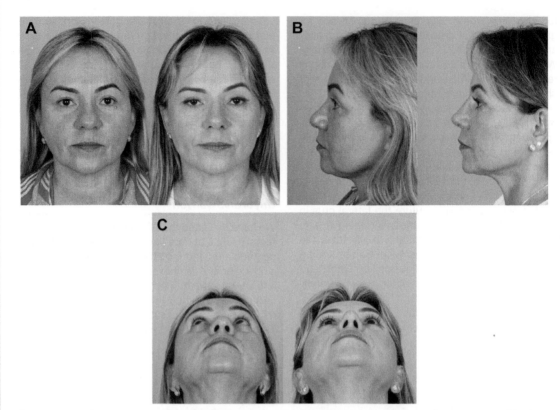

Fig. 24. Pre and 1.5-year post-operative photographs of a 44-year-old female that underwent upper blepharo-plasty and open rhinoplasty with bilateral side-to-side SEGs connected to en-to-end bilateral spreaders grafts, associated LCT and lateral crus repositioning sutures (pulley suture), and internal and external suturing to avoid dead space formation. (*A-C*) preoperative views, left image, Postoperative views, right image.

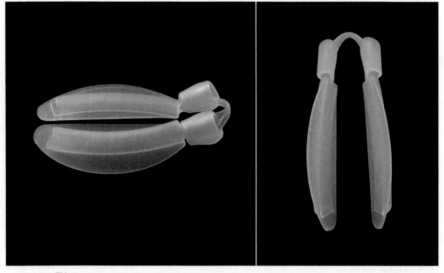

Fig. 25. The BG Splint™ is a new intranasal silicone splint that combines a pair of nostril stents joined to bilateral modified septal splints connected by a bridge anteriorly.

stents as well as that of the typical septal splints. This novel splint has multiple purposes: (1) to aid with elimination of dead space by applying gentle compression from intranasal outward in multiple areas including the nostrils, soft triangle area, and the nasal vestibule, (2) to maintain the nostril shape and vestibule volume, (3) to splint the septum while maintaining an open conduit for the nasal airway, (4) to eliminate the need for suture fixation of the septal splints and thus facilitate removal of both sides with 1 single movement, and (5) to allow long distance patients to easily remove these without the assistance from a trained individual. The BG Splint™ has been especially useful in patients with thick skin to help decrease post-operative edema and promote good apposition of the skin envelope with the underlying framework.

Cobo

In the past 2 years my techniques have not changed dramatically except that some concepts have been reinforced. Today I routinely use oral low dose isotretinoin schemes for most of my thick skin rhinoplasty patients. I routinely prescribe 20 mg isotretinoin 2 to 3 times a week and insist and explain to my patients that it should be used at least for 6 months to be able to see consistent results in the quality and thickness of the skin. I have found that complementing oral isotretinoin with consistent skin regimes helps keep quality of skin in improved conditions.

In addition to this, treating possible dead space formation in a more judicious manner has help reduce swelling and edema in the nasal tip. Today I use a full open approach in a good number of

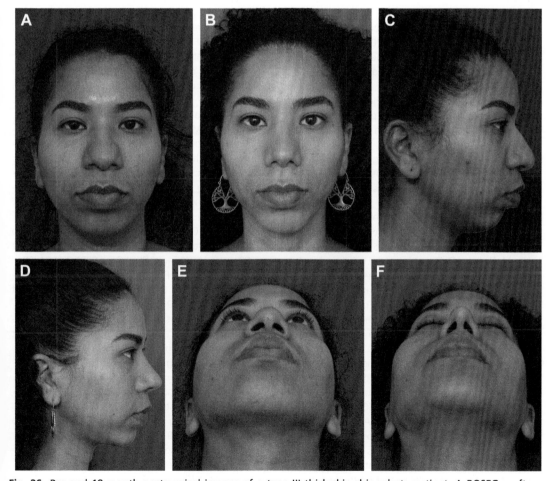

Fig. 26. Pre and 18 month postsurgical images of a type III thick skin rhinoplasty patient. A ROSEG graft was placed to structure the tip, SMAS resection was performed and added definition of the nasal tip was obtained with a bar graft. The patient received an integrated management to the skin soft tissue envelope, and took isotretinoin (low dose schemes) for 6 months. (A-C) preoperative images (D-F) post operative images.

rhinoplasties. In these patients I also routinely leave drains on osteotomy sites.

All thick skin patients are told they need to wait at least 12 months to 18 months post surgically to be able to see final results. Patients need to understand that initially their noses will look big and bulbous and that being patient and consistent with their skin management and diet will help them get improved post surgical results (**Fig. 26**).

DISCLOSURES

B. Guyuron has a direct financial interest PS Devices, LLC in the design and manufacture of the BG Splint™.

REFERENCES

1. Zingaro EA, Falces E. Aesthetic anatomy of the non-Caucasian nose. Clin Plast Surg 1987;14(4): 749–65.

2. Patrocinio LG, Patrocinio TG, Patrocinio JA. Approach for rhinoplasty in african descendants. Facial Plast Surg Clin North Am 2021;29(4):575–88.

3. Patrocinio LG, Patrocinio JA. Open rhinoplasty for African-American noses. Br J Oral Maxillofac Surg 2007;45(7):561–6.

4. Boahene KDO. Management of the nasal tip, nasal base, and soft tissue envelope in patients of African Descent. Otolaryngol Clin North Am 2020;53(2): 309–17.

5. Davis RE. Lateral crural tensioning for refinement of the wide and underprojected nasal tip: rethinking the lateral crural steal. Facial Plast Surg Clin North Am 2015;23:23–53.

6. Patrocinio LG, Patrocinio TG, Barreto DM, et al. Evaluation of lateral crural steal in nasal tip surgery. JAMA Facial Plast Surg 2014;16(6):400–4.

7. Lee M, Guyuron B. Dynamics of the subdomal graft. Plast Reconstr Surg 2016;137:940e–5e.

8. Guyuron B. Rhinoplasty. Elsevier Saunders; 2012.

9. Savetsky IL, Avashia YJ, Rohrich RJ. The five-step rhinoplasty dead space closure technique. Plast Reconstr Surg 2022;149(4):679e–80e. https://doi.org/10.1097/PRS.0000000000008971.

10. Ghavimi MA, Taheri Talesh K, Ghoreishizadeh A, et al. Efficacy of tranexamic acid on side effects of rhinoplasty: A randomized double-blind study. J Cranio-Maxillo-Fac Surg 2017;45(6):897–902.

11. Vasconcellos SJ, Nascimento EM, Aguiar MV, et al. Preoperative tranexamic acid for treatment of bleeding, edema, and ecchymosis in patients undergoing rhinoplasty: a systematic review and meta-analysis. JAMA Otolaryngol Head Neck Surg 2018 Sep 1;144(9):816–23.

12. McGuire C, Nurmsoo S, Samargandi OA, et al. Role of tranexamic acid in reducing intraoperative blood loss and postoperative edema and ecchymosis in primary elective rhinoplasty: a systematic review and meta-analysis. JAMA Facial Plast Surg 2019 May 1;21(3):191–8.

13. Haddady-Abianeh S, Rahmati J, Delavari C, et al. Comparison of the effect of injectable tranexamic acid and inhaled desmopressin in controlling bleeding and ecchymosis in open rhinoplasty. World J Plast Surg 2022;11(3):24–7. PMID: 36694687; PMCID: PMC9840754.

14. Cobo R, Vitery L. Isotretinoin use in thick-skinned rhinoplasty patients. Facial Plast Surg 2016;32(6): 656–61.

15. Sazgar AA, Majlesi A, Shooshtari S, et al. Oral isotretinoin in the treatment of postoperative edema in thick-skinned rhinoplasty: a randomized placebo- controlled clinical trial. Aesthet Plast Surg 2019;43(1):189–95.

16. Yahyavi S, Jahandideh H, Izadi M, et al. Analysis of the effects of isotretinoin on rhinoplasty patients. Aesthet Surg J 2020;40(12):NP657–65.

17. Yigit E, Rakici IT, Seden N, et al. The impact of isotretinoin therapy on the nasal skin thickness and elasticity: an ultrasonography and elastography based assessment in relation to dose and duration of therapy. Aesthetic Plast Surg 2022;46(4):1760–70.

18. Ozucer B, Yildirim YS, Veyseller B, et al. Effect of postrhinoplasty taping on postoperative edema and nasal draping: a randomized clinical trial. JAMA Facial Plast Surg 2016;18(3):157–63.

19. Hanasono MM, Kridel RW, Pastorek NJ, et al. Correction of the soft tissue pollybeak using triamcinolone injection. Arch Facial Plast Surg 2002;4(1):26–30.

20. Aydın C, Yücel ÖT, Akçalar S, et al. Role of steroid injection for skin thickness and edema in rhinoplasty patients. Laryngoscope Investig Otolaryngol 2021;6(4): 628–33.

21. Kridel RW, Castellano RD. A simplified approach to alar base reduction: a review of 124 patients over 20 years. Arch Facial Plast Surg 2005;7(2):81–93.

22. Irvine LE, Nassif PS. Use of 5-fluorouracil for management of the thick-skinned nose. Facial Plast Surg 2018;34(1):9–13.

23. Kovacevic M, Kosins AM, Davis RE, et al. Doxycycline sclerodesis - "Rhinodesis" - for enhanced soft tissue adhesion in rhinoplasty: a preliminary study. Facial Plast Surg 2024. https://doi.org/10.1055/a-2247-5005.

24. Cobo R, Camacho JG, Orrego J. Integrated management of the thick-skinned rhinoplasty patient. Facial Plast Surg 2018;34(1):3–8. Epub 2018 Feb 6. PMID: 29409097.

25. Zouboulis CC. Isotretinoin revisited: pluripotent effects on human sebaceous gland cells. J Invest Dermatol 2006;126:2154–6.

26. Melnik BC. Linking diet to acne metabolomics, inflamma- tion, and comedogenesis: an update. Clin Cosmet Investig Dermatol 2015;8:371–88.

27. Spring LK, Krakowski AC, Alam M, et al. Isotretinoin and timing of procedural interventions: a systematic review with consensus recommendations. JAMA Dermatol 2017;153(8):802–9. https://doi.org/10.1001/jamadermatol.2017.2077.

28. Zaenglein AL, Pathy AL, Schlosser BJ, et al. Guidelines of care for the management of acne vulgaris. J Am Acad Dermatol 2016;74(05):945–73.e33.

29. Gruber Ronald PMD, Zeidler Kamakshi RMD, Berkowitz R, et al. Desmopressin as a hemostatic agent to provide a dry intraoperative field in rhinoplasty. Plast Reconstr Surg 2015;135(5):1337–40. https://doi.org/10.1097/PRS.0000000000001158.

30. Guyuron B, Zarandy S, Tirgan A. von Willebrand's disease and plastic surgery. Ann Plast Surg 1994 Apr;32(4):351–5. PMID: 8210151.

31. Pappas A. The relationship of diet and acne: a review. Dermatoendocrinol 2009;1(05):262–7.

32. Amichai B, Shemer A, Grunwald MH. Low-dose isotretinoin in the treatment of acne vulgaris. J Am Acad Dermatol 2006;54:644–6.

33. Agarwal US, Besarwal RK, Bhola K. Oral isotretinoin in different dose regimens for acne vulgaris: a randomized comparative trial. Indian J Dermatol Venereol Leprol 2011;77:688–94.

34. Akman A, Durusoy C, Senturk M, et al. Treatment of acne with intermittent and conventional isotretinoin: a randomized, controlled multicenter study. Arch Dermatol Res 2007;299:467–73.

35. Saadoun R, Risse EM, Crisan D, et al. Dermatological assessment of thick-skinned patients before rhinoplasty - what may surgeons ask for? Int J Dermatol 2023;62(5):599–603.

36. Kosins AM, Obagi ZE. Managing the difficult soft tissue envelope in facial and rhinoplasty surgery. Aesthet Surg J 2017;37(2):143–57.

37. Guyuron B, Lee M. An effective algorithm for management of noses with thick skin. Aesthetic Plast Surg 2017;41(02):381–7.

38. Naves MM, Sousa RC, Tomé RAF, et al. Evaluation of the ultrasound reproducibility as a method to measure the subcutaneous tissue of the nasal tip. Int Arch Otorhinolaryngol 2011;15(3):346–9.

39. Dey JK, Recker CA, Olson MD, et al. Predicting nasal soft tissue envelope thickness for rhinoplasty: a model based on visual examination of the nose. Ann Otol Rhinol Laryngol 2021 Jan;130(1):60–6.

40. Cho GS, Kim JH, Yeo NK, et al. Nasal skin thickness measured using computed tomography and its effect on tip surgery outcomes. Otolaryngol Head Neck Surg 2011;144:522–7.

41. Lessard ML, Daniel RK. Surgical anatomy of septorhinoplasty. Arch Otolaryngol 1985;111:25–9.

42. Jomah J, Elsafi RA, Ali KSAE, et al. Nasal Skin Thickness Measurements Using Computed Tomography in an Adult Saudi Population. Plast Reconstr Surg Glob Open 2019 Sep 30;7(9):e2450.

43. Zouboulis CC. Acne and sebaceous gland function. Clin Dermatol 2004;22:360–6.

44. Michelson LN, Peck GC Jr, Kuo HR, et al. The quantification and distribution of nasal sebaceous glands using image analysis. Aesthetic Plast Surg 1996 Jul-Aug;20(4):303–9. PMID: 8791568.

45. Robotti E, Daniel R, Leone F. Cone-beam computed tomography: a user-friendly, practical roadmap to the planning and execution of every rhinoplasty-a 5-year review. Plast Reconstr Surg 2021 May 1;147(5):749e–62e.

46. Tasman AJ, Helbig M. Sonography of nasal tip anatomy and surgical tip refinement. Plast Reconstr Surg 2000;105(7):2573–9.

47. Çavuş Özkan M, Yeşil F, Bayramiçli İ, et al. Soft tissue thickness variations of the nose: a radiological study. Aesthetic Surg J 2020;40(7):711–8.

48. Hoehne J, Brandstetter M, Gubisch W, et al. How to reduce the probability of a pollybeak deformity in primary rhinoplasty: a single-center experience. Plast Reconstr Surg 2019;143(6):1620–4.

49. Zholtikov V, Kosins A, Ouerghi R, et al. Skin contour sutures in rhinoplasty. Aesthet Surg J 2023 Mar 15;43(4):422–32.

50. Guyuron B, DeLuca L, Lash R. Supratip deformity: a closer look. Plast Reconstr Surg 2000;105(3):1140–51.

Comparison of Blunt Force (Mechanical), Piezoelectric, and Electric Instruments in Bony Vault Management

Olivier Gerbault, MD[a],*, Nazim Cerkes, MD[b], Emmanuel Racy, MD[c], Vitaly Zholtikov, MD[d]

KEYWORDS

- Rhinosculpture • Osteotomy • Ostectomy • Bone stability • Ultrasonic rhinoplasty
- Preservation rhinoplasty • Rhinoplasty

KEY POINTS

- Blunt force instruments can create unwanted fractures and comminutive fractures that depend on the surgeon's technique, the instruments used and the bones characteristics.
- Piezoelectric instruments and electric instruments don't create unwanted or comminutive fractures.
- PEI and EI can preserve more easily bone stability than blunt force instruments.
- New mechanical instruments tends to avoid blunt force: hand saws, rasps, rongeur, etc.

 Video content accompanies this article at http://www.facialplastic.theclinics.com.

PANEL DISCUSSION

What is your preferred instrumentation for nasal bone surgery? Do you exclusively use it or combine it with other instruments? If so, what other instruments do you use, and under what circumstances? Do you have extensive experience using mechanical, electrical, and piezoelectric instruments?

What is your usual approach to the nasal pyramid? Please explain the positioning of incisions, the dissection plane(s), and the cephalic and lateral extent of the dissection. Under what circumstances do you modify your dissection? Please provide details of these modifications.

Is rasping of the nasal bones (or rhinosculpture) a routine technique you use to treat a dorsal hump? If yes, please specify the instruments used (with a photo if possible) and the exact extent of rasping on the nasal bones. Do you perform the same type of rasping for dorsum preservation techniques as for structural dorsum techniques? Please elaborate.

Are there any limitations to this rasping technique, or does it sometimes pose difficulties? If yes, what are they, and in which cases? How do you correct and avoid these difficulties? Do you observe any differences in rasping based on the type of instruments used (mechanical, electrical, piezoelectric)?

[a] Policlinique Esthetique Marigny Vincennes, Vincennes, France; [b] Cosmed Plastic Surgery, Istanbul; [c] Maxillofacial Department, Clinique saint jean de Dieu, Paris, France; [d] Saint-Petersburg, Russia
* Corresponding author. 3 Cours Marigny, Vincennes 94300, France.
E-mail address: dr.gerbault@gmail.com
Twitter: @dr_gerbault_rhinoplastie_paris (O.G.)

Facial Plast Surg Clin N Am 32 (2024) 495–516
https://doi.org/10.1016/j.fsc.2024.06.001
1064-7406/24/© 2024 Elsevier Inc. All rights are reserved, including those for text and data mining, AI training, and similar technologies.

Regarding lateral osteotomies: What instruments do you use (with a photo if possible)? What approach do you use for this osteotomy? Where does it start and end? Does this trajectory vary based on the appearance of the nasal pyramid or the technique used for dorsal hump correction (bony impaction or cartilaginous resection)?

Are lateral osteotomies with your preferred instruments sometimes a source of difficulties? If yes, what are they, and in which cases? How do you correct and avoid these difficulties? Do you observe any differences in lateral osteotomies based on the type of instruments used (mechanical, electrical, piezoelectric)?

Concerning paramedian or oblique medial osteotomies: What instruments do you use (with a photo if possible)? What approach do you use for this osteotomy? Where does it start and end? Does this trajectory vary based on the appearance of the nasal pyramid or the technique used for dorsal hump correction (bony impaction or cartilaginous resection)?

Are paramedian or oblique medial osteotomies with your preferred instruments sometimes a source of difficulties? If yes, what are they, and in which cases? How do you correct and avoid these difficulties? Do you observe any differences in paramedian or oblique medial osteotomies based on the type of instruments used (mechanical, electrical, piezoelectric)?

Concerning transverse osteotomies: What instruments do you use (with a photo if possible)? What approach do you use for this osteotomy? Where does it start and end? Does this trajectory vary based on the appearance of the nasal pyramid or the technique used for dorsal hump correction (bony impaction or cartilaginous resection)?

Are transverse osteotomies with your preferred instruments sometimes a source of difficulties? If yes, what are they, and in which cases? How do you correct and avoid these difficulties? Do you observe any differences in transverse osteotomies based on the type of instruments used (mechanical, electrical, piezoelectric)?

How have your techniques in this area changed over the last 2 y?

INTRODUCTION

The reshaping of the nasal pyramid has evolved significantly over the past 20 years. Mechanical instruments have been refined to minimize the bone trauma of osteotomies. Fine and sharp instruments are used to allow precise cutting. Highly efficient hand rasps and saws have been designed to avoid the inherent defects of conventional mechanical instruments. Indeed, these instruments can inadvertently cause radiated fractures and comminuted fractures that compromise bone stability and can create surface defects. Other mechanical instruments that do not involve blunt force have also been developed, such as nail clippers, rongeurs, and even the use of a scalpel blade.

Electric and piezoelectric instruments (PEI) have been developed to address these problems of uncontrolled fractures. These 2 types of instruments are similar, but PEI instruments are selective unlike electric instruments. This means that PEI cannot damage adjacent tissues. These instruments not only allow for precise rhinosculpture and osteotomies under direct visual control, but also for precise mobilization and stabilization of the nasal bones.

The article reviews the advantages and disadvantages of each method by comparing them for the most frequently performed procedures on the nasal bone pyramid in rhinoplasty: the necessary approach, removing the bony layer when treating humps, and finally each of the osteotomies.

Experts were invited to defend their preferred method. All but 1 had extensive experience in electric and piezoelectric rhinoplasties; this further validates the choices they have made over the years in reshaping the nasal bone pyramid.

Question 1: What is your preferred instrumentation for nasal bone surgery? Do you exclusively use it or combine it with other instruments? If so, what other instruments do you use, and under what circumstances? Do you have extensive experience using mechanical, electrical, and piezoelectric instruments?

Cerkes

My preferred instruments for nasal bone surgery are No: 15 blade, Cerkes Bone Nipper (Marina Medical İnstruments FL-USA), Cerkes 3-mm straight osteotome (Marina Medical İnstruments FL-USA), Cerkes Curved osteotome (Marina Medical İnstruments FL-USA), 5-mm delicate tip osteotome, and delicate 7 -mm Tastan Rasp (Medisoft Medical-TR). I always use the hand instruments mentioned earlier for bone reduction, osteotomies, and bone reshaping. In rare circumstances, I combine hand tools with the electrical instruments (power burr) particularly in cases with high radix for reduction of radix.

I have experience with electrical and piezoelectric instruments. They are useful tools, but their use elongates the surgery time and need larger periosteal degloving to execute the osteotomies and bone reshaping.

Gerbault

I have exclusively used PEI since 2013, except for septoplasty, where I had to wait until 2017 to have the first prototypes of long inserts to perform piezoelectric septoplasties and endonasal osteotomies. My journey into rhinoplasty began during my internship in 1990, initially using exclusively mechanical instruments in closed rhinoplasty and later in open rhinoplasty. I started with endonasal osteotomies and, from 2005 onwards, incorporated external osteotomies combined with internal or isolated osteotomies.

For nearly 20 years, I used rasps, osteotomes, chisels, bone scissors, and nail clippers while visiting some of the world's best surgeons very early on. On these occasions, I realized the frequent difficulties they could encounter during bone procedures, particularly osteotomies. It was because of the lack of control, reliability, and predictability in my osteotomies that I began using electric instruments in 2010, using burrs first, and then instruments developed by Dr Y Avsar in Turkey in collaboration with the Swiss laboratory Bien Air.[1] The limitations of these instruments, for me, were the lateral osteotomies performed in an enlarged tunnel without being able to precisely visualize the saw and being confined to a straight fracture line. Hence, I frequently continued to combine traditional osteotomes with electric instruments. Moreover, damage to the surrounding tissues with burrs and saws was not infrequent. I then had ultrasonic piezoelectric rhinoplasty instruments developed, first in 2013 with the NSK company, and then from 2014 with the Acteon company. In the end, I have over 20 years of experience with mechanical instruments, 3 years with electric instruments, and finally 12 years with piezoelectric instruments.

Racy

I use Electric power instruments (BIEN AIR RHINOSCULPTURE SET) since 2011(Video 1).
I quit mechanical instruments in 2013.
I use PEI for orthognathic surgery only (in every procedure).

Zholtikov

Since December 2016, I use PEI in 100% of the cases when bony pyramid work is needed. PEI allow me to do all the work on the bones, except for the radix osteotomy when performing Foundation Dorsal Preservation, I use a 2-mm chisel for the oblique osteotomy. Also, in cases of significant bony thickness at the base of the pyramid or in the radix or in cases of post-traumatic deviations or in some secondary rhinoplasties, I use first cylindrical or diamond burr, which allows to remove the necessary bony thickness very quickly, and then PEI for more precise sculpture and osteotomies. I have extensive experience using mechanical and electrical instruments, which I used for 12 years until 2016, and switched to using PEI in 2016, which has allowed me to significantly improve my own results.

Question 2: What is your usual approach to the nasal pyramid? Please explain the positioning of incisions, the dissection plane(s), and the cephalic and lateral extent of the dissection. Under what circumstances do you modify your dissection? Please provide details of these modifications.

Cerkes

Open rhinoplasty approach provides better visualization of nasal dorsum anatomy and easier execution of maneuvers. Using a mid columellar inverted V incision, skin flap elevation is performed on supra perichondral level leaving all subcutaneous soft tissues within the skin flap. To perform basic nasal dorsum maneuvers such as hump removal, spreader flaps or spreader grafts, osteotomies, and onlay grafts, I described a different concept of nasal dorsum dissection called "the perichondro-periosteal flap."[2] In this technique, perichondrium of upper lateral cartilages (ULCs) and periosteum of nasal bone are elevated as a continuous flap on both sides (**Fig. 1**). Periosteal undermining on the bony dorsum is partial subperiosteal degloving. It is limited to the keystone area and on the cephalic part of the bony dorsum wide enough to execute medial oblique, transverse (and intermediate if required) osteotomies under direct vision. On the cephalic part of the bony dorsum, lateral extent of the dissection up to the medial canthal tendon but on the caudal portion of the nasal pyramid, it is limited just a few of milimeters lateral to the level of bony reduction. If an osteoplasty procedure is required to correct irregularities or asymmetries on the nasal bones, I perform a larger periosteal degloving, in particular cases total periosteal degloving for rhinosculpture.

Gerbault

I perform 95% open approaches, with dissection always supra perichondral on the lower lateral cartilages (LLCs) and ULCs, then subperiosteal on the entire or just a part of the nasal pyramid when

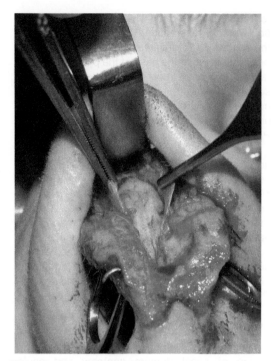

Fig. 1. Periosteal undermining.

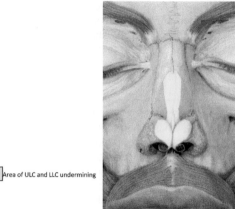

Area of ULC and LLC undermining

Fig. 2. Extent of soft tissues undermining.

bone modifications are necessary, which is the case for almost all patients. The marginal incision usually ends laterally at the turning point (except when transposition of lateral crura is performed, where it is extended externally) and crosses the columella at its midpoint with an inverted V-shaped design at the narrowest part of the columella. Subcutaneous tissue dissection between the medial and intermediate crura is systematically done since 2019 to ensure a robust Pitanguy flap and intercrural ligaments for traction on the supra-tip at the end of the procedure. This dissection continues supra perichondral from the anterior septal angle, lifting the intercrural ligament and interdomal ligament with the subcutaneous tissue flap between the medial crura (**Fig. 2**). Subperiosteal dissection is most often extended over the entire bony pyramid (full open approach), extending about a centimeter beyond the nasofacial groove and ascending beyond the nasofrontal suture in the midline (**Fig. 3**).[3,4] It is important to note that when bone impaction is planned (foundation technique), the procerus insertions are left intact to provide superficial support to the radix bones, meaning that the upper-middle part of the pyramid is not undermined. In cases where only lateral osteotomy and/or lateral rhinosculpture are performed, bone dissection is limited to the ascending branch of the maxilla, with subperiosteal access in continuity with the lateral crus and

extending from the Webster triangle at the bottom to the most cephalic part of the ascending branch, beyond the insertion zone of the internal canthal ligament (**Fig. 4**). Lever-arm movement with a periosteal elevator is necessary to stretch the fibrous ligamentous attachments at the edge of the pyriform aperture, denser in the caudal part.

Racy

- I do a central dissection for the hump with a superior lateral dissection to help for transverse osteotomies.
- I only do extend dorsum dissection for a very croocked nose.
- I do lateral dissections through a 1 cm vertical pyriform incision into the nostril for lateral osteotomies.

Zholtikov

I use open approach rhinoplasty in most cases with combined approach in my practice, and use 3

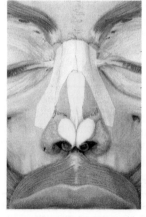

Area of bone undermining

Fig. 3. Extent of bony pyramid undermining in full open approach.

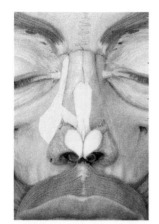

Area of bone undermining

Fig. 4. Extent of bony pyramid undermining in limited lateral approach.

planes of dissection (sub-dermal or supra SMAS plane, sub-SMAS dissection, and dissection in supraperichondrial and subperiosteal plane), depending on the anatomic area where I work. I perform dissection in sub-dermal plane and sub-SMAS plane above the LLC, while keeping SMAS attachment in the scroll area projection, and then the dissection continues supraperichondrially above the ULC until key stone junction and then dissection goes on subperiosteally cranially above the bony vault.[5]

However, access to the bones depends on the dorsal technique I plan to perform. In cases where I perform Dorsal Preservation, I use a limited approach, with no soft tissue envelope (STE) elevation on the dorsum. Dissection performs in the subperiosteal plane over the base of the bony pyramid longitudinally from the keystone junction up to the cephalic part of the radix with a subperiosteal tunnel width of no more than 15 mm. Usually, the lateral pyriform aperture ligaments are stretched to allow wider access to the base of the nasal bony wall along the pyriform aperture (**Fig. 5**) Then, I can extend it in central part of the dorsum, in cases when it is necessary to modify the central dorsum additionally, but necessarily keeping the STE attachments to the lateral walls and to the radix area. That helps me to prevent excessive mobility of the bony pyramid, fully mobilized by circular osteotomies.

Whenever I perform Dorsal Modification or Dorsal Reconstruction techniques, I use a full open approach to the bones.[6] Full subperiosteal dissection of the bony vault performs longitudinally from the keystone junction up to the cephalic part of the radix and transversely from one ascending frontal process of the maxilla to the other side. In addition,

it is necessary to undermine the periosteum beyond the nasofacial groove to achieve the requisite exposure. Usually, the lateral pyriform aperture ligaments are stretched to allow complete access to the nasal bony wall along the pyriform aperture (**Fig. 6**). The using of complete extended periosteum mobilization over the entire osseocartilaginous vault permits direct visual assessment of the deformities as well as piezo rhinosculpture to reduce asymmetries followed by appropriate precise osteotomies.[5]

Question 3: Is rasping of the nasal bones (or rhinosculpture) a routine technique you use to treat a dorsal hump? If yes, please specify the instruments used (with a photo if possible) and the exact extent of rasping on the nasal bones. Do you perform the same type of rasping for dorsum preservation techniques as for structural dorsum techniques? Please elaborate.

Cerkes

Hence, the rasps may damage the ULCs, perichondrium of ULCs, and periosteum on the keystone region; I do not prefer to use them for bony dorsum reduction. My preferred instrument to take the bony cap off is the No. 15 blade in the majority of my cases. In young individuals and females, a No. 15 blade easily takes off the bony cap on the keystone area (**Fig. 7**, Video 2). I found this method as the most delicate and the least traumatic way to remove the bony cap. In some males and some older patients, nasal bones are thicker and cutting the bone with a No. 15 blade can be difficult. In such patients, I use a 5-mm straight chisel which has a blade-like cutting edge to remove the bony cap. After removal of the bony cap using a No. 15 blade or 5-mm chisel, I use specific bone scissors (Cerkes Dorsum Nipper-Marina Medical Instruments, FL, USA) for additional reduction from the nasal bones (**Fig. 8**, Video 3). The tip of the scissors are delicate that can fit into small spaces on the bony dorsum and make very precise cuts (**Fig. 9**). With this bone scissors even after the osteotomies, an additional bony reduction can be performed without destabilizing the nasal bones.

Although the rasps are not my preferred instruments for bony cap removal and bony dorsum reduction, in some cases, I use a 7-mm Tastan fine rasp (Medisoft Medical-TR) for reduction of the cephalic portion of the nasal bones and radix area under direct vision with care (**Figs. 10** and **11**). In cases with significantly high radix disproportion, I prefer to use an electrical instrument (power burr) which eases the procedure and shortens the operating time.

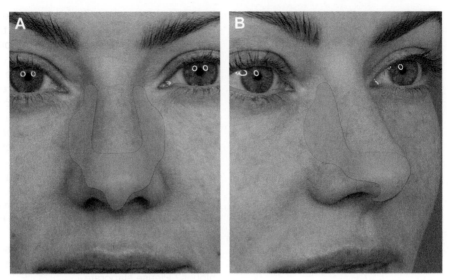

Fig. 5. (*A, B*) Limited dissection. The blue area is dissected part.

Gerbault

Rhinosculpture with piezoelectric instruments has the advantage of being selective, gradually reducing bone thickness without damaging adjacent structures such as cartilage, skin, and muscles.

All areas where the bone is too convex are flattened by rhinosculpture. Exceptions include as follows

- If the bone is thin or has already been refined by rhinosculpture, and the bone color starts to change, indicating significant bone thinning. Osteotomies in 2 perpendicular axes are then performed to flatten the bone without creating a defect (criss cross osteotomies).
- If a bone lowering of the dorsum is planned in the context of an osseocartilaginous surface dorsal preservation (DP) (Ishida and Ferreira-Ishida techniques).[7,8]

If a dorsum structural technique is chosen, the extent of rhinosculpture depends on the type of hump: it involves the dorsal keystone area (DKA) if the hump is mainly marked in profile, the lateral keystone area (LKA) if the hump is mainly marked from three-quarters view, and often both areas.

If a DP surface technique is used, rasping rhinosculpture is essential to avoid irregularities,

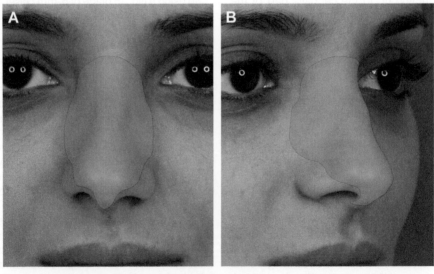

Fig. 6. (*A, B*) Full open approach. The blue area is dissected part.

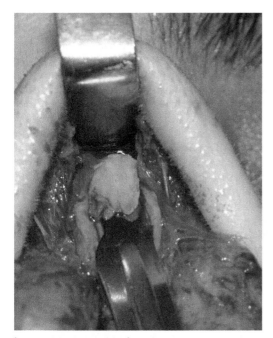

Fig. 7. Bony cap removal.

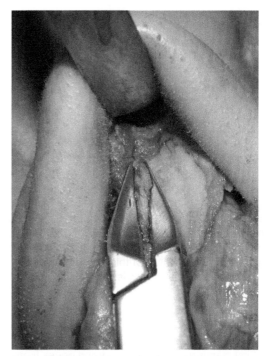

Fig. 9. Additional Bone Reduction with bone scissors.

especially in the LKA areas. However, it is done after the dorsum central and paramedian osteotomies in the Ferreira Ishida technique.

If a DP foundation technique is used, rhinosculpture allows reshaping the bony profile after impaction. This is especially useful when the nasal bones have an S shape, to convert it in a V shape pattern.

In all DPs, dorsum rhinosculpture allows better flexibility of the dorsum to change its shape, but it can also weaken the strength of the dorsum.

The instruments chosen for rhinosculpture are the scraper (RHS1) **(Fig. 12)** in areas where the bone is thick and dense. This instrument actually performs a rapid ostectomy, but less homogeneous than rasps. It is the only instrument that

can damage the ULC when the hump is removed if not used appropriately. In almost all cases, the flat rasp is used after the scraper to smooth out the small irregularities often found after using the scraper.

Conversely, rasps perform a true rhinosculpture by gently and progressively removing bone layers (RHS2 and RHS7) **(Figs. 13** and **14)**. Long rasps are used when a closed approach is performed **(Fig. 15)** Piezo rasps have 2 different grains depending on whether the bone is thick or thin, but also depending on the fineness of the overlying skin. This allows changing bone's characteristics, making the bones more malleable and flexible, allowing in some cases to pass sutures through

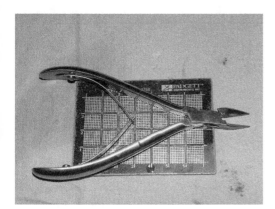

Fig. 8. Bone Nipper.

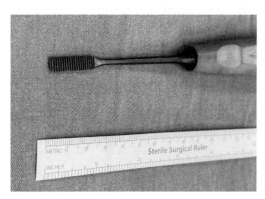

Fig. 10. Tastan fine rasp.

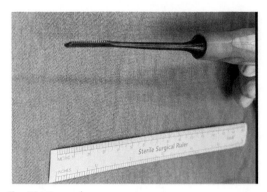

Fig. 11. Power burr.

them without completely removing the bones. Trumpet-shaped rasps are more effective than flat rasps for rhinosculpture of thick bones, especially when treating the lateral walls: they are as efficient as electric burrs.

Racy

For rasping the bone, I use 3 types of rasps.

First rasp is a rough one (for strong bone). It can be used with a rotating alternating saw (the bulldozer way). You always have to move and never stay in the same place to avoid irregularities.

The second one is the diamond rasp. Smoothing bone and cartilage.

The third one is a little one for revision surgery, or little spin.

I rarely do nasal preservation, but I can rasp a residual hump with the diamond rasp.

Zholtikov

As well as access to the bony pyramid, the use of rhinosculpture for the treatment of the dorsal hump depends on the technique of working on the dorsum. I perform rhinosculpture in almost 100% of the cases when work with the bony pyramid is necessary. When performing Dorsal Preservation and there is no need for additional modification of the dorsum, I usually perform rhinosculpture only

to reduce bone thickness and asymmetries at the base of the bony pyramid, but not for the treatment of the dorsal hump. This makes it possible to prevent impairment of breathing due to inward displacement of the thick bones of the base of the bony pyramid. Conversely, in cases where I perform Dorsal Modification or Dorsal Reconstruction techniques, I almost always remove the bony cap and reduce the asymmetries on the entire surface of the bony pyramid with Ultrasound Rhinosculpture. In this case, the rougher work of removing bone thickness is done with the Scraper, and then the bone surface and keystone area is more precisely treated with flat rasps. **Figs. 16** and **17** The main advantage of Ultrasound Rhinosculpture is the ability to remove the bony cap without damaging the upper laterals, which completely eliminates the "open roof" deformity.

Question 4: Are there any limitations to this rasping technique, or does it sometimes pose difficulties? If yes, what are they, and in which cases? How do you correct and avoid these difficulties? Do you observe any differences in rasping based on the type of instruments used (mechanical, electrical, piezoelectric)?

Gerbault

The limits of rhinosculpture are excessively thin bones, where it could create a bone defect. In these cases, correcting a convexity involves osteotomies performed in 2 perpendicular axes called criss-cross osteotomies.[2] Conversely, in the case of very dense bones, the use of a scraper or trumpet-shaped rasp in the first instance allows rapid reduction of bone volume.

Mechanical rasps work perfectly, but they are most effective when bones are thin or medium. It is very challenging to reduce convexities of the sidewalls with this type of instrument. Moreover, these rasps are not selective and can damage the ULC. Electric rasps are also effective, but like mechanical rasps, they are not selective and can damage the ULC and the soft tissues.

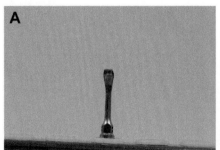

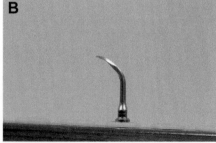

Fig. 12. (*A, B*) The scraper (RHS1).

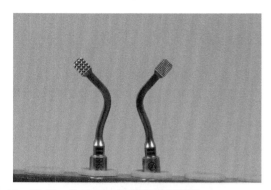

Fig. 13. The flat rasps (RHS2H & RHS2F).

To be comprehensive, the bony cap can be effectively removed on the DKA using an osteotome. This becomes more challenging if one aims to remove the bony cap on the LKA, as it involves a curved surface. The risk is damaging the ULC, hindering preservation of the dorsum in case of DP, or impeding anatomic reconstruction of the dorsum in case of structural dorsum approach.

Ultimately, for removing a bony cap, refining bones, or correcting convexity through rhinosculpture, it seems logical to use piezoelectric instruments, which are particularly precise and only affect the bones while sparing all soft tissues, rather than electric or mechanical instruments that can damage cartilages as well as subcutaneous tissues.

Racy

I am so used to electrical rasp; I cannot imagine using other instruments. I need a little water. I have never had a burn.

Zholtikov

In some cases of severe bone thickness and dense bone tissue, using only PEI for rhinosculpture may take longer than desired. In such cases, I first use electro power instruments, in particular cylindrical or diamond burr, which allows to remove the required bone thickness very quickly,

and then PEI for more precise bone processing and osteotomies with flat rasps. In all other cases, the use of PEI allows to solve almost all the problems, including rhinosculpture and all variants of osteotomies.

Question 5: Regarding lateral osteotomies: What instruments do you use (with a photo if possible)? What approach do you use for this osteotomy? Where does it start and end? Does this trajectory vary based on the appearance of the nasal pyramid or the technique used for dorsal hump correction (bony impaction or cartilaginous resection)?

Cerkes

I perform the lateral osteotomies after the medial oblique (or paramedian) and transverse osteotomies. I always do internal low to low lateral osteotomies using a 3-mm straight (without guard) osteotome (Cerkes Micro Osteotome-Marina Medical Instruments, FL-USA) (**Fig. 18**). I do not elevate the periosteum off the maxillary bone on the osteotomy line while performing the lateral osteotomy except in the cases where I do bony resection from the base of the nasal pyramid. The lateral osteotomy starts from the pyriform aperture and extends in the cephalic direction along the base of the bony pyramid. The low to low osteotomy extends up to the medial canthus level, about 1 to 2 mm medial to the medial canthal tendon to avoid damage to the tendon. The lateral osteotomy is performed as a complete osteotomy to mobilize the base of the nasal bones medially. After completion of lateral osteotomies, the bones are mobilized medially using the thumb. The hinge of the fracture is the medial oblique and transverse osteotomy line which is usually a greenstick fashion fracture.

Although I perform low to low lateral osteotomy up to the medial canthal tendon in majority of cases, in patients with a narrow upper bony vault and radix, it is not necessary to extend the lateral osteotomy up to the medial canthal tendon. In

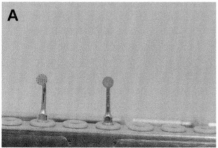

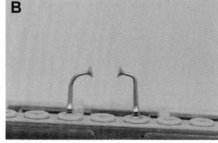

Fig. 14. (*A, B*) The trumpet rasps (RHS7H & RHS7F).

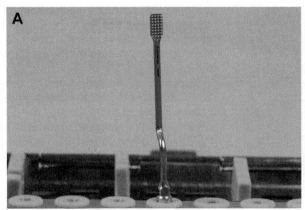
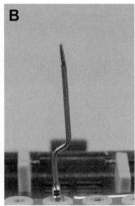

Fig. 15. (*A, B*) The long rasp (RHL2).

these types of bones, the medial oblique and/or transverse osteotomies are also placed caudal to medial canthus level in order to perform a caudal fracture line to avoid additional narrowing of the radix.

Gerbault

Lateral osteotomies are performed to narrow the width of the nasal pyramid base, which is often necessary when reducing, refining the nose, correcting a hump, or addressing asymmetry. The approach for open lateral osteotomies is usually through an extended open approach or a limited open approach to the dissection of the ascending branch of the maxilla as described in question number 2, performed if this lateral osteotomy is done alone without a planned surface modification on the dorsum. The same applies to the closed approach. These osteotomies are usually performed with rounded fan-shaped saws (RHS3R and L) (**Fig. 19**) that easily reach low on the maxilla at the Webster triangle and rise very high on the lateral wall while following the contours of the nasofacial groove. Indeed, it is mainly at the level of this natural relief where the maxillary

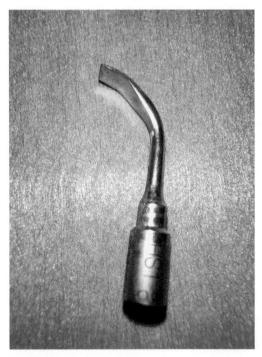

Fig. 16. Piezo head Scraper.

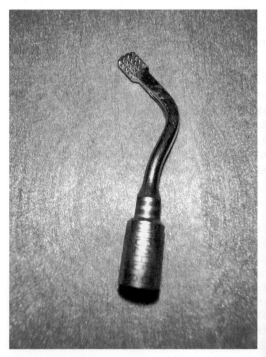

Fig. 17. Piezo head flat Rasp.

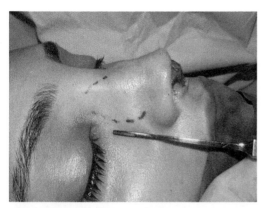

Fig. 18. Low to low lateral osteotomy with a 3-mm straight (without guard) osteotome.

bone begins to turn vertically to form the lateral wall of the nose that the lateral osteotomy is made in rhinoplasties that are not foundational DPs. It is therefore a lateral osteotomy that goes from very low to very low cranially (**Figs. 20** and **21**). The orientation of the saw defines the ease of the rotational bone movement: the more sagittal this orientation, the more easily the bone moves (**Fig. 22**). When a significant narrowing of the bony base is planned, it is preferable to perform a partial low ostectomy before completing the osteotomy to avoid the risk of obstructing the nasal fossa.

Closed lateral osteotomies are usually performed with small straight saws at the bottom (RHS5 or RSD1) (**Fig. 23**) and a long straight saw upwards (RHL5, RHL3) (**Fig. 24**).

When a foundational DP technique is performed, the path of the lateral osteotomy is different: it is more medial by about 1 cm and has a curvilinear shape upwards, to locate its cephalic part where the bone is usually less thick and without an angle between the lateral and transverse osteotomies (**Fig. 25**).

An ostectomy of the Webster triangle can be performed with a straight saw (RHS5) if the bony pyramid needs to descend more than 2 to 3 mm, to avoid obstruction of the nasal fossa (**Fig. 26**). This ostectomy can be continued upwards when one wants to significantly lower the bony pyramid or avoid any risk of obstruction, but this also increases bone instability.

Racy

I use an angulated lateral saw. It is a straight saw for a low-to-low osteotomy. For Structural rhinoplasty, the axis of sawing is horizontal to avoid a step.

The hand piece used has to be the rotating alternating saw (Bulldozer way).

For asymmetric push down, the side that has to be impacted needs a vertical cut to help the push down.

Zholtikov

I use 2 different approaches for osteotomies: Limited for Dorsal Preservation and Full Open for Dorsal Modification (DM) and Dorsal Reconstruction (DR). The lateral osteotomies are also performed differently. In Dorsal Preservation, I perform lateral osteotomies at the level of the nasofacial groove, smoothly transitioning in the area of the intercantal line cranially into transverse osteotomies without sharp angles (Banana types), most often double on each side, to remove a strip of bone and perform Let Down technique. This osteotomy technique makes it easier to perform bony impaction. In Dorsal Modification and Dorsal Reconstruction, I perform lateral osteotomies 2 to 3 mm below the nasofacial groove and thus on the ascending portion of the frontal process of the maxilla. The lateral osteotomies perform 2 to 3 mm cranial to the intercantal line, which allows giving the bony pyramid more stability and prevent excessive verticalization of the lateral walls (**Fig. 27**). In both cases, I use a PEI straight saw for the osteotomies (**Fig. 28**).

Question 6: Are lateral osteotomies with your preferred instruments sometimes a source of difficulties? If yes, what are they, and in which cases?

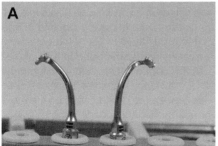
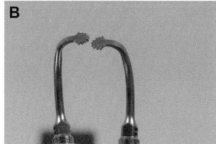
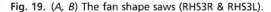

Fig. 19. (A, B) The fan shape saws (RHS3R & RHS3L).

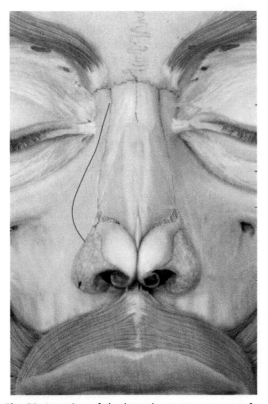

Fig. 20. Location of the lateral osteotomy except for foundation techniques.

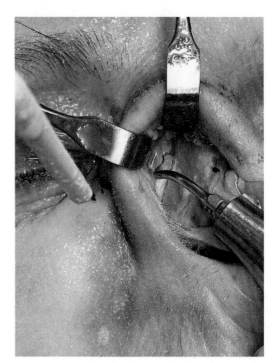

Fig. 22. Lateral osteotomy with the fan shape saw.

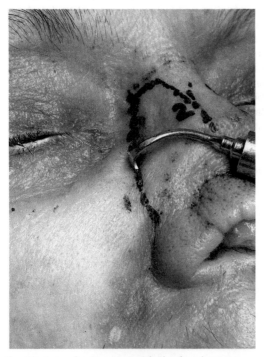

Fig. 21. Lateral osteotomy with the fan shape saw.

How do you correct and avoid these difficulties? Do you observe any differences in lateral osteotomies based on the type of instruments used (mechanical, electrical, piezoelectric)?

Gerbault

Lateral osteotomies performed with piezoelectric instruments do not cause comminution at the fracture line or radiated fractures, regardless of the characteristics of the bone. The bone is selectively cut without damaging the underlying periosteum and mucosa that maintain bone stability from below. This is fundamental to explain the differences with mechanical instruments.

The mechanical instruments use blunt force (pounding blows) to cut the bone, creating micro or macro comminutions and unintentional radiated fracture lines. These 2 phenomena depend largely on bone's characteristics but also on the quality of the osteotomes and the gestures made by the surgeon. To avoid these 2 problems, surgeons using osteotomes tend to place the osteotomy paths in positions where the bone is thinner, reducing the risk of comminution and unintentional fracture. This, however, increases bone instability and the risk of stairstep demarcation on the nasal pyramid, creating often a residual hump.

Furthermore, when mechanical instruments are used, bone stability relies on preserving a connection on the lateral walls between very loose and

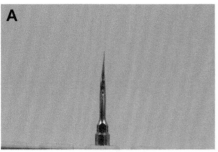
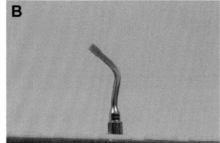

Fig. 23. (*A, B*) The straight short saw (RHS5).

mobile skin and the bones, and performing greenstick fractures between the different osteotomies. These greenstick fractures are difficult to control as they largely depend on the bone's characteristics (thickness, hardness, brittle appearance…).

Lateral osteotomies performed with electric instruments do not have this risk of comminution and radiated fracture, but the shape of the lateral saws allows only a straight fracture line ignoring the contours of the nasofacial groove, with an endonasal approach that places this osteotomy more medially than piezo osteotomies.

The use of piezo for lateral osteotomies allows easy and controlled cutting under direct vision of all types of bones, even the thickest and most brittle ones. Unlike lateral osteotomies with an osteotome, there remains elasticity of the cut bone and a more or less marked spring effect depending on the bone's characteristics, but also on the positioning of the osteotomy and the use of other osteotomies afterward. When the lateral osteotomy is done in isolation (partial osteotomy) and a spring effect persists, a graft, usually taken from the vomer, is placed at the caudal part of the fracture line to block the bone in a more internal position. This graft is called doorstop interposition graft.

Racy

I never had to use mechanical instruments for 11 years.

The learning is quite long and the cut became easy since I use the rotating alternating saw.

Zholtikov

This very lateral location of the lateral osteotomy would be virtually impossible if a conventional osteotomy were utilized. Consequently, the use of mechanical instruments, in my opinion, allows less control over the horizontal displacement of the base of the pyramid and can create excessive verticalization and asymmetries.

Question 7: Concerning paramedian or oblique medial osteotomies: What instruments do you use (with a photo if possible)? What approach do you use for this osteotomy? Where does it start and end? Does this trajectory vary based on the appearance of the nasal pyramid or the technique used for dorsal hump correction (bony impaction or cartilaginous resection)?

Cerkes

For paramedian osteotomies, I use a 2-mm delicate tip straight osteotome. I generally perform

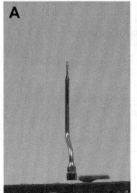
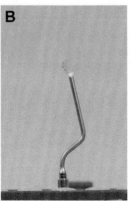
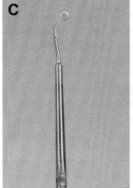
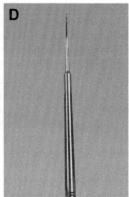

Fig. 24. (*A–D*) The straight long saws (RHL5 and RHL3).

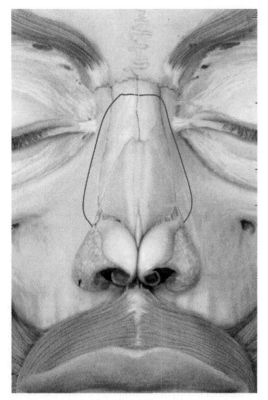

Fig. 25. Location of the lateral osteotomy for foundation techniques.

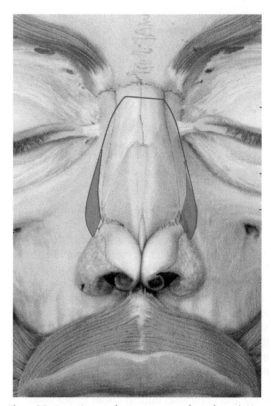

Fig. 26. Location of ostectomy for foundation techniques.

paramedian osteotomies in cases with wide bony pyramid or in cases with asymmetric bony dorsum without bony hump. The osteotomy starts from the most caudal point of the nasal bones. Location of the paramedian osteotomies will determine the width of the dorsal aesthetic lines on the bony dorsum.

For medial oblique osteotomy, I use a 4-mm specifically designed curved tip osteotome with a very sharp cutting edge (Cerkes Medial Oblique Osteotome, Marina Medical Instruments, FL, USA) (**Fig. 29**). This delicate tool is less traumatic to the adjacent tissues, produces less swelling compared to larger osteotomes, and does not produce heat as power instruments do. Using this tool, a controlled incomplete osteotomy can be done to perform a greenstick fashion fracture.

Medial oblique osteotomies help to define dorsal aesthetic lines while preserving the nasal bone on the radix area and prevents from the Rocker deformity. With open rhinoplasty approach, the osteotomies are performed under direct vision. The medial oblique osteotomy starts from the lateral inferior point of the remaining bony cup. The angle of the osteotomy is about 20° to 30° from the midline. The osteotomy usually continues

up to the level of the medial canthus, but in cases with wide radix, it extends about 2 to 3 mm superior the medial canthus level. However, in cases with narrow radix, the osteotomy may end caudal to the medial canthus level.

When I do medial oblique osteotomy with the curved tip osteotome, I first score the osteotomy line with the tip of the osteotome, then the bone is penetrated step by step with the osteotome

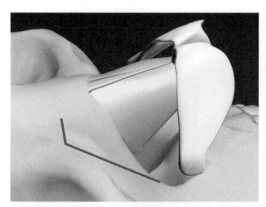

Fig. 27. Scheme of low to low lateral osteotomy and a partial length transverse osteotomy.

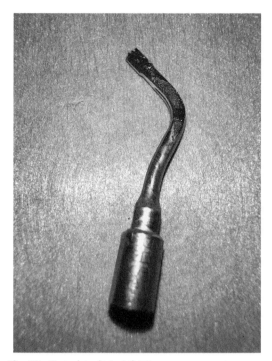

Fig. 28. Piezo head straight Saw.

using hand power (without using a mallet) from inferior to superior up to the level of the medial canthus (**Fig. 30**, Video 4). In most cases, I perform an incomplete osteotomy with partial penetration of the tip of the osteotome into the bone for a greenstick fracture on the osteotomy line. In cases with thick nasal bones, a mallet can be used to facilitate the osteotomy. However, to prevent the cracking of the nasal bones, careful and gentle hits should be done with the mallet. Cracking on the nasal bone can be the complication of this technique, but if the osteotomy is performed with care, it happens rarely. I have not experienced a complete fragmentation on the nasal bones in any of my cases so far.

Gerbault

Paramedian osteotomies are performed to reduce the width of the top of the nasal pyramid. This osteotomy is frequently necessary not only when the upper part of the pyramid is wide and cannot be reduced by simple rhinosculpture, but also when a hump is moderate or significant. I perform paramedian osteotomies (I do not use medial oblique osteotomies) after a medial or extended subperiosteal dissection of the bony pyramid, with very fine straight saws (RHS5) starting from the area of the dorsal keystone where the cartilaginous dorsal aesthetic lines (DAL) is located. The fracture line ascends vertically, diverging slightly outward (toward the medial eyebrow) as it progresses (**Figs. 31** and **32**). The end of this osteotomy is usually above the internal canthal line, at a location that is forbidden when osteotomes are used to avoid rocker deformity. Indeed, the higher this osteotomy goes, the thicker the bone, the harder it is to break with regular osteotomes or chisels, and prevents the medialization of the bone flap with this characteristic appearance of a wide remaining root.

Piezoelectric instruments, like electric instruments, are not affected by this issue because they cut very precisely through very thick bones.

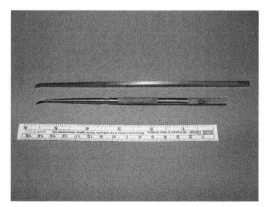

Fig. 29. A 4-mm curved tip osteotome for medial oblique osteotomy.

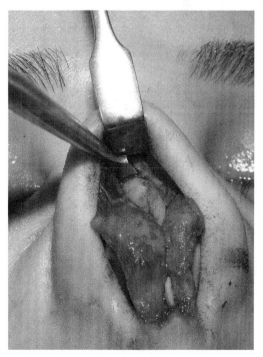

Fig. 30. Medial oblique osteotomy.

In the rare cases where the radix is very wide, this paramedian osteotomy must be a little wider, either by making a fine ostectomy with the same saw (RHS5), or by using a wider saw (RSD1) to create a larger bony defect.

Racy

After separating septum from the ULC with a 15 blade, the specific paramedian blade is introduced vertically with the rotating alternation saw (running for bottom to the top) and this is where I can break easily the blade because of the hardness of the frontonasal Beak which can be large.

If necessary, a slice of bone is cut in 1 side to help in fracturing a laterally deviated bone.

Zholtikov

For paramedian or oblique medial osteotomies, I also use the PEI straight saw. **Fig. 28** In many cases, however, I do not perform these osteotomies at all because there is no need for them. In those cases where it is necessary, such as with a wide dorsal part of the bony pyramid, I almost always perform paramedial instead of medial oblique osteotomies. Paramedial osteotomies are most often performed longitudinally from the dorsal

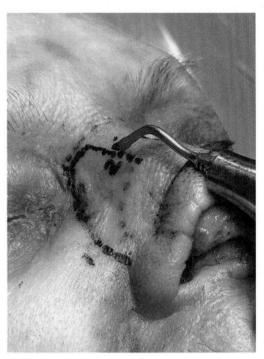

Fig. 32. Paramedian osteotomy with the straight saw.

keystone area up to the intercantal line usually 1 to 2 mm from the septum. **Fig. 33** They can be single or double on one or both sides, for example, to reduce the width of the central part of the bony pyramid or to create slots, to fix high spreader grafts in reconstructive dorsal augmentation.[9]

Question 8: Are paramedian or oblique medial osteotomies with your preferred instruments sometimes a source of difficulties? If yes, what are they, and in which cases? How do you correct and avoid these difficulties? Do you observe any differences in paramedian or oblique medial osteotomies based on the type of instruments used (mechanical, electrical, piezoelectric)?

Gerbault

The paramedian osteotomy is, for me, the most unforgiving, as the skin above it is usually thin. Well-positioned and performed with a very fine saw, preserving bone stability, this osteotomy generally does not cause problems. If its path is more lateral, especially for medial oblique osteotomies, the underlying bone support by the ULC is less. The bone fragment is then more unstable, with a significant risk of a visible stairstep deformity, which needs to be corrected by 4/0 polydioxanone sutures on either side of the osteotomy line after drilling holes with the ultrasonic drill. In case of a step deformity, the bony median fragment can also be rasped to smooth its visible edge.

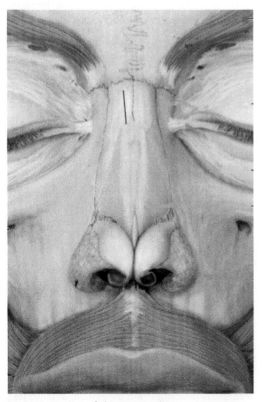

Fig. 31. Location of the paramedian osteotomy.

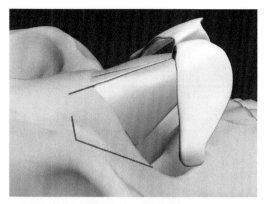

Fig. 33. Scheme of low to low lateral osteotomy and a partial length transverse osteotomy + paramedial osteotomy. However, there remains an intact bony segment between the anterior transverse and paramedial osteotomies.

Paramedian osteotomy can be combined with push-down/let-down osteotomies when the bony pyramid is wide. It is necessary not to lateralize this paramedian osteotomy, to avoid the risk of a stairstep deformity due to strong instability of the lateral wall bony flap.

Paramedian osteotomies can be performed closed using usually small straight saws at the bottom (RHS5 or RSD1), and a long straight saw upwards (RHL5).

Paramedian osteotomies can be performed with electric saws as precisely as with piezoelectric instruments. Narrow burrs or drills are sometimes used for these osteotomies, but with a more noticeable bone defect and therefore less bone stability with longer healing.

Finally, fine osteotomes are used for these paramedian or medial oblique osteotomies, but there are notable risks of radiated fractures at the caudal part (where the bone is thin), and significant risks of comminuted fractures at the cephalic part if this osteotomy is raised high. This is why it is usual to stay below the intercanthal line when osteotomes or bone chisels are used.

Split thickness osteotomies are sometimes attempted with osteotomes to avoid destabilizing the bones with the risk of uncontrolled bone sinkage creating a residual dent or hump at the level of the adjacent bone. However, they are very difficult to perform reliably without PEI because their success depends on the thickness and characteristics of the bones, and not only on the surgeon and osteotome used.

Racy

Paramedian and Transverse osteotomies are simple, but this is where the blades could break more.

Zholtikov

The use of PEI allows performing any variants of medial osteotomies very precisely and quickly without any difficulties, to remove any, even very thin strips of bone (up to 1 mm in width) in paramedial osteotomies without destroying the surrounding bony and cartilage structures, which, in my opinion, is difficult to perform precisely with conventional instruments.

Question 9: Concerning transverse osteotomies: What instruments do you use (with a photo if possible)? What approach do you use for this osteotomy? Where does it start and end? Does this trajectory vary based on the appearance of the nasal pyramid or the technique used for dorsal hump correction (bony impaction or cartilaginous resection)?

Cerkes

For transverse osteotomy, I use a 4-mm curved tip Cerkes Medial Oblique Osteotome, which is the same osteotome I use for the medial oblique osteotomy. The curved tip of the osteotome enables to perform the osteotomies internally under direct vision with a limited periosteal undermining when open approach is used. I believe that this delicate tool is the least traumatic to the adjacent tissues and very useful for transverse osteotomy. With this tool, an incomplete osteotomy can be done to perform a greenstick fracture.

The osteotomy usually starts at the superior end of the medial oblique/paramedian osteotomy. Its direction toward the medial canthus and it ends just above the medial canthal tendon (**Fig. 34**). An incomplete or complete transverse osteotomy can be performed depending on the case. The osteotomy can be performed as an incomplete osteotomy with partial penetration of the tip of the osteotome into the bone using the power of hand or a mallet. When mallet is used, the osteotomy should be done with gentle hits to avoid unwanted fragmentation of the nasal bones. In cases with

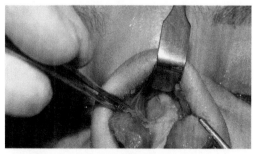

Fig. 34. Transverse osteotomy with a 4-mm curved tip Cerkes Medial Oblique Osteotome.

wide bony pyramid and asymmetric nasal bones, complete mobilization of the nasal bones is required. In this situation, a full cut (complete) transverse osteotomy should be performed instead of incomplete osteotomy using the same osteotome.

In cases with narrow radix, it is not necessary to do the transverse osteotomy at the medial canthus level or above. In such cases, the osteotomy can be placed more caudal to medial canthus to avoid additional narrowing of the radix.

Gerbault

Transverse osteotomies join lateral and paramedian osteotomies at their cephalic part (**Fig. 35**). They are necessary when the bony pyramid remains too wide despite lateral and paramedian osteotomies. Unlike the previous ones, they are simple to perform and do not create instability if performed very high on the nasal pyramid, above the intercanthal line. However, if performed too low, they can promote a depression of the bony flap with a visible stairstep deformity. These osteotomies are performed, after a generally extensive subperiosteal dissection, with very fine saws, one for the right side (RHS4L), the other for the left side (RHS4R) (**Figs. 36** and **37**). The same transverse osteotomies are performed with thicker

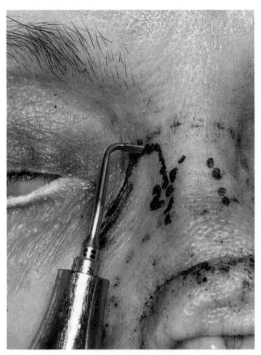

Fig. 36. The short-angled saws (RHS4R & RHS4L).

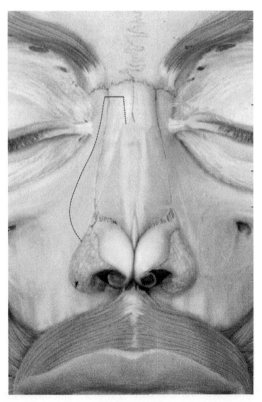

Fig. 35. Location of the transverse osteotomy.

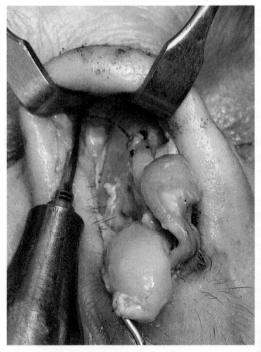

Fig. 37. Transverse osteotomy with the angulated saw.

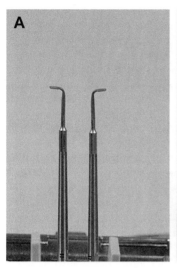
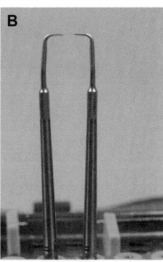

Fig. 38. (*A, B*) The long-angled saws (RHL4R & RHL4L).

saws (RHS3L and RHS3R) when more bone insta-bility is desired, that is, in impaction bone tech-niques (foundation techniques). However, in these cases, the most medial part of these osteotomies is made through the non-dissected procerus mus-cle with fine saws (RHS4 L and R) to avoid depres-sion of the radix. Those transverse osteotomies can be done through a closed approach with long saws (RHL4 R & L) (**Fig. 38**).

Racy

Transverse osteotomies are done with a specific oscillating hand piece for the upper part of the par-amedian osteotomy to the upper part of the lateral osteotomy. It can be a complete cut or an incom-plete cut for a greenstick fracture.

It is always a horizontal cut from the nasion to the anterior lachrymal crest.

Zholtikov

For transverse osteotomies, I use PEI right and left curved saws **Fig. 39**. Access, as I described earlier, depends on the dorsal technique. Limited approach for Dorsal Preservation and Full Open approach for DM and DR. In Dorsal Preservation, the transverse osteotomies continue smoothly from the lateral (Banana type) at the level of the intercanthal line and are combined with radix osteotomies on both sides. This allows mobiliza-tion of the entire nasal pyramid and bony impac-tion. In DM or DR, I most often perform partial transverse osteotomies that perform 2 to 3 mm more cranially than the intercanthal lines, con-necting laterally with the lateral osteotomies and ending medially approximately 5 to 7 mm from the central (dorsal) part of the bony pyramid. The partial-length transverse osteotomy leaves a short

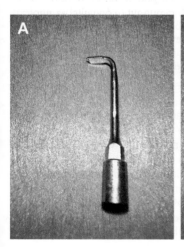
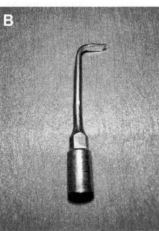

Fig. 39. (*A, B*) Piezo heads right and left curved Saws.

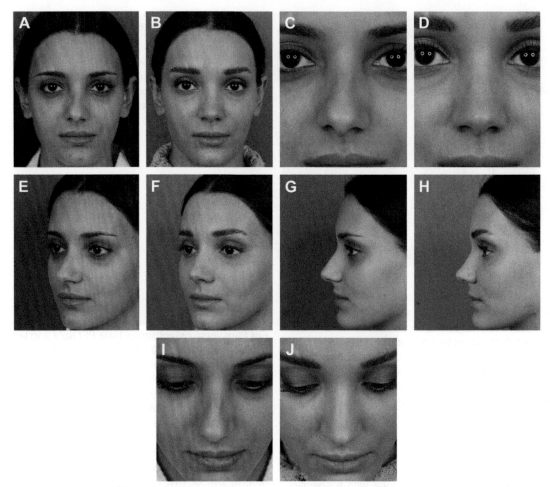

Fig. 40. This 25-year-old woman complained of having a deviated dorsum with a small hump as well as a bulbous, asymmetric tip. Following elevation of the skin envelope through an open approach, a full subperiosteal dissection of the bony vault was performed longitudinally from the keystone junction up to the radix, and transversely from one ascending frontal process of the maxilla to the other side. Then, ultrasonic RS of both sides of the bony pyramid was performed. The bony thickness was removed more from the lateral part of the bony pyramid on the left side (on the frontal process area of the maxilla) and from the medial part of the right bony side (on the area over the nasal bones). This maneuver shortened the length of the bony wall on the left side and elongated the bony wall on the right side. Next, the bony cap was removed with a piezo flat rasp and the cartilaginous vault was exposed cephalically for approximately 5 mm. Were no done osteotomies, only rhinosculpture. Then, following release of the ULCs, the dorsal septum and ULCs were lowered 2 mm. Next, elongated asymmetric pedestal spreaders (right side thinner, left side thicker) were inserted 1 mm below the ULCs and were then sutured to the septum above the spreaders. A septal extension graft was fixed between the spreaders. Lateral crura transposition with lateral crura strut grafts and tip sutures were utilized for tip reconstruction. Alar base reduction was performed to reduce alar flare. (*A, C, E, G, I*) Preoperative images; (*B, D, F, H, J*) 25 months postoperatively. RS, rhinosculpture; ULC, upper lateral cartilage.

segment of intact bone between the anterior end of the transverse osteotomy and the dorsum, thereby providing stability. This combination of osteotomies allows me to shift the bony pyramid base medially by several millimeters moving the base inward by straight elevator. In those cases in which mobilization of the lateral bony wall is inadequate, an additional paramedial or medial oblique osteotomy is performed. It should be noted that this additional osteotomy does not connect with the transverse osteotomy, and a bony bridge of at least 5 mm is maintained between them. In the cases when all of the performed manipulations were not enough to achieve symmetric and correct width of the bony pyramid, or in the cases of initially severe deviated bony pyramid when a complete osteotomy could not be avoided, then a combined lateral, transverse, and paramedial osteotomy performs, resulting in a U-shaped osteotomy.[10]

Question 10: Are transverse osteotomies with your preferred instruments sometimes a source of difficulties? If yes, what are they, and in which cases? How do you correct and avoid these difficulties? Do you observe any differences in transverse osteotomies based on the type of instruments used (mechanical, electrical, piezoelectric)?

Gerbault

Transverse osteotomies are the simplest and safest to perform as long as they are performed high enough. They can be partial or complete depending on the range of movement desired. These osteotomies are a bit more complicated to perform closed with RHL4 R and L inserts and require an extended closed approach to be performed, keeping only the central part of the nose where the procerus is respected as the only non-dissected part.

Racy

It could be difficult if the bone is very thick.

Zholtikov

Difficulties arise only with limited visibility, when using a limited approach for Dorsal Preservation, when the saw itself is not visible and the work is performed as close as possible to the dorsal part of the bone pyramid, in such cases, it is sometimes necessary to slightly widen the access to the sides for better visualization. In all other cases, difficulties arise very rarely, as the possibility of visual control allows osteotomies to be performed very precisely.

Question 11: How have your techniques in this area changed over the last 2 years?

Cerkes

In the last few years, I am using power instruments less frequently for bone reshaping. The 7-mm Tastan rasp is very delicate and powerful, and can fit into small spaces. It is a very useful tool in reshaping the nasal bones and correct irregularities on the surface of the nasal bones. Recently, I prefer it to power instruments in most cases.

Gerbault

In the last 2 years, I have used more dorsum preservation techniques (40% of cases in primary rhinoplasty). As a result, osteotomies have changed to adapt to Dorsal Preservation osteotomies. The bony pyramid was necessarily less stable in foundational techniques. I had to develop bone

restabilization techniques with sutures and grafts placed in the fracture sites.

But above all, what has most changed my practice is the routine use of long piezo inserts, to perform any type of septoplasty, very precise septal resections particularly for dorsal preservation while keeping the ability of significant septal harvesting for structural use without septal destabilization, and to do more ultrasonic rhinoplasties via the endonasal route.

Racy

No changes.

Zholtikov

Over the last 2 years, I have started to use electro power instruments, particularly cylindrical or diamond burr, more frequently as the initial part of rhinosculpture to speed up the operation, especially in patients with thick bones at the base of the bony pyramid and in secondary cases. In addition, by using Dorsal Preservation and DM more frequently, the number of Dorsal Reconstruction I perform has decreased from 50% to 20% of all primary rhinoplasties (**Fig. 40**).

DISCLOSURES

Consultant for Acteon.

SUPPLEMENTARY DATA

Supplementary data to this article can be found online at https://doi.org/10.1016/j.fsc.2024.06.001.

REFERENCES

1. Avsar Y. Nasal hump reduction with powered micro-saw osteotomy. Aesthet Surg J 2009;29(1):6–11.
2. Cerkes N. Concurrent elevation of upper lateral cartilage perichondrium and nasal bone periosteum: the perichondrium-periosteal flap. Aesthetic Surg J 2013;33:899.
3. Gerbault O, Daniel RK, Kosins AM. The role of piezoelectric instrumentation in rhinoplasty surgery. Aesthet Surg J 2016;36(1):21–34.
4. Gerbault O, Daniel RK, Palhazi P, et al. Reassessing the surgical management of the bony vault in rhinoplasty. Aesthet Surg J 2018;38(6):590–602.
5. Neves JC, Zholtikov V, Cakir B, et al. Rhinoplasty dissection planes (Subcutaneous, Sub-SMAS, Supra-perichondral, and Sub-perichondral) and soft tissues management. Facial Plast Surg 2021;37(1): 2–11.
6. Gerbault O, Daniel R, Palhazi P, et al. Reassessing surgical management of the bony vault in rhinoplasty.

Aesthetic Surg J 2018;38. https://doi.org/10.1093/asj/sjx246.

7. Ishida LC, Ishida J, Ishida LH, et al. Nasal hump treatment with cartilaginous push-down and preservation of the bony cap. Aesthet Surg J 2020;40:1168–78.

8. Ferreira MG, Ishida LC, Ishida LH, et al. Spare roof technique B. step-by-step guide to preserving the bony cap while Dehumping. Plast Reconstr Surg 2022 May 1;149(5):901e–4e.

9. Zholtikov V, Ouerghi R, Daniel RK. Composite dorsal augmentation. Aesthet Surg J 2022;42(8):874–87.

10. Zholtikov V, Golovatinsky V, Palhazi P, et al. Rhinoplasty: a sequential approach to managing the bony vault. Aesthetic Surg J 2019;40(5):479–92.

Managing the Midvault - Autospreaders, Spreader Grafts or What?

Fred G. Fedok, MD[a,b,*], Enrico Robotti, MD[c,d,e], Benjamin Marcus, MD[f]

KEYWORDS

• Midvault • Spreader graft • Autospreader flaps • Rhinoplasty

KEY POINTS

• Some form of midvault stabilization or maintenance should be considered in every rhinoplasty where a dorsal hump is taken down.
• Spreader grafts and autospreader flaps are reliable methods to stabilize the midvault to prevent and correct midvault collapse.
• Midvault collapse after rhinoplasty results in distortion of the brow-nasal aesthetic line and nasal obstruction.

 Video content accompanies this article at http://www.facialplastic.theclinics.com.

PANEL DISCUSSION

How do you prepare and treat the patient with contracted S-STE?

How do you manage the contracted inner lining (nasal stenosis)?

What techniques do you use to lengthen the overshortened nose?

What techniques do you use to support the dorsum?

Do you use any special techniques to prevent vestibular stenosis?

How have your techniques in this area changed over the last 2 years?

Question 1: When Do You Use Autospreader Flaps?

Fedok

What are autospreader flaps? For clarification, let me first describe what my concept of autospreader flaps are. Autospreader flaps [1] as described and popularized by H.Steve Byrd, MD were described as a method to maintain the midvault after a dorsal hump is taken down during a rhinoplasty. Autospreader flaps are fashioned for the stabilization of the midvault and the lateral nasal sidewall. This is particularly important when the relationship between the upper lateral cartilages and the septum has been disrupted. Midvault collapse is commonly seen when a dorsal hump has been taken down, especially when the hump is taken down as a complete unit, as was performed routinely in earlier rhinoplasty techniques. The hump was frequently removed en-bloc including portions of the dorsal nasal bones, the dorsal septum, and the medial portions of the bilateral upper lateral cartilages, including the keystone area. After that method of hump reduction, if the lateral nasal wall support is not maintained or reconstructed there is a greater risk of midvault collapse, thus, resulting in distortion of the brow-nasal aesthetic lines and causing

[a] Department of Surgery, University of South Alabama Mobile, AL, USA; [b] Fedok Plastic Surgery, 113 East Fern Avenue, Foley, AL 36535, USA; [c] Rhinoplasty Society of Europe; [d] Italian Society of Plastic Surgery; [e] Ospedale Papa Giovanni XXIII, Bergamo, Italy; [f] Department of Surgery, Division of Otolaryngology-Head & Neck Surgery University of Wisconsin School of Medicine and Public Health, K4/719 CSC, 600 Highland Avenue, Madison, WI 53792-7375, USA
* Corresponding author. Fedok Plastic Surgery, 113 East Fern Avenue, Foley, AL 35653.
E-mail address: drfredfedok@me.com

Facial Plast Surg Clin N Am 32 (2024) 517–532
https://doi.org/10.1016/j.fsc.2024.06.013
1064-7406/24/© 2024 Elsevier Inc. All rights are reserved, including those for text and data mining, AI training, and similar technologies.

nasal obstruction. This midvault collapse is more prevalent when the patient has short nasal bones, and a large hump is taken down. The risk is greater when a larger hump, that is, greater than 4 mm in height is taken down. The unsupported lateral nasal wall will have the propensity to collapse medially toward the septum overtime, thus, negatively affecting both the contour of the nose, as well as the nasal airway.

My autospreader technique is as follows:

Typically, I take a patient's dorsal convexity or hump down in a component manner. This may be performed using either an open or endonasal approach. Usually, the patient will have undergone a septoplasty with elevation of the lining on both sides of the septum. The upper lateral cartridges are submucosally divided from the midline septum. The upper lateral cartridges are divided away from the underside of the nasal bones centrally with the aid of a Freer elevator. The cartilaginous central dorsal septum is reduced with the aid of an 11 or 15 scalpel blade or an angled dorsal scissors. The planned reduction of the nasal bones is performed with either a Rubin osteotome, a motorized device, or a rasp. The edges of the reduced bones are rasped with a 2 to 4 rasp to smooth the edges. The remaining portions of the upper lateral cartridges are then trimmed to accommodate the planned dorsal height. Finally, the upper lateral cartridges are manipulated into the midline adjacent to the remaining septum and sutured in place using 2 to 3 horizontal mattress sutures using 4-0 polydioxanone (PDS) suture material.

In my practice, autospreader flaps are performed when candidates possess a dorsal hump or convexity and there is the intent for the dorsal convexity to be taken down. The shape and height of the dorsal convexity must include an adequate surplus of upper lateral cartilage, so that when the hump is taken down there is adequate remaining amount of the upper lateral cartilages so that they can be used for creating autospreader flaps possessing the necessary horizontal and vertical characteristics.

Patients that are less favorable candidates for autospreader flaps include those without a dorsal convexity or those without an excess of upper lateral cartilage or those with such a minimal dorsal convexity that taking down the dorsal hump would not leave an adequate amount of upper lateral cartilage to carry out the autospreader flap technique. Also, anatomic distortion and scarring from previous injury or surgery on the midvault area may prevent the use of any suitable residual upper lateral cartilage. (**Figs. 1** and **2**)

Autospreader flaps can be executed and created effectively via both the external and endonasal approach.[2] I frequently use the autospreader flap technique in primary rhinoplasty. Because of the points made in the previous paragraph I use the technique less frequently in revision rhinoplasty cases. In general, I use them in patients with noses that are straight and have not undergone previous significant nasal surgery.

Robotti

My answer to this question in my current practice is essentially: hardly ever. Indeed, we recently looked at our last 2 years series of primary rhinoplasties and pure "structural" dorsal management by component separation-incremental reduction (where we may need autospreaders, spreaders, or a combination of those), is now done in less than 5% of cases. The reason is that in the vast majority of my primary rhinoplasties, I now use a "modified dorsal split" technique followed by either (a) a cartilaginous push down or (b) a full letdown (symmetric or asymmetric)[3,4] The Dorsal Keystone Area (DKA) is preserved, but the middle vault is opened along the anatomic plane between the edges of the "Septal T" or "T bar" and the upper lateral cartilages. Then, the middle vault will be adjusted as needed by differential trimming of the upper laterals, overlap of the septal T to one side to compensate deviation, or using an underlay "pedestal" spreader. This allows me to achieve symmetry in the dorsal aesthetic lines (DALs) and expands significantly the indications of the traditional push-down or let-down procedure where the whole middle vault is, by definition, left intact. Indeed, relatively few patients, at least in our practice, enjoy the luxury of a symmetric middle vault to be left untouched.

No Lateral Keystone Area (LKA) release or "ballerina maneuver" will be needed, since the vertical excess of the upper lateral cartilages will be trimmed as necessary and then tensioned distally at the W point (where the upper laterals anatomically join to the distal septum). Independently, on whether a cartilaginous pushdown or a full letdown maneuver will subsequently follow, splitting the dorsum anatomically along the septal T will allow to reshape the middle vault appropriately and reestablish aesthetic DAL's. We previously published this concept, its rationale and its technical details.[3,4]

There is, however, a specific instance in which I use autospreader flaps even within a "modified dorsal split" scenario. This relates to the case where the bony cap is still small, but not so small as to be manageable just by osteoplasty (with burr or Piezo) followed by a cartilaginous pushdown. In those cases, which refer to bony caps measuring about 4 or 5 mm in height, we are recently using a

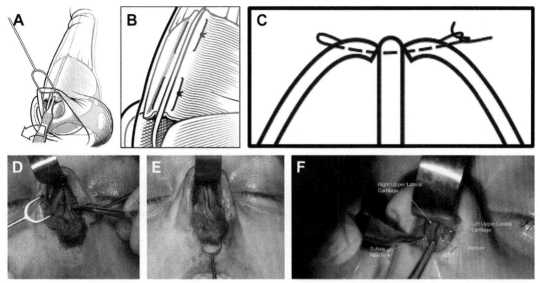

Fig. 1. (*A–C*) Illustration depicting endonasal autospreader flaps, (*D*) Clinical intraoperative photograph depicting endonasal autospreader flaps technique. Midline septum is taken down to level of planned dorsal reduction. Upper lateral cartilage height is preserved. (Note–this photograph from external approach case), (*E*) Clinical intraoperative photograph depicting endonasal autospreader flap technique. Midline septum has been taken down to level of planned dorsal reduction. Upper lateral cartilage height is preserved and adjusted prior to suturing. (Note–this photograph from external approach case), (*F*) Clinical intraoperative photograph depicting endonasal autospreader flap technique. Upper lateral cartilage is sutured to the septum. (Note–this photograph is from endonasal case). (Note (labels): visualized through retracted left nostril after upper lateral cartilages have been divided from the septum–right upper lateral cartilage, suture needle engaging right upper lateral cartilage with intent to place needle from right to left through right upper lateral cartilage, septum (that is temporally caudally defected) and left upper lateral cartilage.). (*From:* Management of the Middle Vault in Endonasal Rhinoplasty Fred G. Fedok, Frank Garritano, Facial Plast Surg 2014;30:204 to 212 (see **Fig. 7**).)

modification of our original cartilaginous pushdown dorsal split technique,[3] which has been independently developed by Ali Khazaal from Iraq[5] and Sergio Furtado from Brazil.[6]

The residual portion of the bony cap is circumscribed by paramedian Piezo osteotomies, which follow the DALs as well by a transverse greenstick fracture by Piezo, positioned at the start of the bony hump. An ostectomy of a triangular bony wedge just lateral to the paramedian osteotomy is performed of the same width as the planned transverse reduction of the bony dorsum. The septal T is pushed down after removal of a high-middle strip of septal cartilage. As an alternative to trimming the cranial edge of the upper laterals, autospreaders can then be advantageously used to stabilize the "shoulders "of this pushed-down combination of residual bony cap and septal T. Then, the middle vault is re-sutured in the same way as the original "modified dorsal split" technique. Interestingly,

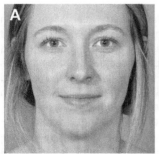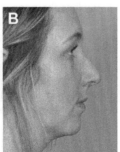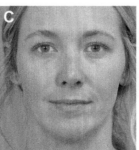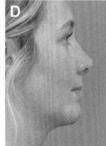

Fig. 2. Clinical images of patient who underwent primary open rhinoplasty incorporating autospreader flaps. (*A, B*) Preoperative, (*C, D*) Postoperative.

the use of autospreader flaps in a hybrid dorsal preservation procedure with dorsal split and a Cottle septoplasty had also been previously published by Sousa Viera.[7]

Marcus

I think of auto-spreader flaps as a type of preservation technique. In contrast to a pure joseph reduction–the use of auto-spreader flaps by definition preserves the upper lateral cartilage. This choice alone provides several unique options for dorsal reconstruction.

My choice to use this option is triggered by one of several findings in the patient examination. The main indication is the patient with a dorsal hump of at least 3 mm who desires dorsal reduction. As previously described–I would first asses if this patient was a candidate for dorsal preservation rhinoplasty (DPR). In my patient population, there is a high incidence of severe nasal septum pathology. In my hands–these cases are not good candidates for DPR. When DPR is not an option my next choice would be to use spreader flaps in these cases (**Fig. 3**).

Another common scenario where I use auto-spreader flaps is in revision functional rhinoplasty. I routinely see patients who have had septoplasty at an outside hospital and need nasal valve reconstruction. While autologous rib cartilage is always my preferred option, there are many patients who are over 50, have significant ossification of their chest, and have limited grafting material. Turn-in flaps of the upper lateral cartilages can be very helpful to preserve grafting material for other areas of the repair.

During midvault reconstruction, I tend to use spreader flaps in one of 2 main ways. The most common technique is the turn-in flap.[8] When this technique was introduced, I was concerned that the softer nature of the upper lateral cartilage would not be suitable to maintain strength long-term. The functional outcomes of this technique have now been well-established in the short-term[9] and long-term.[10] While most surgeons associate the use of spreader flaps–hump reduction itself is not a true prerequisite for the technique.[11,12] While a hump is not required, I certainly find it easier to create the flaps when a cartilaginous hump of at least 3 mm is present. Spreader flaps have a unique nature that also allows fine tuning of the brow-tip-aesthetic line (BTAL). After creation of the flap and suturing to the septum, additional mattress sutures can be placed with 5-0 PDS to precisely shape the BTAL. This is a real advantage over standard spreader grafts that tend to be a singular width. I tend to avoid using auto-spreader grafts in thin noses that have a significant mid-vault narrowing. Tall narrow noses with very narrow midvault are quite common in the upper Midwest. From both a functional and an aesthetic standpoint, I find it difficult to shape the spreader flaps precisely to correct the pinched mid-vault.

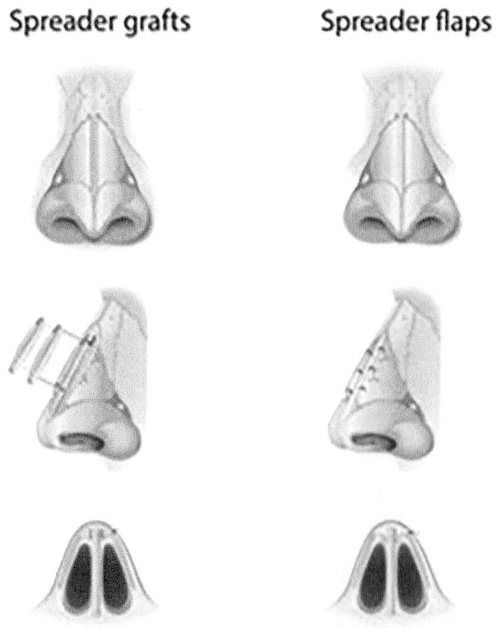

Question 2: When Do You Use Spreader Grafts?

Fedok

The popularization of spreader grafts changed rhinoplasty results.[13] Nasal contour was improved. The brow-nasal aesthetic line could be maintained and recreated. More importantly after rhinoplasty, patients did not suffer the midvault collapse that was frequently typical of rhinoplasty results before the use of spreader grafts, extended spreader grafts, and other methods of managing the midvault of the nose.

Spreader grafts have been extremely helpful in the management of the patient with a crooked nose, which is frequently coupled with a crooked septum. In my experience, the addition of this additional structure to aid in "bracing" the repaired septum in the midline of the nose serves as an adjunct in straightening the crooked nose.

I use some form of midvault stabilization whenever I approach the surgery of a patient with: a dorsal hump that will be taken down, the patient with a crooked nose, the patient with a saddle nose deformity, the patient who complains of nasal

Spreader grafts   Spreader flaps

Fig. 3. Spreader grafts and Spreader flaps.

obstruction and shows evidence of lateral nasal wall dysfunction, the patient who has avulsion of an upper lateral cartilage, and the patient without satisfactory brow–nasal aesthetic lines. Thus, either spreader grafts or autospreader flaps techniques are utilized in most of my rhinoplasty cases. I will utilize spreader grafts for both functional and cosmetic indications. At times the placement of spreader grafts is performed for the correction of a preexisting problem, and at times they are placed prophylactically to prevent a problem. I use spreaders grafts and create autospreader flaps for various similar reasons. Whether I use spreader grafts or autospreader flaps has to do whether my surgical maneuvers will allow me to retain sufficient excess of upper lateral cartilage to fold over and create autospreader flaps, if not, I will resort to spreader grafts. In the case of crooked nose deformity; however, I usually find spreader grafts to be more reliable in buttressing the septum into the central midline (**Fig. 4**).

In my early rhinoplasty experience middle vault stabilization was not well emphasized (I am referring to the late 80's early 90's). I noted that many patients displayed a nasal contour issue with collapse of the midvault. Even when they did not complain of nasal obstruction, one could recognize the problem in their postoperative examination. The need of some form of stabilization of the midvault appears to be particularly an issue in patients with short nasal bones. In the patient with short nasal bones there is less support of the lateral nasal wall. If there is violation of the keystone area, the nasal bones and the upper

lateral cartilages as in hump reduction, midvault collapse is at risk.

Studies have universally advocated the use of spreader grafts and autospreader flaps for the stabilization of the midvault lateral nasal wall in rhinoplasty. Nasal contour is fairly accurately maintained, but the efficacy in airway improvement is controversial. The author's personal experience with this is consistent with these reports.[14–17]

My evaluation of patients who are candidates for either autospreader flaps or spreader grafts includes visual inspection of the nose and preoperative images looking for signs of short nasal bones, 8 midvault narrowing, and midvault collapse. I will also inspect their nose during inspiration looking for signs of midvault insufficiency. I will judge the effect of performing a modified cottle maneuver and solicit their history of nasal breathing problems or their spontaneous application of the cottle maneuver or other adjuncts.

My standard technique for placing spreader grafts is as follows. In rank order of use, I will create and place spreader grafts with the use of septal, auricular, and rib cartilage. Spreader grafts can be placed with either an open or endonasal rhinoplasty approach. The open approach is significantly easier than the endonasal approach to perform this technique. Spreader grafts are usually placed after appropriate septal work is completed, dorsal height is adjusted, and the upper lateral cartridges are divided away from the septum. When using septal cartilage, usually the intrinsic thickness of the cartilage is appropriate to be placed as a spreader graft. When using auricular cartilage

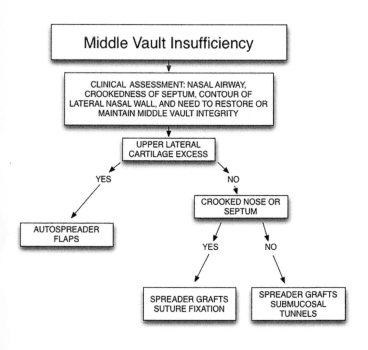

Fig. 4. Schematic depicting suggested algorithm. The clinical assessment involves the recognition or anticipation of midvault insufficiency. Parameters to be considered include the need to straighten the nose or septum, the intrinsic size and strength of the upper lateral cartilages, the contour of the lateral nasal wall, the airway patency, and whether there will be excess upper lateral cartilage height after dorsal reduction. (*From:* Management of the Middle Vault in Endonasal Rhinoplasty Fred G. Fedok, Frank Garritano, Facial Plast Surg 2014;30:204–212 (see **Fig. 9**).)

or rib cartilage, some sculpting of the graft may be necessary to achieve this dimension. Usually, the width or height of the spreader graft must be on the order of at least 3 to 4 mm to be of practical use. The length will vary according to the dimensions of the cartilage harvested and the length of the upper lateral cartilages. I have found this will vary from 15 to 20 mm in most patients and can extend easily to up to 30 mm depending on the need and placement when one is contemplating the creation of extended spreader grafts. At times the extended spreader graft will extend superiorly under the cut edge of a nasal bone to enlarge the width of the bony vault. At times, they will extend caudally to the nasal tip to engage a septal replacement graft or septal extension graft where the length may be 35 mm (**Figs. 5** and **6**).

Robotti

In my current primary rhinoplasty practice, I use spreader grafts in 2 occasions: (a) when I do purely structural rhinoplasty by component separation–incremental reduction of the dorsum, which is, as I said previously, very rare in my current practice, since it happens exclusively in some crooked noses and (b) when I need to symmetrize the middle vault in my "modified dorsal split" cartilaginous pushdown or full letdown technique[3,4] This occurs when the middle vault is asymmetric and although still preserving the DKA, I will still need some considerable surface modification of the middle vault. Here, I use spreader grafts whenever trimming the vertical excess of the upper laterals and tensioning them at the W point will not be enough to provide symmetry of the middle vault. In such cases, I use finely shaped spreaders, at times of differential thickness, unilateral or bilateral, gently beveling the edges and placing them just below the upper edge of the septum (**Fig. 7**). The upper lateral cartilage will then be sutured to the septum, on top of the spreader graft, which is, thus, placed in a "pedestal" fashion (Video 1). Occasionally, I will instead need the upper edge of the spreader graft to actually bridge a desirable gap between the upper laterals and the septum, when I need to reestablish some transverse distance in between.

Although I think this may be beyond the original scope of the question, I should mention that the matter becomes totally different in secondary rhinoplasty. Here, I liberally and extensively use spreader grafts from fine rib laminations, to rebuild the horizontal element of the L-strut, and reconstruct a dorsal plateau of correct width.[18,19] It is a variegated scenario in which, as needed, I will use long extended spreaders or, rather, staggered shorter spreaders (**Fig. 8**). Piezo will serve to develop slots on the bone on either side of the residual septum at the DKA (Video 2), then I will raise the spreaders on top of the residual septum, if needed, to start reestablishing dorsal height, and I will use transosseous sutures to stabilize the rib spreaders-septum unit to each bone laterally, usually after osteoplasty.[20]

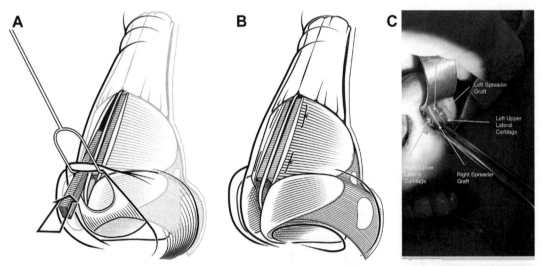

Fig. 5. (*A, B*) Illustration depicting endonasal suturing of spreader grafts, (*C*) Clinical intraoperative photograph depicting endonasal suturing of spreader grafts. (Note [labels]: visualized through retracted left nostril after upper lateral cartilages have been divided from the septum–right upper lateral cartilage, bayonet forceps positioning right spreader graft, septum, left spreader graft positioned between septum and left upper lateral cartilage.) (*From*: Management of the Middle Vault in Endonasal Rhinoplasty Fred G. Fedok, Frank Garritano, Facial Plast Surg 2014;30:204–212 (see **Fig. 3**).)

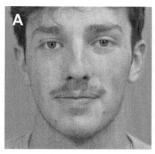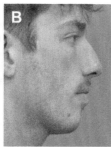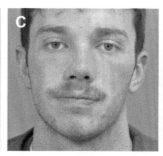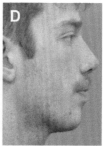

Fig. 6. Clinical images of patient who underwent primary open rhinoplasty incorporating spreader grafts. (*A, B*) Preoperative, (*C, D*) Postoperative. (Note: The patient presents with midvault narrowing and short nasal bones)

Marcus

Spreader grafts remain a staple of my rhinoplasty practice. There are multiple clear indications for this time-tested technique. In my patient population, nasal obstruction is an element in at least 2/3 of my cases. The presence of nasal trauma, prior surgery or lateral wall insufficiency is quite common. Traditional spreader grafts are a key tool for mid-vault reconstruction in this group. Nasal valve compromise is often multi-factorial, but the creation of a strong and open mid-vault is a key step to restore breathing. My functional indications for spreader grafts include: (1) a narrowed internal nasal valve, (2) creating a strong and straight L-Strut after trauma, and (3) use of extended spreader grafts to control position of a caudal septum extension graft (CSEG). Correction of the internal nasal valve with spreader grafts is well-documented.[21] In addition to dynamic nasal valve collapse (which is outside this discussion), many of my functional nasal cases have narrowed internal nasal valves. This static narrowing is efficiently corrected with open placement of traditional spreader grafts. While there are several reports that endonasal spreader graft placement is effective,[22] I have not found that to be the case in my hands. In many ways I think these are different procedures. Endonasal placement (without detachment of the upper lateral cartilages) is less likely to increase the cross-sectional area of the nasal valve. The detachment of the upper lateral cartilages and placement of variable size spreader grafts is a more definitive way to open the internal nasal valve. When trauma has left a patient with a weakened or distorted L-strut, extended spreader grafts are very useful to restore the proper

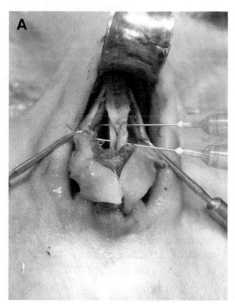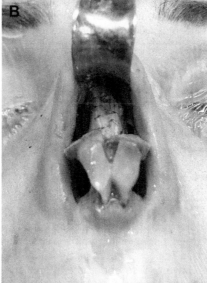

Fig. 7. (*A, B*) spreader grafts to symmetrize the middle vault in a modified dorsal split.

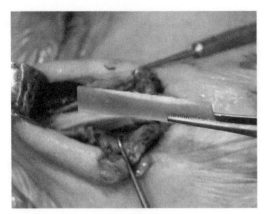

Fig. 8. Extended spreader graft from rib lamination to reconstruct the horizontal portion of the L-strut in secondary rhinoplasty.

architecture.[23] Even after corrective septoplasty, many post-traumatic noses have residual and intrinsic bend to the L-strut. Rather than further thinning or scoring (which would lead to further weakness and distortion), I like the stability of long and strong extended spreader grafts.[24]

Spreader grafts can be very helpful in aesthetic surgery as well. I am not yet at a stage where DPR can be used to treat cosmetic asymmetries of the mid-vault. While DPR can certainly be done in these cases by more advanced surgeons–I find the use of precisely sized spreader grafts (often of different sizes) allow me to create a more symmetric mid-vault. The utility of spreader grafts in the cosmetic patient has been demonstrated to be a successful long-term strategy.[25]

Revisions rhinoplasty is another clear indication for traditional spreader grafts. Many of these patients are poor candidates for DPR and often the septum has been significantly altered during their prior surgery. Spreader grafts are a useful tool in these cases to restore dorsal support and often improve nasal valve patency. Many of these cases are done using autologous rib cartilage. Costal cartilage can make ideal spreader grafts for revision surgery.[26] The grafts tend to have significant rigidity, as well as the volume to allow precise carving size.

Question 3: Can You Perform the Combined Approach to Treat the Middle Vault

Fedok
I will use a combined or hybrid approach, that is, using both the autospreader flaps and the spreader grafts in some situations. A prerequisite is that the patient must have excess upper lateral cartilage material, available to create autospreader flaps. This will have to be the case after a dorsal convexity

is taken down. The autospreader flaps are created from the residual bilateral upper lateral cartilage, so that is an obvious necessity. The reasons to add another midvault stabilization method are somewhat varied. These include: the patient with a high septal deviation, causing distortion in the brow-nasal aesthetic line and the patient with crooked nose deformity. In cases where there is a need to lengthen the over -rotated nasal tip with the use of extended spreader grafts or the patient with a cartilaginous saddle where you may need extended spreader grafts would be another situation. Although I have simultaneously used both autospreader flaps and spreader grafts in primary rhinoplasty, I have done it more often in cases of revision rhinoplasty, where the amount of scarring and difficulty in dissecting out the septum is managed by adding cartilage in a midline that is asymmetric. In some cases, the spreader graft may only have to be applied unilaterally to accommodate for a high septal deviation.

Robotti
We need to clarify here. I use the term "hybrid" to actually designate structural reediting on the tip and preservation on the dorsum. This structural tip work is; however, accomplished with a new perspective, stemming from the "preservation anatomy" concepts, with attention on preserving–reconstructing ligaments and on proper dissection planes. This has been a significant, progressive mental change, which I derived from studying, and then uniformly applying, preservation concepts.

However, I subsequently "hybridize" further, since I commit the "heresy" (as could be considered by "pure preservationists") of splitting the middle vault before proceeding to a cartilaginous pushdown or a full letdown (symmetric or asymmetric).[3,4] I split the middle vault along that anatomic plane along the edges of the septal T, which anybody can easily see when using loupes while doing a rhinoplasty (**Fig. 9**). This distinctive plane separates the edge of the keel-shaped septal T from the upper lateral cartilages and a semi-sharp elevator can just by a pushing maneuver, easily spread it open. In this sense, I am not only a pure preservationist of the dorsum, but also I am not using a structural approach since I'm not doing a conventional reduction and reconstruction of the dorsal hump. I also demonstrated this further hybrid concept my recent "Primary hybrid Rhinoplasty "live surgery course.[27] I leave intact what matters most to me, and what is most difficult to reconstruct, that is, the DKA. As I mentioned previously, I will then "play" with the upper laterals also, potentially, inserting unilateral, bilateral, or asymmetric spreaders to symmetrize

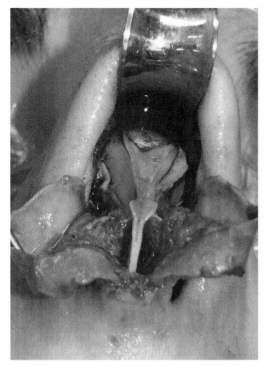

Fig. 9. Splitting the dorsum along the septal T is demonstrated.

the middle vault. Then, after my high-middle strip excision, I will suture-fixate the septal T to the residual septum below under direct vision, in an end-to-end or end-to-side configuration (**Fig. 10**) and finally re-suture the middle vault (**Fig. 11**). This comes together with osteoplasty, as needed or differential osteotomies (**Fig. 12**). It is interesting that other surgeons who seemed initially to be pure preservationist to me have embraced the concept of surface modifications to the dorsum.[28,29] Such surface modifications consist of both osteoplasty maneuvers to convert the S-shaped bony cap to

a more manageable V-shaped structure, better suited to push down–let down, as well as of shaving cartilaginous horns at the keystone and even of partially opening the middle vault. Although our techniques differ, I surely concur with Carlos Neves when he emphasized the need of additional maneuvers to the dorsum in a "mixed" approach to dorsal preservation[30]

Regarding my personal approach, as well as treating the middle vault as stated above, I will also often reshape the bony cap and bony sidewalls by osteoplasty in the vast majority of cases, I do this for conversion of the S-shaped bony cap to a V-shape prior to full letdown, for lowering a small bony cap, and thus, allowing me to perform a cartilaginous pushdown only, and often, as a final touchup, after the dorsum is completed, just before closure. Currently, I have turned away in most cases from the use of Piezo for osteoplasty since I find the use of cylindrical burrs (of different shapes and sizes but all, importantly, with a flat surface) faster, more efficient, and not provoking any damage to cartilage if used carefully and at a low rotation per minute (RPM).[31] Readers could benefit from the table with a step-by-step recapitulation of the modified dorsal split procedure, which is found in our recently published paper in this same journal.[4]

Marcus

There are certainly cases where I will use a combined or hybrid approach. The most common

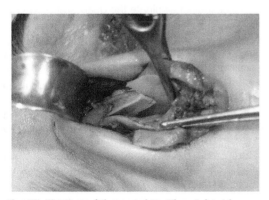

Fig. 10. Fixation of the septal T with a right-side overlap is shown.

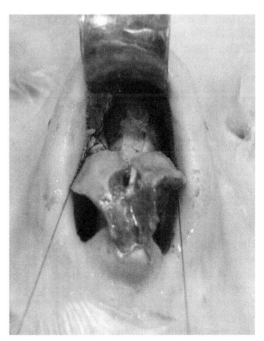

Fig. 11. The middle vault is re-sutured.

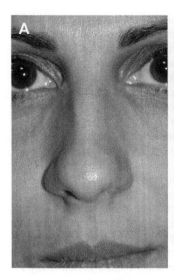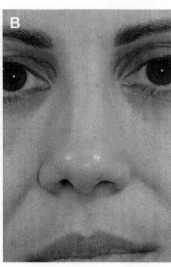

Fig. 12. (*A*, *B*) Pre-and post-zoomed frontal view at 1 year follow up demonstrating the improvement of the middle vault in a modified dorsal split.

scenario for me is the patient who has a dramatic narrowing at the mid-vault. The combination of a spreader flap with a spreader graft is useful to widen the mid-vault effectively, but without the more geometric appearance of overly wide solid spreader grafts. The spreader flap can be shaped allow for greater width but with a more natural gentle slope to the sidewall of the nose. The upper lateral cartilage allows me to add further width with less apparent bulk.[32] The hybrid approach has also proved useful in straightening the crooked nose as well.[33]

Question 4: When You Do Not Have Enough Septal Cartilage, What Are Your Other Grafting Options at the Middle Vault?

Fedok

My preference in all rhinoplasty grafting procedures is to use autogenous tissue. I usually find that there is ample native cartilage available from the patient. In the patient population I have been privileged to take care of, I have been able to avoid the use of alloplastic or cadaver materials in the nose, except in rare temporary situations. The limited morbidity of harvesting septal cartilage, auricular cartilage, and even rib cartilage obviates the need to use non-autogenous tissues in most rhinoplasty cases. The use of autogenous issue eliminates other concerns and complications, intolerance, extrusion, and infection.

To provide structure to the midvault with the use of spreader grafts, I find that I normally have an adequate supply of septal cartilage to use. If I am only limiting my comments to grafting materials necessary to manage the midvault then my next candidate is usually the pinna. Although auricular

cartilage has its own challenges because of its intrinsic curvature and other less desirable characteristics, for simply managing the midvault, it is usually adequate. Auricular cartilage is brittle and at times fragile and hard to carve. Depending on the patient, I usually harvest the cartilage from a posterior approach to the ear. I will harvest portions of the cymba concha and the concha cavum.

In a lesser proportion of patients, depending on the shape of the ear, and what I need in the shape and dimensions of my harvest material, I may approach the ear from an anterior approach. In that situation I make the incision along the inner aspect of the antihelix, elevate the skin, and remove the segment of cartilage I need while maintaining the posterior skin intact. In this case, I usually am harvesting a portion of the cymba concha.

When I harvest cartilage from the ear, I am always careful to use through and through mattress sutures when closing to suture the 2 cutaneous sides together to eliminate the dead-space where the cartilage was removed. This eliminates the possibility of the development of a postoperative hematoma, which although is relatively small, is usually quite painful and hard to manage in the outpatient clinic.

My third choice of donor site for cartilage material is the rib. Although this discussion is focused on managing the midvault, in cases of revision rhinoplasty and after trauma, where more grafting material may be necessary, I may find myself going to the rib before going to the ear. Here at the chest wall, one has essentially all the possible grafting material you possibly could need in the management of the person's nose.

Robotti

One of the assets of dorsal preservation, even if interpreted, as I do, in a hybrid way via a "modified dorsal split" approach, is that one does not need as much grafting as would be required in a purely structural dorsal resection-reconstruction. For this reason, the answer to this question is that I use hardly any septal cartilage for the middle vault and if I do, this happens rather seldom (as mentioned previously, I occasionally employ small spreader grafts, placed symmetrically or asymmetrically, to improve the symmetry of the DALs). So, I do not usually need any grafting material to the dorsum in primary rhinoplasties, while I still need grafting to my tip. While I use autologous rib grafting extensively to the dorsum in my secondaries, I have used rib for my primaries in 5 or 6 cases only over the last 2 years. Those are rare circumstances in which one is dealing with traumatic severely crooked noses, where I find it easier to harvest rib and use fine rib laminations as extended or staggered spreaders rather than differently reassemble the complex puzzle of multiple septum elements derived from a severely deviated septum.

Obviously, circumstances vary in a wide spectrum. There are often cases where a perforated ethmoid plate may be useful, and actually works both as a strong splint to straighten a deviated middle vault, as well as a spreader in providing some needed extra width on whatever side. Likewise, we sometimes use a composite graft, including a portion of the quadrangular cartilage, as well as its attached portion of perpendicular plate of the ethmoid (PPE), for the same reason (**Fig. 13**), and the cartilaginous portion can of course be also used as a septal extension graft (**Fig. 14**). In such cases, the ethmoid portion is reshaped with the use of cylindrical burrs at low RPM and ice-cold irrigation, then perforated with a conical Piezo insert, and then sutured in position (Video 3). Sometimes

people ask the question of what happens to perforated ethmoid splints. I do not have an answer based on studies, but on multiple occasions, while performing a revision rhinoplasty, I encountered previously placed splints of ethmoid bone, which I actually often could previously see in the sagittal view of the cone beam computed tomography (CT) scan, which I request prior to any surgery,[34] I am quite certain that perforated ethmoid splints stay and essentially do not resorb. When using ethmoid splints or composite grafts that include a portion of PPE, an important detail is the use of a long Piezo insert for harvesting ethmoid bone and for posterior septal work (Video 4). I find this a crucial point, since it will avoid the risk of mucosal lacerations bilaterally, even in presence of a significant septal spur. The use of a double-action septal scissor is simply not comparable.

Of course, the answer to the key question of this paragraph will be totally different when I do not have enough septal cartilage in secondary rhinoplasty, as is usually the case. I will touch only briefly on this since I do not think it is within the scope of this section. My tolerance level to harvesting rib will be very low in those circumstances, and I strongly prefer the use of rib laminations to harvesting what finally happens to be a usually very modest portion of residual quadrangular plate. If I work on the septum in those contingencies, it is usually to correct a residual deviation. I find rib much more useful and efficient to design proper spreaders to reconstruct the L-strut, and symmetrize the middle vault.[18] One of the aspects I care about in those circumstances is to use thin rib laminations, although they have to be strong enough to allow support and provide adequate width (**Fig. 15**). In fact, I believe that a common mistake here is to use excessively thick rib segments, which obviously ends up in providing excessive dorsal width that patients essentially dislike.

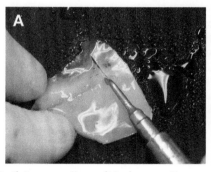 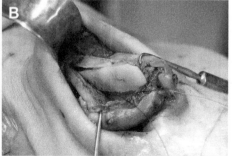

Fig. 13. (*A, B*) A composite graft is shown acting as a spreader after a modified dorsal split cartilaginous push-down. Piezo is used both for cutting the ethmoid plate portion of the composite graft, as well as for perforating it for subsequent suturing.

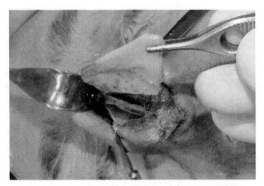

Fig. 14. A composite graft is shown which will act as a septal extension graft while at the same time splinting the septum anteriorly.

Marcus

The lack of adequate septum cartilage is a common occurrence. There are 2 main sources that I use for grafting material: autologous rib and autologous ear cartilage (**Fig. 16**). There are some limited cases when I need costal cartilage, but the patient is too old or objects to rib harvest. In these limited cases, I will consider the use of irradiated rib cartilage. I am personally comfortable using these tissues in the spreader graft position. Their utility in other areas has been shown to be variable. While I worry about the use of irradiated rib cartilage for a CSEG, lateral crural graft or a strut–Kridel[35] showed excellent long-term outcomes with a 5% resorption rate in his study. Auricular cartilage is less commonly used as a spreader graft. In my practice–if I need a lot of grafts to reconstruct a nose–I will consider the use of ear cartilage for spreader grafts. They can be layered and appear to have long-term stability.[36]

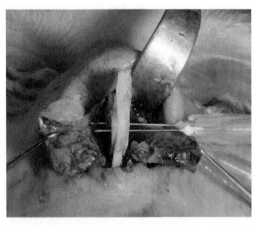

Fig. 15. Rib laminations should be thin, although strong. The thickness of rib spreaders can be compared here to the septum in between.

Question 5: Are There Other Alternatives to Manage The Middle Vault in Addition to Spreader Flaps or Grafts

Fedok

There are other alternatives available that many other rhinoplasty surgeons use. Although I personally have had satisfactory success with spreader grafts and autospreader flaps, I have also found flaring sutures to be helpful in some patients.[37] They are relatively easy to accomplish. I have rarely used them as my primary method to stabilize or reconstruct the integrity of the midvault. I have added them as an adjunct when I am not totally satisfied with the configuration of the midvault after placing spreader grafts or creating autospreader flaps.

Other methods that can be successfully applied include butterfly grafts[38] and alar batten grafts[39] and various suspension sutures.

Robotti

I will be short in replying to this question, since essentially it brings me back again to the concepts, which I discussed previously. My current technique in managing the nasal dorsum is a "modified dorsal split" preservation,[3,4] which means separating the septal T from the upper lateral cartilages anatomically, preserving the DKA and then using one of these 3 options: (a) a cartilaginous push down, in

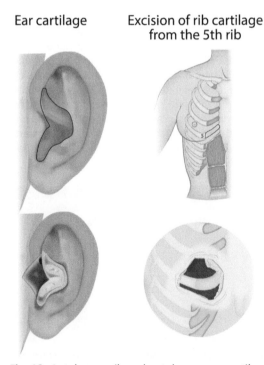

Ear cartilage   Excision of rib cartilage from the 5th rib

Fig. 16. Autologous rib and autologous ear cartilage used as graft.

which the dorsal is managed by osteoplasty and a high middle strip used to push down the cartilaginous dorsum. Vertical release incisions in the Vitruvian man manner.[40] In that vertical short portion of septum left attached to the septal T are used to allow better flexion at the chondro-osseous DKA joint. Direct suturing is easily done under direct vision, after overlap or end-to-end approximation and the midvault is resutured. (b) A modified cartilaginous push down, recently described independently by Furtado and Khazaal,[5,6] which is an interesting modification of option (a), in which a residual portion of the bony cap after osteoplasty is included in the pushed-down section. The portion of the bony cap, together with the septal T is pushed down after having been delimitated by paramedian short osteotomies and a transverse cut, which allows a controlled greenstick like fracture. (c) A full letdown procedure, in which circumferential osteotomies are done by Piezo (symmetrically or asymmetrically, meaning with the differential resection of a bone strip at the base of the nasal bones, which will be wider on the side of greater bony length and obliquity). We then currently perform the carefully controlled transverse osteotomy at the radix with a fine burr disc, under direct vision (**Fig. 17**).

Thus, as I mentioned previously, I almost have no remaining indications for spreader flaps, while spreader grafts are used, though infrequently, in combination with the dorsal split preservation technique when one needs to provide better symmetry of the middle vault.

Marcus

For many years–the deconstruction of the midvault was a standard in almost every case. With the explosion of preservation rhinoplasty–I simply look at the dorsum and mid-vault differently. Preservation rhinoplasty is truly a range of techniques.

In aesthetic cases, the surface techniques[41] from DPR have been very easy to integrate into my practice. Using powered instrumentation, I shape the bone and even the cartilaginous midvault without any deconstruction. It has really been a change in mindset (**Fig. 18**).

Question 6: How Have Your Techniques in This Area Changed Over The Last 2 Years?

Fedok

Most of my rhinoplastic experience has been with using the midvault stabilization methods discussed in this article. My management of the dorsum hump has typically been as a component reduction and restoration of the midvault. This is in contrast with the dorsal preservation techniques that are becoming more popular. At this point of time, I have performed only a limited number of dorsal preservation procedures, although my technique continues to evolve.

Robotti

To provide an honest answer, I have to look back a little further, at least 5 or 6 years.

Since the end of 2017, we started using the "modified dorsal split preservation" approach and we applied this to the cartilaginous pushdown concept. We had several problems in the beginning, which were essentially undercorrections of the hump. We were not understanding fully the need of proper fixation, either end-to-end or end-to-side, after removing the high middle strip and of gently extending the chondro-osseous junction. We were not using initially vertical incisions, according to the "Vitruvian man" concept[40] and fixation of the septal T was at times imperfect. This led to some issues, those being essentially minor residual humps, well-tolerated by men and less by young females. Over the following 3 years, we perfectioned the technique by improving the fixation,

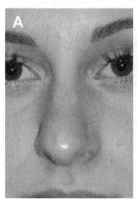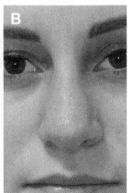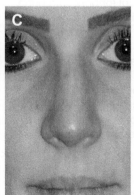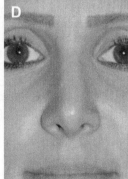

Fig. 17. (*A–D*) Examples of "modified dorsal split" hybrid procedure to the dorsum and structural tip (1 year follow-up).

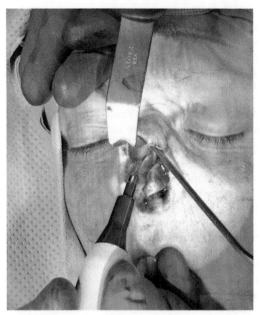

Fig. 18. Use of powered instrumentation to shape the bone and the cartilaginous midvault without any deconstruction.

done precisely under direct vision, as easily allowed by a full dorsal split, and by using the overlap concept, in most occasions, in preference to an end-to-end fixation. The overlap will indeed help to correct small residual deviations and asymmetries of the middle vault and will also strengthen and stabilize the horizontal element of the L-strut, thus, in a way, acting in the same support manner as a spreader graft would do.[3]

Over the last 2 to 3 years, we then transitioned to applying the "modified dorsal split" method even to full letdown and asymmetric letdown procedures.[4] This came together with a better understanding of using specific Piezo inserts in combination with an array of burrs. Essentially, we use Piezo as a cutting tool for bone and burrs as a shaping tool, combining the 2 without any issue and to a significant advantage. Progressively, we also understood the importance of the "blocking points", and this allowed us to avoid residual humps.

In addition to all this, I should mention that, even though my tips remain structural, I now essentially almost never split my tips, preserving the interdomal ligament unless distal septal deviation is severe. I identify the vertical and horizontal scroll areas, I use a 3-points compartmentalization technique,[42] and I also re-suture the Pitanguy as a supratip defining anchor. Importantly, the bony management has completely changed for me, with a preoperative assessment in every single

case by a cone beam CT scan, including its 3-dimension views.[34] Piezo and Burrs are used in combination together with usually incomplete osteotomies, asymmetric osteotomies, and bone fixation transosseous sutures. Again, this is outside the scope of the question of this paragraph, but current rhinoplasty is indeed multifaceted and interrelated in all the parts of the nose.

Briefly stated, I can surely state that although I was hesitant at the beginning toward preservation concepts and actually quite uninspired by the surrounding resonant social media, I have now come to the conclusion that preservation concepts are what truly matters. If properly understood, they will allow each rhinoplasty to become customized, by understanding its specific anatomy in detail and by combining a vast array of tools in the preservation-structural toolbox.[43] I can also surely say, with some adequate follow-up now available to me, that my results are now definitely better. So, the learning curve and the related effort were justified, even in a surgeon like me who was reasonably satisfied with purely structural technique.

Marcus
When evaluating the midvault in nasal surgery the analysis I perform has really changed in the last 4 years. Prior to 2020, I was a pure structural rhinoplasty surgeon. With the resurgence of Let-down techniques and the creation of DPR,[44] I have a larger set of tools for how I will approach the midvault and dorsum. Rather than be dogmatic and perform only one technique or the other–I have enjoyed having an alternative to standard joseph reduction. Indications for DPR are well-covered in several articles.[45] As a general rule, if can preserve any element of the dorsum, I try to do so. It has become clear that future structural deformation may be reduced with this approach.[46] Because my practice involves a large amount of revision functional nasal surgery DPR is not often a viable option.

SUPPLEMENTARY DATA

Supplementary data to this article can be found online at https://doi.org/10.1016/j.fsc.2024.06.013.

REFERENCES

1. Byrd HS, Meade RA, Gonyon DL Jr. Using the autospreader flap in primary rhinoplasty. Plast Reconstr Surg 2007;119(6):1897–902.
2. Fedok FG, Garritano F. Management of the middle vault in endonasal rhinoplasty. Facial Plast Surg 2014;30(2):205–13.

3. Robotti E, Chauke-Malinga NY, Leone A. Modified Dorsal Split Preservation Technique for Nasal Humps with Minor Bony Component: A Preliminary Report. Aesthetic Plast Surg 2019 Oct;43(5):1257–68.

4. Robotti E, Cottone G, Leone F. Modified Dorsal Split Preservation Hybrid Rhinoplasty for Cartilaginous Pushdown and Full Letdown Applications: A PROM-Based Review of 100 Consecutive Cases. Facial Plast Surg 2023 Aug;39(4):441–51.

5. Khazaal A. A modified dorsal split push down technique , including a portion of the bony cap. Cairo: Presented at the 27th RhinoEgypt conference; 2021.

6. Furtado S. Hybrid Preservation Rhinoplasty with Dorsal Split Modification" Presented at Seventh Bergamo Open Rhinoplasty Course, 2022 March 24-26, Bergamo, Italy.

7. Sousa Vieira A, Milicic D, Torrão Pinheiro C, et al. Extended Dorsal Preservation in a New Concept of Preservational Rhinoplasty. Adv Plast Reconstr Surg 2020;4(2):1055.

8. Humpectomy and spreader flaps, Gruber RP, Perkins SW. Clin Plast Surg 2010 Apr;37(2):285–91. https://doi.org/10.1016/j.cps.2009.12.004.

9. Saedi B, Amali A, Gharavis V, et al. Spreader flaps do not change early functional outcomes in reduction rhinoplasty: a randomized control trial. Am J Rhinol Allergy 2014 Jan-Feb;28(1):70–4.

10. Barone M, Cogliandro A, Salzillo R, et al. Role of Spreader Flaps in Rhinoplasty: Analysis of Patients Undergoing Correction for Severe Septal Deviation with Long-Term Follow-Up. Aesthetic Plast Surg 2019 Aug;43(4):1006–13. Epub 2019 Mar 13.

11. Sowder JC, Thomas AJ, Gonzalez CD, et al. Use of Spreader Flaps Without Dorsal Hump Reduction and the Effect on Nasal Function. JAMA Facial Plast Surg 2017 Jul 1;19(4):287–92.

12. Sazgar AA, Razmara N, Razfar A, et al. Outcome of rhinoplasty in patients undergoing autospreader flaps without notable dorsal hump reduction: A clinical trial. J Plast Reconstr Aesthet Surg 2019 Oct; 72(10):1688–93. Epub 2019 Jun 28.

13. Sheen JH. Spreader graft: a method of reconstructing the roof of the middle nasal vault following rhinoplasty. Plast Reconstr Surg 1984;73(2):230–9.

14. Camirand A, Doucet J, Harris J. Nose surgery: how to prevent a middle vault collapse–a review of 50 patients 3 to 21 years after surgery. Plast Reconstr Surg 2004;114(2):527–34.

15. Kern EB. Surgical approaches to abnormalities of the nasal valve. Rhinology 1978;16(3):165–89.

16. Larrabee WFCC. Advanced Nasal Anatomy. Fac Plas Clin 1994;2(4):393–416.

17. Yoo S, Most SP. Nasal airway preservation using the autospreader technique: analysis of outcomes using a disease-specific quality-of-life instrument. Arch Facial Plast Surg Jul-Aug 2011;13(4):231–3.

18. Robotti E, Penna WB. Current Practical Concepts for Using Rib in Secondary Rhinoplasty. Facial Plast Surg 2019 Feb;35(1):31–46.

19. Robotti E, Leone F. The SPF-SPLF Graft: Building the Ideal Dorsum in Revision Rhinoplasty. Plast Reconstr Surg 2020 Jun;145(6):1420–4.

20. Haack S, Hacker S, Mann S, et al. Bony Fixation of the Nasal Framework. Facial Plast Surg 2019 Feb; 35(1):23.

21. Schlosser RJ, Park SS. Functional nasal surgery. Otolaryngol Clin North Am 1999 Feb;32(1):37–51.

22. Talmadge J, High R, Heckman WW. Comparative Outcomes in Functional Rhinoplasty With Open vs EndonasalSpreader Graft Placement. Ann Plast Surg 2018 May;80(5):468–71.

23. Kim L, Papel ID. Spreader Grafts in Functional Rhinoplasty. Facial Plast Surg 2016 Feb;32(1):29–35. Epub 2016 Feb 10.

24. Toriumi DM. Subtotal septal reconstruction: an update. Facial Plast Surg 2013 Dec;29(6):492–501. Epub 2013 Dec 10.PMID: 24327248.

25. Al Abduwani J, Singh A. Impact of osteotomies and structural grafts in the management of severe twisted or deviated nasal deformity: a critical analysis of 179 patients with open rhinoplasty. Am J Otolaryngol 2015 Mar-Apr;36(2):210–6. Epub 2014 Nov 5.

26. Fedok FG. Costal Cartilage Grafts in Rhinoplasty. Clin Plast Surg 2016 Jan;43(1):201–12. Epub 2015 Oct 24.PMID: 26616708 (This is listed as reference 26 and 32).

27. Robotti E. "Primary Hybrid Rhinoplasty" Live surgery Course: combining Preervation and Structural. Bergamo, Nov29-Dec 2, 2023.

28. Kosins AM. Expanding indications for dorsal preservation rhinoplasty with cartilage conversion techniques. Aesthet Surg J 2021;41:174–82.

29. Toriumi DM, Kovacevic M, Kosins AM. Structural Preservation Rhinoplasty: A Hybrid Approach. Plast Reconstr Surg 2022. May 1;149(5):1105–20.

30. Neves JC, Arancibia-Tagle D. Avoiding Esthetic Drawbacks and Stigmata in Dorsal Line Preservation Rhinoplasty. Facial Plast Surg 2021;37(1):65–75.

31. Ilhan E. The use of cylindric burrs for osteoplasty. Mad-Rhinoplasty Course 2022.

32. Fedok FG. Costal Cartilage Grafts in Rhinoplasty. Clin Plast Surg 2016 Jan;43(1):201–12. Epub 2015 Oct 24. PMID: 26616708.

33. Apaydin F. Lateral crural turn-in flap in functional rhinoplasty. Arch Facial Plast Surg 2012 Mar-Apr;14(2): 93–6. Epub 2011 Oct 17.PMID: 22006234.

34. Robotti E, Daniel RK, Leone F. Cone-Beam Computed Tomography: A User-Friendly, Practical Roadmap to the Planning and Execution of Every Rhinoplasty-A 5-Year Review. Plast Reconstr Surg 2021 May 1; 147(5):749e–62e.

35. Kridel RW, Ashoori F, Liu ES, et al. Long-term use and follow-up of irradiated homologous costal cartilage

grafts in the nose. Arch Facial Plast Surg 2009 Nov-Dec;11(6):378–94.

36. Murrell GL. Auricular cartilage grafts and nasal surgery. Laryngoscope 2004 Dec;114(12):2092–102. PMID: 15564827.

37. Jalali MM. Comparison of effects of spreader grafts and flaring sutures on nasal airway resistance in rhinoplasty. Eur Arch Oto-Rhino-Laryngol 2015;272(9):2299–303.

38. Stacey DH, Cook TA, Marcus BC. Correction of internal nasal valve stenosis: a single surgeon comparison of butterfly versus traditional spreader grafts. Ann Plast Surg 2009;63(3):280–4.

39. Becker DG, Becker SS. Treatment of nasal obstruction from nasal valve collapse with alar batten grafts. J Long Term Eff Med Implants 2003;13(3):259–69.

40. Neves JC, Arancibia Tagle D, Dewes W, et al. The split preservation rhinoplasty: "the Vitruvian Man split maneuver". Eur J Plast Surg 2020;43:323–33.

41. Ferreira MG, Santos M. Surface Techniques in Dorsal Preservation. Facial Plast Surg Clin North Am 2023 Feb;31(1):45–57. PMID: 36396288.

42. Robotti E, Leone F, Malfussi VA, et al. The "3 Points Compartmentalization" Technique in Subperichondrial-Subperiosteal Dissection in Primary Rhinoplasty to Reduce Edema and Define Contour. Aesthetic Plast Surg 2022 Aug;46(4):1923–31.

43. Patel PN, Kandathil CK, Buba CM, et al. Most SP Global Practice Patterns of Dorsal Preservation Rhinoplasty. Facial Plast Surg Aesthet Med 2022;24(3):171–7.

44. Daniel RK. The Preservation Rhinoplasty: A New Rhinoplasty Revolution. Aesthet Surg J 2018;38(2):228–9.

45. Patel PN, Most SP. Overview of Dorsal Preservation Rhinoplasty. Facial Plast Surg Clin North Am 2023 Feb;31(1):1–11. doi: 10.1016.

46. Saman M, Saban Y. Long-Term Follow-Up with Dorsal Preservation Rhinoplasty. Facial Plast Surg Clin North Am 2023 Feb;31(1):13–24. doi: 10.1016.

Management of the Crooked Nose: Structural, Preservation, or Camouflage Techniques

Steven J. Pearlman, MD[a], Sebastian Haack, MD[b],
Monica K. Rossi Meyer, MD[c], Sam P. Most, MD[c],*

KEYWORDS

- Crooked nose • Nasal asymmetry • Structural rhinoplasty • Preservation rhinoplasty
- Facial plastic and reconstructive surgery • Selfies • Osteotomies • Septoplasty

KEY POINTS

- The septum contributes to midvault deviations and the position of the high septum in relation to the nasal bones is an important relationship to recognize.
- In the right patient, dorsal preservation techniques can be successfully employed in the treatment of the crooked nose.
- With the advent of social media, patients are more aware of nasal and facial asymmetry.
- Crooked noses can be treated by either an endonasal or an open approach depending on the complexity of the deformity.
- Severely deviated noses and septums might best be treated with an extracorporeal approach.

PANEL DISCUSSION

Open or endonasal approach?
Management of the septum in the crooked nose
Is it only structural approaches or is there a role for preservation techniques? If so which?
In the severely damaged septum what harvesting options do you use?
Treatment options for facial asymmetries in the crooked nose
How have your techniques in this area changed over the last 2 years?

OPEN OR ENDONASAL APPROACH

Pearlman: Sociologic Background for Surgical Choices on the Crooked Nose

I utilize both open and endonasal, or closed, approaches for treating the crooked nose. Over the past decade, I have changed to applying the open approach more than prior strictly due to changes in patient self-evaluation and expectations. With the advent of selfies and social media, patients are looking at themselves with heightened scrutiny, both preoperatively and postoperatively.[1]

Selfies have been around for decades but became more prevalent in the last decade. Facebook began in 2004 and Instagram, a more prevalent tool utilizing selfies, in 2010. Selfie was the word of the year by the Oxford dictionary in 2013.[2]

[a] Pearlman Aesthetic Surgery, Department of Otolaryngology–Head and Neck Surgery, Columbia University New York, 110 East 60th Street, Suite 908, New York, NY 10022, USA; [b] Department for Facial Plastic Surgery, Marienhospital Stuttgart, Böheimstr. 37, Stuttgart 70199, Germany; [c] Division of Facial Plastic and Reconstructive Surgery, Department of Otolaryngology–Head & Neck Surgery, Stanford University School of Medicine, 801 Welch Road, Stanford, CA 94305, USA
* Corresponding author. Division of Facial Plastic and Reconstructive Surgery, Department of Otolaryngology–Head & Neck Surgery, Stanford University School of Medicine, 801 Welch Road, Stanford, CA 94305.
E-mail address: smost@stanford.edu

Facial Plast Surg Clin N Am 32 (2024) 533–550
https://doi.org/10.1016/j.fsc.2024.06.002
1064-7406/24/© 2024 Elsevier Inc. All rights are reserved, including those for text and data mining, AI training, and similar technologies.

We conducted an in-house study reviewing the presenting complaints for 100 consecutive patients in 2017 compared with 100 consecutive consultations in 2012.[3] We chose 2012 as our control group, which is 1 year before selfies became a commonly used term. The primary presenting issues were reviewed and compared in the 2 cohorts. Patients seen in 2017 more commonly reported a crooked nose as one of their primary reasons for seeking rhinoplasty when compared to 2012. Interestingly, patients with crooked noses in the 2017 cohort were more likely to report crookedness as one of their presenting complaints if they took more frequent selfies.

Another manifestation of selfies is the patient's postoperative self-evaluation. It is not uncommon for patients to come in for a postoperative visit and they scroll through a series of selfies from multiple angles and with different lighting to find the ones that best demonstrate asymmetries and irregularities. It is well documented that cellphone photos and selfies distort facial features creating a fisheye effect.[4] Structures in the center of the photo, like the nose, are more exaggerated than the surrounding photo. There is also more distortion when compared to standardized before and after photos with a macro portrait lens in the surgeon's office.

In a 2018 in-house study, we evaluated 200 consecutive rhinoplasty patients at the time of consultation.[5] We recorded how patients rated their photographic image compared to a mirror image. The photograph was flipped back and forth from a standard frontal photograph to a reversed mirror image using a Canfield Mirror program (Canfield Scientific Inc Parsippany, N.J.). The vast majority of patients preferred their mirror image. Anecdotally, when the patient had a significant other present for the consultation, they almost always chose the photographic image as their favored photo. This provides more evidence for the impact of selfies on patient self-evaluation. With selfies, patients now see photos of themselves several times a week or more, as compared to a decade prior when patients saw photos of themselves only from special events and holidays. They are now exposed to their crooked noses much more often than in the preselfie era.

Because of this heightened scrutiny and lower acceptance rates of minor postoperative deformities, we use the open approach much more often than prior to the selfie era.

Surgical treatment

For a straight-line dorsal angulation or angulation of the bony dorsum to one side or a straight-line angulation of the lower two-thirds of the nose to the opposite side of the bony dorsum, an endonasal approach is utilized (**Fig. 1**). When there is a more complex deviation, an open approach is used so the crooked or curved middle vault can be more precisely addressed, often requiring separation of the upper lateral cartilages. We also apply the open approach for very overprojected noses and complex revision rhinoplasty (**Fig. 2**).

Haack

For the severely crooked nose, I prefer the open approach. There are several reasons for that. The open approach facilitates a direct and less-restricted access to pathologies of the bony sidewalls and the cartilaginous vault. Bony convexities, spiculas, or fracture lines can be smoothened easily by the help or powered instruments, which can be brought in place more easily by an open approach.[6] Another benefit of the open approach is that by more extensive dissecting of the soft tissue attachments from the cartilaginous-bony framework, the memory effect of the soft tissue envelope is reduced. This asymmetry of the soft tissue envelope may often influence the long-term result.

Meyer/Most

The debate surrounding open versus endonasal surgical approaches to rhinoplasty is an old one; clearly, advantages and disadvantages exist for both techniques. Proponents of the endonasal approach feel that preserving the skin-soft tissue envelope over the nasal tip prevents destabilization and loss of tip support caused by disruption of these attachments from the underlying cartilaginous support.[7] However, in the setting of the asymmetric nose, full soft-tissue/bony-cartilaginous vault dissociation, the superior visualization, and ability to manipulate the bones using piezoelectric instruments make the external approach the preferred method for the senior author (SPM).[8]

Open rhinoplasty utilizes the columellar incision connected to bilateral marginal incisions at the caudal border of the lower lateral cartilages. Dissection of the skin and soft tissue envelope is performed in a supraperichondrial avascular plane directly over the lower lateral cartilages then the upper lateral cartilages and continued to the caudal aspect of the nasal bones where subperiosteal elevation is continued over the nasal bones to the nasion.[7] The full open approach provides complete exposure of the entire bony vault, as well as the cartilaginous skeleton, to identify and surgically correct deviations from midline and thus makes it the ideal surgical approach for the treatment of the crooked nose.

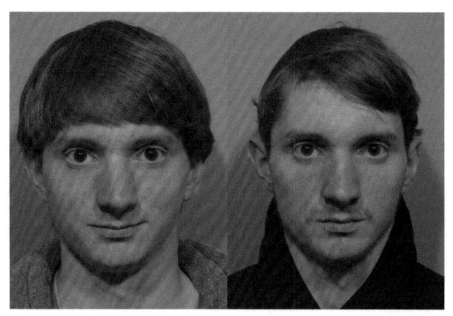

Fig. 1. Endonasal rhinoplasty crooked nose.

MANAGEMENT OF THE SEPTUM IN THE CROOKED NOSE
Pearlman

A systematic approach to the septum is important for obtaining a straight nose. Not every patient requires the entire nose to be taken apart. As each step is performed, the septum and nose is evaluated to see how much it has straightened out.

A. When performing open rhinoplasty for a crooked nose, the upper lateral cartilages are separated from the dorsal septum to maximize exposure. Dorsal reduction is performed before submucous resection or septoplasty. This maximizes the amount of cartilage that can be removed and available for grafting in a structural approach.

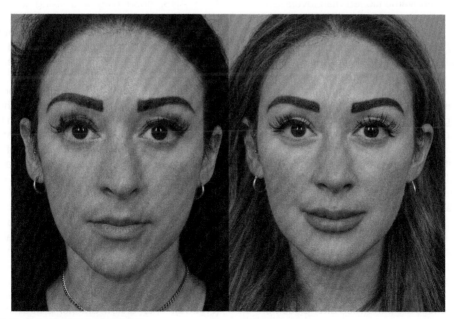

Fig. 2. Open rhinoplasty crooked nose.

B. Depending on the amount of cartilage required for reconstruction, the septum is cut parallel to the maxillary crest. Along with release of the bony/cartilaginous junction up to 1 cm from the dorsum, this often straightens the septum. The height of the horizontal incision is determined by the amount of cartilage needed for later grafting. At least 1 cm of dorsal and caudal septum is preserved for support.

C. Treatment of a crooked or curved caudal septum depends on the position of the nasal spine. A curved caudal septum is often too long. When cut flush with the spine, it often straightens out (**Fig. 3**). Osteotomy of a crooked nasal spine can also bring this junction into the midline. Alternatively, the caudal septum is separated from the nasal spine and fixed to the side of the crooked spine in the midline. To maintain the caudal septum in its new position, a drill hole is made through the spine with an 18 or 20 gauge needle. Once through the spine, the tip of the needle on a 4-0 polydioxanone (PDS) suture is placed into the 18 gauge needle and threaded through the hole with retrograde withdrawal of the needle (composite photo of caudal septum and needles).

D. If the caudal septum remains curved, a shim can be sutured to the concave side with a thin piece of perforated septal ethmoid bone, thin piece of septal cartilage, or 0.25 mm perforated PDS Plate (Ethicon, Inc Somerville, N.J.). Placement of a side-to-side caudal septal extension graft is an alternative treatment.

E. Curvature of the dorsal septum that remains after the abovementioned maneuvers is most commonly treated with bilateral spreader grafts. The spreader grafts are fixed approximately 1.5 mm below the dorsum of the septum and will not significantly widen the middle vault, unless widening is desired, then they are placed flush with the dorsal septum. More aggressive treatments can include a thin piece of septal cartilage or 0.25 mm PDS plate placed through a dorsal cut from underneath where the submucous cartilage resection was performed, but not through the dorsal septal strut (**Fig. 4**). This cut is made at the most convex part of the septal curvature. The PDS plate is sutured to the side of dorsal remnant on the convex side of the curvature caudally toward the tip, placed through the cut to the concave side of the dorsal remnant, and sutured to the dorsal septum on the portion cephalic to the maximum curvature. Some surgeons advocate cutting and overlapping a long, curved dorsal septal strut.[9]

F. Osteotomies are performed after placement of spreader grafts. This yields more stability during manipulation of the dorsal septum and reduces the chance of disarticulating the dorsal bony and cartilaginous septum.

G. If the dorsal septum still has a minor tilt to one side, clocking sutures are utilized to bring the lower dorsum into the midline. A 5-0 PDS suture is placed through the upper lateral cartilage on the side away from the deviation, then through the septum at a more superior point, and then parallel through the other upper lateral cartilage. The suture is then reversed parallel through the side of the deviation, straight through the septum and superiorly on the first side. This will help bring the dorsum into the midline.

H. For an extremely crooked nose and/or severely crooked septum in multiple directions, see section "In the severely damaged septum, which harvesting options do you use?"

Haack

The septum determines the axis of the septum essentially. The goal is a straight and stable septum. The pathology determines the technique. We have to differentiate between fixed breaks, sharp-angled deviations (eg, after trauma; **Figs. 5 and 6**) and, on the other hand, smooth curvatures caused by tension after overly growth of the septum in relation to a too small frame of the bony skeleton. And we have to analyze which part of the septum is affected. Is the anterior leading edge affected, resection of a central septal piece (**Fig. 7**), disconnecting the anterior pillar from ANS, shortening and fixing it in midline without tension will do the job (**Fig. 8**). If there are fixed deflexions, the aforementioned techniques with additional gentle scoring and splinting with a thinned ethmoid plate are successful strategies (**Fig. 9**).

Another situation is given, when the dorsal leading edge of the septum is affected. If the dorsal axis presents only a small aberration from the ideal orientation, spreader grafts will help to straighten the dorsal septum (**Fig. 10**). The same effect may be achieved by clocking sutures.[10] An additional optical effect will be achieved by the use of asymmetric spreader grafts/flaps (**Fig. 11**).

Often, we see a dorsal edge that is more deflected and cannot easily bended to midline. But, frequently, cranial parts of the dorsal edge of the septum come back more to midline. In such situations, a partial extracorporeal septoplasty can be performed. Thereby, the anterior caudal septum is resected leaving parts of the dorsal pillar in situ (**Fig. 12**). Then a new anterior L-strut is created and replanted (**Fig. 13**). The dorsal edge of the

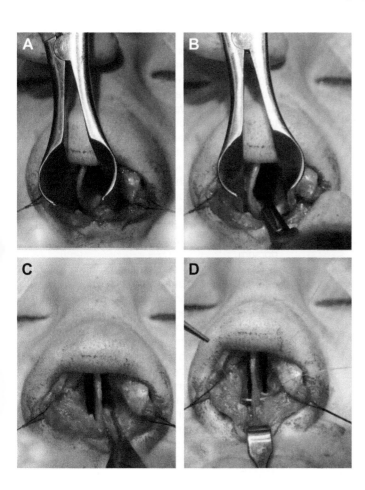

Fig. 3. Caudal septal treatment. (*A*) Crooked caudal septum. (*B*) Cutting caudal septum flush with the nasal spine. (*C*) Straightening out of the caudal septum. (*D*) Fixation of the caudal septum to the nasal spine.

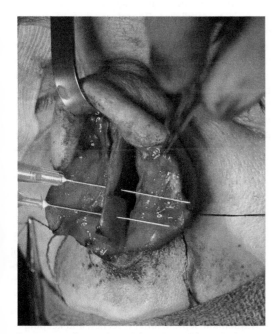

Fig. 4. Dorsal septal straightening with PDS plate.

new septum is fixed to the remaining dorsal pillar from the concave side, so the result is a straighter dorsal leading edge (**Fig. 14**). Then the dorsal esthetic lines (DALs) and the inner valve are shaped by applying spreader grafts/flaps.

If the dorsal pillar is extremely harmed with breaks and severe intrinsic deflections, we perform a complete extracorporeal septoplasty, where the whole septum is resected and a completely new septal plate or L-strut is created (**Fig. 15**). By a sufficient 3 point fixation, a reliable repositioning can be achieved.[11] The great advantage of this technique is that by primarily complete resection and consecutive complete reconstruction and refixation, all bending forces and memory effects of the septal cartilage and its attachments are diminished.

Meyer/Most

Septal deviations contribute to asymmetries observed in the middle vault. Deformity of the septal cartilage has been classified into 6 different types: septal tilt deformity, C-shaped anteroposterior deviation, S-shaped anteroposterior deviation,

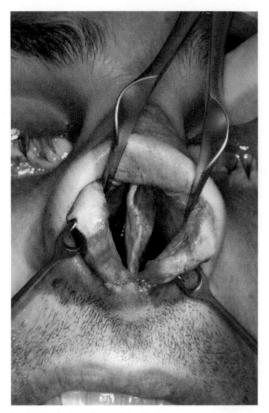

Fig. 5. Intrinsic s-shaped deviation.

localized deviations or spurs, C-shaped cephalo-caudal deformity, and S-shaped cephalocaudal deformity.[12] In our estimation, these classifications, as well as others, are not as important as determination as whether or not the L-strut is deviated, and whether it is dorsal, caudal, or both.[13] In addition, the etiology of the deviation, such as a flexion deformity due to trauma, or simply a tension deformity, is important, as the former needs replacement and the latter may be corrected with full septal release. Once the area of deviation is identified, operative approaches include structural and camouflage techniques. The first step in correction of septal deviation is to separate the upper lateral

cartilages from the dorsal septum. This simple step functions to release asymmetric tension, allow for trimming of asymmetric dorsal cartilage projection, and give space for the positioning of spreader grafts. Spreader grafts serve to stabilize and widen the internal nasal valve for patients with concomitant nasal obstruction.[14] Autologous cartilage is the preferred material for spreader grafts, which can be placed either bilaterally or unilaterally. Placement of a thicker spreader graft or thinner double grafts on the concave side of a deviation can provide support and straightening, and if the deviation continues from the middle vault into the tip, an extended spreader graft can be used to help further straighten the caudal nasal dorsum.[15,16]

The clocking or septal rotation suture is a further refined method to straighten dorsal deviation.[12] An asymmetric horizontal mattress suture is placed between the upper lateral cartilages at the point of maximal deviation. Different placements of the suture can affect the degree of septal rotation, it does not widen the middle vault, and can be combined with other deviation correction techniques allowing for adaptability in addressing deviation.[10] Placement of a suture between the nasal bones and upper lateral cartilages with a unilateral spreader graft combined with a suture spanning the sidewalls to lift a depressed upper lateral cartilage to the opposite nasal bone have also been described.[17,18]

Another important principle of mobilization of the nasal vault with traditional osteotomies is that once mobilized, the natural tendency of the nasal bones is to medialize. Therefore, it is of utmost importance to determine the position of the high septum in relation to the axis of dorsal deviation.[19] When the position of the septum is deviated in the same direction as the external deviation, it will tend to block medialization of the deviated nasal bone on that side and is referred to as an unfavorable dorsal septal gap (DSG).[20] In our practice, the unfavorable configuration is addressed by resecting a small triangle of nasal bone above this to

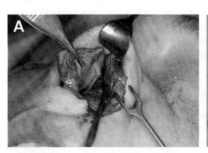
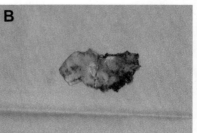
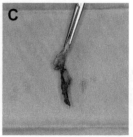

Fig. 6. (*A*) Posttraumatic septum with multiple breaks (*B, C*) posttraumatic septum (after resection and keeping a dorsal septal column).

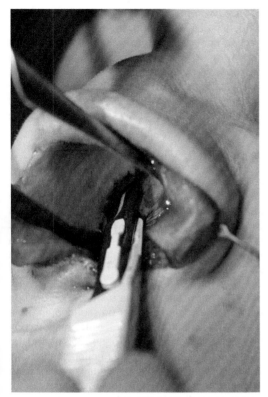

Fig. 7. Removing the central deviated part. Performing a round incision line.

promote medialization and using an extended spreader graft on the opposite side to promote lateralization of the opposite nasal bone. In some cases, a double-layered spreader graft may be required. Suturing of the nasal bones can be easily accomplished if required, using either a piezo drill or an 18 gauge needle. This method avoids

disruption of the keystone area and risk of injury to the cribriform plate, which can occur with full extracorporeal septoplasty and mobilization of the perpendicular plate of the ethmoid. When the high nasal septum is deviated away from the axis of external deviation it is referred to as a favorable DSG, which allows for more complete straightening of the dorsum.[20]

IS IT ONLY STRUCTURAL APPROACHES OR IS THERE A ROLE FOR PRESERVATION TECHNIQUES? IF SO, WHICH?
Pearlman

The concept of preservation rhinoplasty is a very attractive alternative to structural rhinoplasty of the nasal dorsum. The upper lateral cartilages and septum embryologically fuse into one contiguous structure during embryonic growth.[21] Instead of unroofing the bony dorsum and destroying the dorsal complex of the septum and upper lateral cartilages, then restructuring them with osteotomies and spreader grafts or flaps, the inborn dorsal structures are preserved and lowered from below.

Preservation rhinoplasty has a number of techniques that can be applied to crooked noses. The bony dorsum is treated by a larger low ostectomy on the longer side, or the side away from the deviation[22] along with full mobilization and let down of the nasal pyramid. Goncalves-Ferriera[23] described a higher ostectomy on the nasal bones that defines the dorsal lines called a spare roof-B. The cartilaginous dorsum can be straightened by a high subdorsal triangular flap described by Kovacevic and Toriumi[24] (**Fig. 16**) or a rectangular midvault flap, called the Tetris by Nevis.[25] The

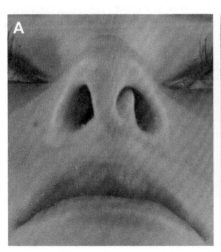

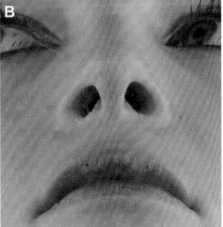

Fig. 8. (*A*) Luxation of the anterior septum (*B*) after septoplasty with anterior shortening, relocation, and fixation at the anterior nasal spine.

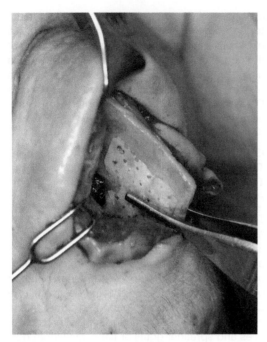

Fig. 9. Straightening and stabilizing of the septum with a thinned ethmoid plate.

mobilized dorsal flap is overlapped and sutured on the side away from the dorsal deflection to pull the lower dorsum into the midline. The Tetris flap is more useful when you wish to lower the supratip.

Correction of a more severely deviated septum and nose might require more mobilization than can be achieved by preserving or altering the dorsal L-strut. This is the Cottle low strip technique.[26] The septum is disarticulated off the maxillary crest along its entire length and separated from the bony septum up to the dorsum. This flap is trimmed, straightened, or flattened, then rotated inferiorly to aid in lowering the dorsum, and then fixed to the nasal spine.

I have performed the subdorsal triangle and Tetris techniques with good success, but for more crooked noses, I prefer to rely more on structural techniques. This is not because either technique is superior, rather, I am more comfortable and have vast experience with structural rhinoplasty for complex changes. I favor this method instead of entering an entirely new learning curve for a more aggressive preservation technique.

Haack

Dorsal preservation techniques may be perfectly used in situations, when the dorsum itself is nice and the axis rather straight, but the whole nose is tilted to one side and is not matching the axis of the face. In such cases push over techniques can perfectly applied. Thereby a larger bony banana wedge is resected on the longer side of the sidewall (the side to which the nose should be shifted; **Fig. 17**). On the shorter side a smaller one. When the dorsal height should not be reduced, in most of the cases, no wedge needs to be resected on the shorter side and a simple bone cut is adequate. To prevent a complete disconnection of the bony pyramid from the facial skeleton, it is advisable to keep a bony hinge by performing the transverse osteotomy on the shorter side as a discontinuous fracture.

The septum can be corrected by Cottles technique (and its variations) or by an extracorporeal septoplasty, where the septum is completely harvested, transformed in a new L-shaped frame, and then replanted and fixed at 3 points (ANS, w-point of the cartilaginous vault, bony pyramid).

Meyer/Most

Application of dorsal preservation to the crooked nose is possible with variations based on the location of deviated aspects of the bony and

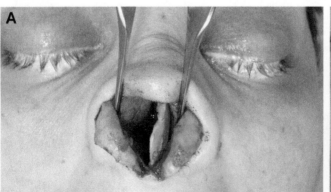
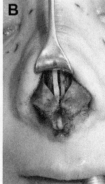

Fig. 10. (A) C-shaped deviated dorsal edge of the septum (B) creation of straight DALs with a spreader graft (rib) on the right side.

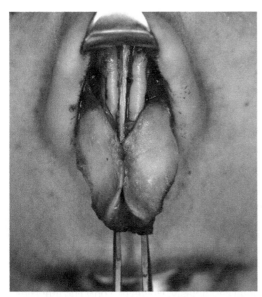

Fig. 11. Deviation of the dorsal edge of the septum to the right. Creation of straight DALs with asymmetric spreader grafts.

cartilaginous dorsum. Preservation of the bony vault allows its movement to one side or the other en bloc, which avoids the undermobilization or overmobilization of the nasal bones that can occur with traditional osteotomies. The best patients for this method have upper and middle nasal third deviations along the same axis. For mild axis deviations, the subdorsal flap (we prefer the modified subdorsal strip method) may be placed on the side opposite the deviation, with symmetric bony cuts (**Fig. 18**).[20] For asymmetric bony pyramid, the dorsal preservation letdown techniques can be modified to adjust differential bony vault length with asymmetric bony resection (**Fig. 19**). When an I-shaped deformity characterized by a longer nasal bone on the contralateral deviation side

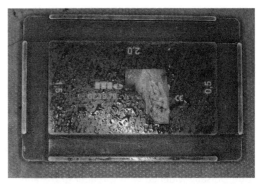

Fig. 13. Extracorporeal created anterior septal replacement graft.

and a shorter bone on the ipsilateral side exists, a combination of the letdown technique for the longer side and pushdown technique for the shorter side can accomplish suitable correction.[27] In this instance, a larger amount of bone is resected from the side contralateral to the deviation (longer nasal bone) so that when the nasal bones descend, they will rotate to the side where greater bone has been removed. This position is then fixated by securing the subdorsal strip to the septum on the side that had the larger wedge of bone resected, as shown in **Fig. 20**.[20]

An important pitfall to avoid is that dorsal preservation may result in a dorsal let down with an unplanned axis deviation of the dorsum. When this occurs, additional deviation correction is done

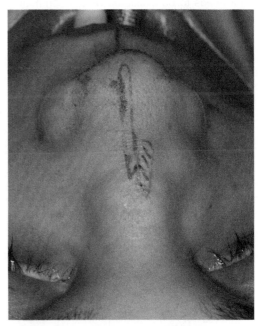

Fig. 14. Drawing of the replantation and refixation of the new anterior septum.

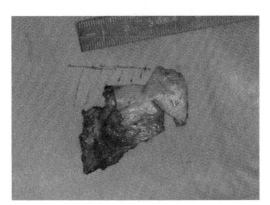

Fig. 12. Severely harmed septum after resection, leaving a dorsal column in situ.

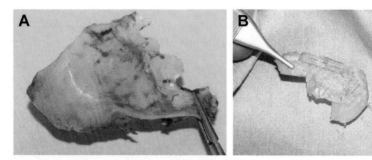

Fig. 15. (*A*) Total resection of a severely deviated septum with a harmed dorsal column and (*B*) the new septal L-strut. Dorsally widened with spreader grafts and stabilized with a thinned ethmoid plate.

with correction of the anterior septal angle position when needed. When the caudal septum is so severely deviated that it requires excision and reconstruction, often referred to as anterior septal reconstruction (ASR),[13] the senior author (SPM) recommends avoiding dorsal preservation techniques because of the inability to secure and properly tension the trimmed nasal septum without introducing additional destabilizing forces onto the reconstructed caudal strut. The technique may be used in dorsal reduction techniques with very mild humps that do not require large amounts of dorsal flexion.[28]

IN THE SEVERELY DAMAGED SEPTUM, WHICH HARVESTING OPTIONS DO YOU USE?
Pearlman

For an extremely crooked septum and nose, the L-strut needs to be evaluated before committing to a technique. I open the nose, separate the upper lateral cartilages and elevate the mucoperichondrial flaps over the maxillary crest. If a straight L-strut can be visualized with the technique in "Management of the septum in the crooked nose" section, I will work with the septum in situ. If there are multiple angulations or fractures or complex deviations, then I perform an extracorporeal septoplasty. However, I only find that I need to use this technique a few times a year (**Fig. 21**). For a more comprehensive description of the extracorporeal septoplasty, I defer to the senior panelist in this section, Dr Most, since he has published on this topic.[13]

Haack

Sometimes it is possible, even in a severely damaged septum, by following the principles of an extracorporeal septoplasty, to reconstruct a sufficient L-shaped septal frame. Thereby cartilaginous fragments as well as pieces of the ethmoid plate are used (**Figs. 22** and **23**).

If the septal material is not suitable, our favorite donor material is autogenous rib cartilage (**Fig. 24**).

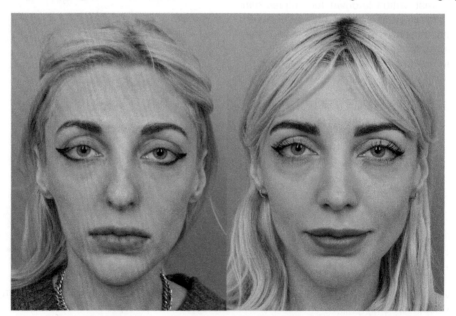

Fig. 16. Preservation rhinoplasty crooked nose.

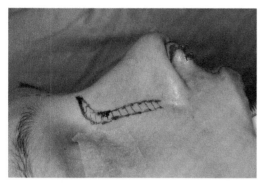

Fig. 17. Banana resection in dorsal preservation. Performing a large resection transversally to allow a horizontal closing of the bony gap, that is needed for a push over.

The standard solution are extended spreader grafts, which are fixed to a remaining dorsal septal remnant. These are fixing an anterior septal replacement graft, which is fixed to the anterior nasal spine (ANS) (**Fig. 25**).

Also ear cartilage can be used for complete L-strut reconstruction (**Fig. 26**).[29] Anyhow, in most of the cases, we prefer rib cartilage, since mostly additional grafts in these severe cases are required.

Meyer/Most

Costal cartilage provides the largest amount of cartilage for grafting when septal cartilage reserve is inadequate.[30] However, this must be balanced with the morbidity of graft harvest, which is greater than those of auricular and septal cartilages. The likelihood of costal cartilage warping is higher compared to other graft sources and special attention must also be paid to graft processing techniques.[31] For example, obliquely cut rib cartilage has been shown to minimize warping compared to concentric slices,[32] and in our practice, the cut grafts are submerged in saline for a minimum of 20 minutes; only pieces that remain straight are used for grafting. However, costal cartilage has been shown to have a very low resorption rate in other types of head and neck reconstruction and offers significant volume for reconstruction without the drawbacks of other homologous or synthetic graft materials.[33]

Auricular cartilage is typically used in situations in which insufficient septal cartilage is available and only a modest amount of cartilage is still needed. However, the curvature of the cartilage may present challenges in areas where straight grafting material is necessary.[34] Split calvarial bone is an option in situations where maximal structural integrity is desired with minimal potential for warping.[35] The major drawback is donor site morbidity and potential for dural exposure or tears during harvest.[36] Homologous graft material such as irradiated or fresh frozen cadaveric cartilage and synthetic graft material such as porous polyethylene have also been described[37–39] but are not routinely used in the senior author's

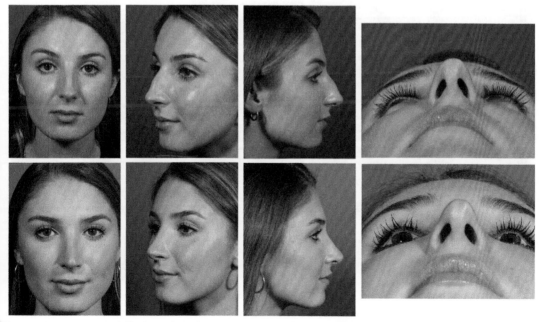

Fig. 18. Pre/post 12 mo follow-up (f/u) after let-down, modifed subdorsal strip method (MSSM). Notice mild preoperative axis deviation to the left. Placement of the sub dorsal flap (MSSM-flap) on the right side can correct mild deviations such as this.

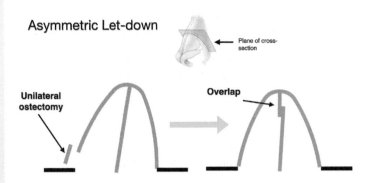

Fig. 19. An asymmetric bony resection (asymmetric let-down) can be used to adjust differential bony vault length.

(SPM) practice. However, when homologous cartilage is necessary, fresh frozen cadaveric cartilage is the preferred homologous grafting material of the senior author (SPM) because of its reduced resorption rate compared with irradiated cartilage.[40]

TREATMENT OPTIONS FOR FACIAL ASYMMETRIES IN THE CROOKED NOSE
Pearlman

From personal observations and evaluating thousands of faces, it is clear that the vast majority of patients have asymmetric faces. In the literature, as many as 85% to 97% of patients presenting

for rhinoplasty have measurable facial asymmetry.[41,42] When facial asymmetry is obvious and affects the nose, we point it out at the time of consultation. As discussed in "Open or endonasal approach" section, switching back and forth from the photographic to mirror image helps make that point with patients.

In a recent in-house study, we looked at nasal asymmetry and the relationship to facial disproportion.[43] We studied nasal deviation and correlated it with midface length, comparing the length from the lateral canthus with the ipsilateral oral commissure between the 2 sides of the patient's face as the benchmark for midface asymmetry. The nasal bones were most deviated

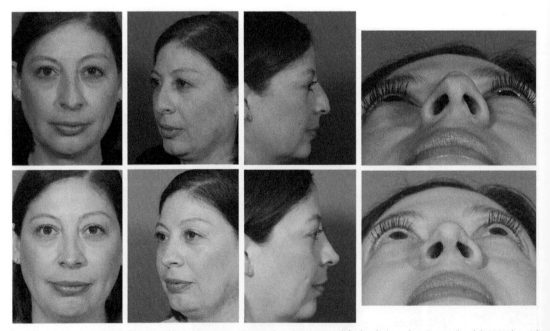

Fig. 20. Pre/post 12 mo follow-up (f/u) after asymmetric let-down, modifed subdorsal strip method (MSSM), with right septal extension graft (R SEG). In this case, the deviation was more severe, so in addition to asymmetric suturing of the subdorsal flap, the bony vault was treated asymmetrically as well. A unilateral ostectomy (let-down) was performed on the right side.

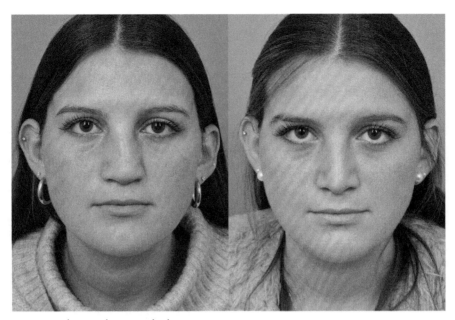

Fig. 21. Extracorporeal septoplasty crooked nose.

toward the side of midface hypoplasia. Once a nose is surgically straightened, cartilaginous and soft tissue memory has been attributed to the nose partially reverting to its deviated shape during the healing process.[44] However, this may also be because of underlying facial deficiency on the side the nose is tilted to.

Preventing redeviation of the nose following rhinoplasty might be aided by addressing the nasal musculature after rhinoplasty. Wong and D'Souza[45] felt that the nasal muscles on the convex side of the nose will hypertrophy over time due to an increased load. Postoperative botulinum toxin injections can be used to block the overaction of the stronger side, allowing the nose to heal in a more central position.

Another manifestation of facial and nasal asymmetry is the height of insertion of the ala on the face. In crooked noses, one ala is frequently higher than the other. This often parallels tilt in the oral commissures. This asymmetry relates to the underlying bony skeleton and is only partially correctable during rhinoplasty. Partial improvement can be achieved by placing diced cartilage under the base of the higher ala to push it inferiorly.[46]

As discussed in "Management of the septum in the crooked nose" section, when discussing potential results and expectations with patients, it is extremely important to point out and document any and all asymmetries before surgery. To quote E. Gaylon, McCollough, MD heard early in my career: "pointing out something before surgery is an explanation, pointing it out after surgery is an excuse."

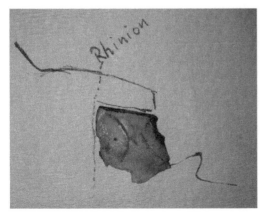

Fig. 22. Secondary case with anterior septal loss. Harvesting a caudo-central cartilage piece for ASR.

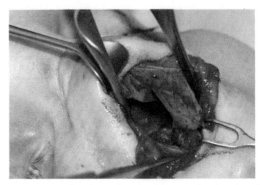

Fig. 23. ASR fixed on the anterior nasal spine (ANS) and dorsally stabilized with short spreader grafts.

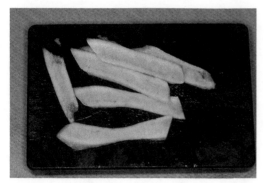

Fig. 24. Rib cartilage slices, ready for further preparation.

Haack

The most important thing is to inform the patient about these asymmetries and their impact on the nose.

Lack of anterior support to the ala base can be corrected by infiltrating free diced cartilage in a subcutaneous pocket (**Fig. 27**). If more support is required, solid cartilage grafts (mostly from the rib) can be placed in epiperiostal pocket directly under the deficient ala base (**Fig. 28**). The grafts could be placed in place via an oral approach or via the rhinoplasty access. Midfacial volume asymmetries can addressed by lipostructuring.

Patients with asymmetries in the lower face, especially in combination with malocclusions, are referred to our maxilla facial colleagues.

Meyer/Most

The foundation of the bony-cartilaginous pyramid must also be evaluated, including the entirety of the midface structure. Occult midface asymmetry (OMA) is a common contributor to the appearance of nasal deviation, and this must be identified and discussed with the patient as surgical corrections to the nose will not address OMA.[41,47] In one previous study, as many as 97% of patients referred for the consideration of esthetic rhinoplasty had significant degrees of facial asymmetry with the greatest variation at the midline to ala distance.[41] Of this group, only 38% of patients were considered asymmetrical through subjective assessment, showing that differences may be subtle and still affect ultimate postoperative outcomes.[41] Therefore, the rhinoplasty surgeon must perform an in-depth analysis and discuss all asymmetries noted with the patient preoperatively.

The nose must be placed in the middle of the asymmetric face so that it will be centered on a line from the midglabellar region to the middle of Cupid's bow on the upper lip.[48] This occasionally requires ASR with movement of the septum off the anterior nasal spine. In cases where the spine is only slightly off center, a new notch may be created in the midline to accept the ASR graft. Whereas, in cases of severe deviation of the nasal spine, it may be salvaged by cutting it free at its base, repositioning it along this line and securing it with 2 miniplates.[49]

Perhaps, the most common scenario for rhinoplasty in the setting of significant facial asymmetry is in the cleft nose patient. In these patients, septal reconstruction with a new midline is often required. In addition, most all cleft rhinoplasty patients present with ipsilateral premaxillary deficiency, even in the setting of prior alveolar bone grafting. In these cases, we routinely augment the premaxilla on the affected side. Options include solid pieces of rib cartilage as well as diced rib wrapped in temporalis fascia.

HOW HAVE YOUR TECHNIQUES CHANGED OVER THE PAST 2 YEARS?
Pearlman

I will take the liberty of expanding my answer to address how my techniques for the crooked nose have changed over the past 4 years. Getting the dorsum straight has always been challenging. Approximately 4 years ago, I started using the en bloc technique described by Wayne.[50] This procedure has been performed on all the before and after patient photographs presented other than the preservation case in this study. With or without hump reduction, a lateral osteotomy is performed on the side away from the dorsal tilt. A medial osteotomy is then executed with a 7 or 10 mm straight osteotome on the side the nose is angled to, and the dorsum torqued toward the side of the first osteotomy. This leaves a partial open

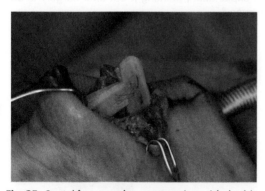

Fig. 25. Septal framework reconstruction with double-layered anterior septal replacement graft. Dorsal reconstruction with spreader grafts fixed side-to-side to the remaining septum. Anterior fixation end-to-end, resting on a small step.

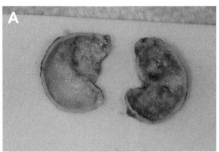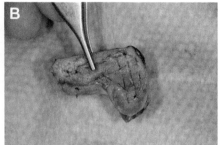

Fig. 26. (*A*) Two resected concha cartilage pieces and (*B*) reconstructed L-strut with 2 conchae.

roof. Lastly, a lateral osteotomy is performed on the side of the nasal tilt and the bone in-fractured to close the roof. If there is a significant dorsal incline and the side away from the tilt is longer, a double osteotomy is performed on that side as well. This has yielded more consistent results for treating the crooked bony dorsum.

Another technique I have utilized occasionally is via dorsal preservation rhinoplasty (DPR). The procedures are discussed in "Is it only structural approaches or is there a role for preservation techniques? If so, which?" section.

Overall, over the past few years, I have also been spending more time during the rhinoplasty consultation discussing nasal and facial asymmetry and the impact of selfies on how patients view themselves. Unfortunately, even after setting expectations, the revision rate for my own rhinoplasties has increased. The average patient has higher expectations and is less tolerant of minor postoperative deformities. Even when their major presenting concerns have been met, minor deficiencies are more visible to them, more likely to be pointed out and no longer tolerated by patients.

Haack

In the last 2 years, I included the push over technique for the straight, but tilted noses in my surgical armamentarium. This reduced significantly the use of the total extracorporeal septoplasties.

Meyer/Most

Over the past few years, the use of piezoelectric instruments has largely supplanted the use of traditional rasps and osteotomies in the senior author's treatment of the crooked nose. The technology has allowed for more precise osteotomies and ostectomies to be performed, as well as the ability to do additional contouring of bone edges after they have been mobilized postosteotomy. For example, this can be used to good effect to narrow the bony vault (**Fig. 29**). With this technology, it is also possible to secure the bones easily with sutures. Additionally, the precision with which piezoelectric saws can fully mobilize the entire bony pyramid makes it a particularly useful tool for performing DPR techniques in patients with upper and middle third deviations in same direction without severe caudal deviation. In instances where there is significant caudal deviation and ASR is required, dorsal preservation techniques have been used less frequently in the senior author's practice because control of the tensioning forces on the trimmed septum are not as reliable when secured to a reconstructed caudal strut.

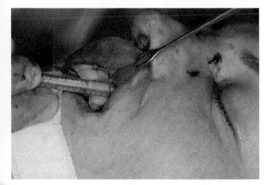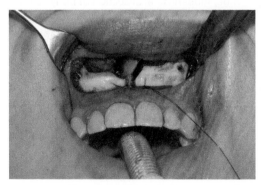

Fig. 27. Augmentation of the left maxilla with free diced cartilage positioned in a soft tissue pocket.

Fig. 28. Maxilla augmentation with 2 (asymmetric) crescent shaped rib cartilage pieces.

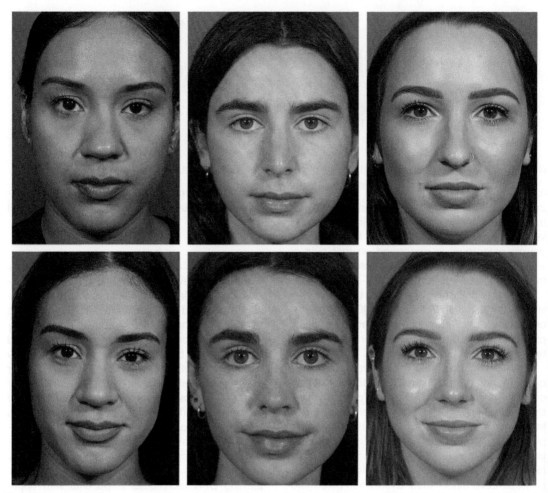

Fig. 29. Several before and after frontal views demonstrating patients treated with structural rhinoplasty techniques. In the first case, osteotomies as well as dorsal augmentation/camouflage with diced rib was performed. In the second and third cases, the DALs were narrowed using piezo osteotomy and osteotomy of the dorsum.

CLINICS CARE POINTS

- Use of piezoelectric instruments requires wide, subperiosteal dissection of bony vault.[51]
- Fine piezoelectric saws perform more precise osteotomies compared to traditional osteotomes.[52]
- Piezoelectric rasps and saws can be used to contour the nasal bones after osteotomies are made.[52]

REFERENCES

1. Ziltzer RS, Mora RM, Mehta P, et al. Analysis of online videos on facial feminization surgery: what are patients watching on TikTok and You-Tube? Facial Plast Surg Aesthet Med 2023; 25(6):528–30.
2. Selfie N., Oxford English Dictionary, 2023, Oxford UP. https://doi.org/10.1093/OED/1169100505.
3. Poster Presented at COSM (Combined Otolaryngology Society Meeting) May 15-June 15, 2020. Virtual Poster Presentation.
4. Ward B, Ward M, Fried O, et al. Nasal distortion in short-distance photographs: The selfie effect. Jama Facial Plas Surg 2018;20(4):333–5.
5. Araslanova R, Pearlman S. Prevalence of Self-photography in patients presenting for primary aesthetic rhinoplasty. Am Journal of Cosmetic Surgery 2022;00(0):1–6.
6. Gerbault O, Daniel RK, Palhazi P, et al. Reassessing Surgical Management of the Bony Vault in Rhinoplasty. Aesthetic Surg J 2018;38(6):590–602. PMID: 29432541.

7. Totonchi A, Guyuron B. Rhinoplasty, in Plastic Surgery: Principles and Practice. Amsterdam, The Netherlands: Elsevier Inc; 2022. p. 1082–95.

8. Akkina S, Most SP. Treatment of the Asymmetric Nose. In: Comprehensive rhinoplasty: Structural and preservation concepts. St. Louis, MO: Quality Medical Publishing, Inc.; 2023.

9. Song HM, Kim J-S, Lee B-J, et al. Deviated nose cartilaginous dorsum correction using a dorsal L-strut cutting and suture technique. Laryngoscope 2008;118(6):981–6.

10. Keeler JA, Moubayed SP, Most SP. Straightening the crooked middle vault with the clocking stitch: an anatomic study. JAMA Facial Plast Surg 2017; 19(3):240–1.

11. Rezaeian F, Gubisch W, Janku D, et al. New suturing techniques to reconstruct the keystone area in extracorporeal septoplasty. Plast Reconstr Surg 2016; 138(2):374–82.

12. Guyuron B,UCD, Scull H. A practical classification of septonasal deviation and an effective guide to septal surgery. Plast Reconstr Surg 1999;104:2202–9.

13. Most S. Anterior septal reconstruction: outcomes after a modified extracorporeal septoplasty technique. Arch Facial Plast Surg 2006;8(3):202–7.

14. Chen YY, Kim SA, Jang YJ. Centering a deviated nose by caudal septal extension graft and unilateral extended spreader grafts. Ann Otol Rhinol Laryngol 2020;129:448–55.

15. Shipchandler TZ, Papel ID. The crooked nose. Facial Plast Surg 2011;27:203–12.

16. Moubayed SP MS. Correcting deviations of the lower third of the nose. Facial Plast Surg 2017; 33(2):157–61.

17. Pontius AT, Leach JL. New techniques for management of the crooked nose. Arch Facial Plast Surg 2004;6:263–6.

18. Dayan SH, Shah AR. A suture suspension technique for improved repair of a crooked nose deformity. Ear Nose Throat J 2004;83:743–4.

19. Patel PN, Mohamed A, Most SP. A review and modification of dorsal preservation rhinoplasty techniques. Facial Plast Surg Aesthet Med 2020;22(2):71–9.

20. Most SP. Comprehensive rhinoplasty structural and preservation concepts. St. Louis, MO: Quality Medical Publishing Inc; 2023.

21. Palhazi P, Daniel RK, Kosins AM. The osseocartilaginous vault of the nose: anatomy and surgical observations. Aesthetic Surg J 2015;15(3):242–51.

22. East C. Preservation rhinoplasty and the crooked nose. Facial Plast Surg Clin North Am 2021;29: 123–30.

23. Goncalves Ferreira M, Isisa LC, Ishida LH, et al. Ferreira-Ishida technique: spare roof technique B. Step by step guide to preserving the bony cap while dehumping. Plast Reconstr Surg 2022; 149(2):901–4.

24. Toriumi D, Kovacevic M. Dorsal preservation rhinoplasty, measures to prevent suboptimal outcomes. Facial Plast Surg Clin N Am 2021;29:141–53.

25. Neves JC, Tagle DA, Dews W, et al. A segmental approach in dorsal preservation rhinoplasty: The tetris concept. Facial Plast Clin N Am 2021;29:85–99.

26. Cottle MH, Loring RM. Corrective surgery of the external nasal pyramid and the nasal septum for restoration of normal physiology. Ill Med J 1946;90:119–35.

27. Özücer B, Ç OH. The Effectiveness of asymmetric dorsal preservation for correction of I-shaped crooked nose deformity in comparison to conventional technique. Facial PLastic Surgery Aesthetic Medicine 2020;22:286–93.

28. Patel PN,MS. Combining open structural and dorsal preservation rhinoplasty. Clin Plast Surg 2022;49: 97–109.

29. Haack S, Gubisch W. Reconstruction of the septum with an autogenous double-layered conchal L-strut. Aesthetic Plast Surg 2014 Oct;38(5):912–22.

30. Fedok F. Costal cartilage grafts in rhinoplasty. Clin Plast Surg 2016;43:201–12.

31. McGuire C, Samargandi OA, Boudreau C, et al. Prevention of autologous costal cartilage graft warping in secondary rhinoplasty. J Craniofac Surg 2020;31: 1246–50.

32. Taştan E, Yucel OT, Aydin E, et al. The oblique split method: a novel technique for carving costal cartilage grafts. JAMA Facial Plastic Surgery 2013;15:198–203.

33. Brent B. Technical advances in ear reconstruction with autogenous rib cartilage grafts: personal experience with 1200 cases. Plast Reconstr Surg 1999; 104:309–34.

34. Lee M, Callahan S, Cochran CS. Auricular cartilage: harvest technique and versatility in rhinoplasty. Am J Otolaryngol 2011;32:547–52.

35. Cheney M, Gliklich RE. The use of calvarial bone in nasal reconstruction. Arch Otolaryngol Head Neck Surg 1995;121:643–8.

36. Young V, Schuster RH, Harris LW. Intracerebral hematoma complicating split calvarial bone-graft harvest. Plast Reconstr Surg 1990;86:763–5.

37. Gürlek A, Ayse E-O, Celik M, et al. Correction of the crooked nose using custom-made high-density porous polyethylene extended spreader grafts. Aesthetic Plast Surg 2006;30:141–9.

38. Boccieri A,MC, Pascali M. The use of spreader grafts in primary rhinoplasty. Ann Plast Surg 2005;55:127–31.

39. Mendelsohn M. Straightening the crooked middle third of the nose using porous polyethylene extended spreader grafts. Arch Facial Plast Surg 2005;7:74–80.

40. Mohan R, Shanmuga Krishnan RR, Rohrich RJ. Role of fresh frozen cartilage in revision rhinoplasty. Plast Reconstr Surg 2019;144:614–22.

41. Chatrath P, De Cordova J, Nouraei SA, et al. Objective assessment of facial asymmetry in rhinoplasty patients. Arch Facial Plast Surg 2007;9(3):184–7.

42. Carvalho B, Ballin AC, Becker RV, et al. Rhinoplasty and facial asymmetry: Analysis of subjective and anthropometric factors in the Caucasian nose. Int Arch Otorhinolaryngol 2012;16(4):445–51.

43. Presented at AAFPRS fall meeting Las Vegas, NV. October 23-26, 2023. Submitted for publication. DMT solutions, St. Louis: Quality Medical Publishing, Inc.

44. Loyo M, Wang TD. Revision rhinoplasty. Plastic Surg Clin North Am 2016;43(1):177–85.

45. Chih Wong EH, D'Souza A. Myomodulation using botulinum toxin in septorhinoplasty for crooked noses: introducing the concept and application of nasal muscle inbalance theory. Facial Plast Surg 2024;40:52–60.

46. Toriumi DT. Managing the deviated/asymmetric nose deformity. In: Structure rhinoplasty. Chicago: DMT Solutions; 2019. p. 461–605.

47. Hafezi F, Naghibzadeh B, Nouhi A, et al. Asymmetric facial growth and deviated nose: a new concept. Ann Plast Surg 2010;64:47–51.

48. Rohrich RJ VN, Small KH, Pezeshk RA. Implications of facial asymmetry in rhinoplasty. Plast Reconstr Surg 2017;140(3):510–6.

49. Mittermiller P, Sheckter CC, Most SP. Efficacy and safety of titanium miniplates for patients undergoing septorhinoplasty. JAMA Facial Plastic Surgery 2018; 20:82–4.

50. Wayne I. Osteotomies in rhinoplasty surgery. Curr Opin Otolaryngol Head Neck Surg 2013;21(4): 379–83.

51. Gerbault O, Daniel RK, Kosins AM. The role of piezoelectric instrumentation in rhinoplasty surgery. Aesthet Surg J 2016;36(1):21–34.

52. Göksel A, Patel PN, Most SP. Piezoelectric osteotomies in dorsal preservation rhinoplasty. Facial Plast Surg Clin North Am 2021;29(1):77–84.

Septal Extension Graft Versus Columellar Strut

Roxana Cobo, MD[a],*, Brian Wong, MD, PhD[b], Edwin F. Williams, MD[c], Matthew J. Urban, MD[c]

KEYWORDS

- Rhinoplasty • Septal extension graft • Columellar strut • Nasal tip support • Undefined nasal tip
- Nasal tip projection • Nasal tip rotation

KEY POINTS

- Septal extension grafts and columellar struts are used frequently to define position of nasal tip and help define nasal tip shape.
- Septal extension grafts and columellar struts are fashioned from cartilage that can be harvested from the nasal septum, conchal cartilage, or rib cartilage.
- Septal extension grafts and columellar struts will have an impact on nasal tip rotation, projection, or both.
- Columellar struts are rectangular pieces of cartilage placed between the medial crura. This can be done through an endonasal or external approach.
- Septal extension graft is a relatively straight piece of cartilage that is placed end to end or overlapping the existing caudal septum.

 Video content accompanies this article at http://www.facialplastic.theclinics.com.

PANEL DISCUSSION

1. How do you design your septal extension graft or your columellar strut?
2. How do you place your septal extension graft or columellar strut? End to end or Overlapping, Extended to the nasal spine? Why?
3. How do you define nasal tip position? How do you measure it?
4. If septal cartilage is not enough for your septal extension graft or columellar strut, what other cartilage options do you use and do you have any special techniques
5. What are the complications of using septal extension graft or a columellar strut?
6. How have your techniques in this area changed over the last 2 years?

How Do You Design Your Septal Extension Graft or Your Columellar Strut?

Wong

I started using septal extension grafts (SEGs) shortly after the publication of the Dean Toriumi's[1] articles in 2006, though I had seen this presented by Kridel[2] and Byrd[3] many years earlier. The design of my grafts has changed over the years, and presently, I use templates in order to specify the precise shape and size required. I will use a template every single time for an end-to-end graft,

[a] Facial Plastic Surgery, Department of Otolaryngology, Clinica Imbanaco, Carrera 38A #5A-100 cons 222 Torre A, Cali 760042, Colombia; [b] Department of Otolaryngology–Head and Neck Surgery, University of California Irvine, 1002 Health Sciences Road East, Irvine, CA 92617, USA; [c] The Williams Center for Plastic Surgery, 1072 Troy-Schenectady Boulevard, Suite 201, Latham, NY 12110, USA
* Corresponding author.
E-mail addresses: Roxana.cobo@quironsalud.com; roxanacobo@gmail.com

Facial Plast Surg Clin N Am 32 (2024) 551–563
https://doi.org/10.1016/j.fsc.2024.06.005
1064-7406/24/© 2024 Elsevier Inc. All rights are reserved, including those for text and data mining, AI training, and similar technologies.

and I shaped these like a "boomerang" and envelop the anterior septal angle (ASA).[4] The approach I use is illustrated in **Fig. 1**. In **Fig. 1A**, a template is made using remnant cardboard typically used for sutures or pledgets. The cardboard is placed against the septum, and an imprint (see **Fig. 1B**) is made from the trace blood that is on the septum, and the silhouette of the ASA and caudal septum is traced out with a marker. From this template, an SEG is drawn (see **Fig. 1C**). The shape is reminiscent of a "boomerang." This cardboard template is then cut to shape and placed in position (see **Fig. 1D**). The skin is reflected over the cardboard template, which is held in position with a forceps. The cartilage graft is then cut to this specification (see **Fig. 1E**) and sutured in position with a series of vertical figure of 8 suture (see **Fig. 1F**). On each side, a very thin bridge graft (~0.5 mm thickness, 6 × 10 mm) is placed (see **Fig. 1G, H**) to secure and stabilize the graft. In terms of side-to-side placement, I will first determine if there is a deviation of the ASA off midline. If one exits, I will secure the SEG on the side opposite to the deviation to restore midline position of the central tip support structure.

Design is very important of a side-to-side graft because that graft can significantly enhance the stability of the axial nasal support. That is extremely important in particular in patients with weak quadrangular cartilages, such is Asian and many South American patients. For either side to side or end to end, the shape of the SEG determines the tip defining point as well as much of the infratip contour.

Williams/Urban

As of yet, I have not adopted the use of an SEG as one of my key surgical maneuvers in rhinoplasty. I do, however, use a columellar strut (CS) on a somewhat regular basis via the endonasal approach. See the attached case in **Fig. 2A–I**, Video 1 as a demonstration. The CS is easily carved from septal cartilage on a back table and the size is much smaller than the early years of my career. The amount of cartilage to achieve the desired effect is much less through the endonasal approach, particularly when adopting the narrow pocket principle. The senior author will typically design the CS in the order of 12 to 15 mm in length and 2 to 3 mm in width from a straight and strong piece of nasal septal cartilage. If nasal cartilage is not available, rib cartilage is preferred because it retains strength even when thinly carved. In years past, the senior author has utilized conchal cartilage, but because it tends to lack tensile strength, it is a distance third option in the senior author's hands.

Cobo

I have been using SEGs for the past 10 to 15 years. SEG were first described by Dean Toriumi in 1995 as caudal septal replacement grafts for deformities in the caudal septum and by Steve Byrd in 1997.[3,5] Since this time, numerous articles have been published on the topic.

Even though I have placed CSs for many years, today I am placing SEG exclusively. The reason for this is my mestizo patient population where most of the nasal tip problems have to do with poor

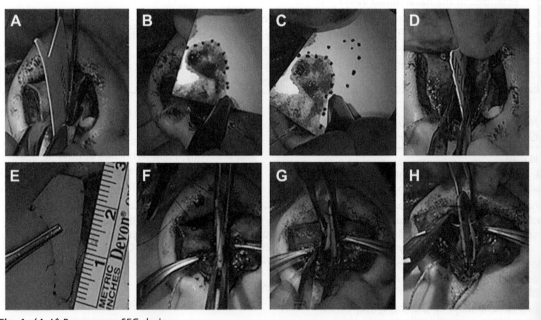

Fig. 1. (*A–H*) Boomerang SEG design.

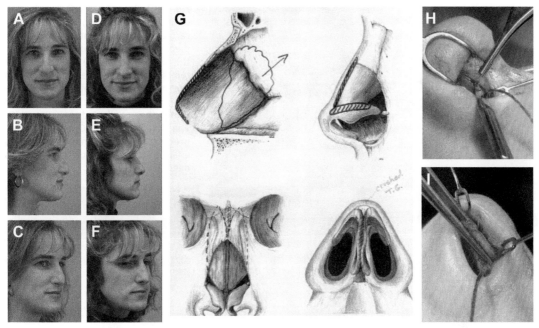

Fig. 2. Case analysis. This young woman presented with complaints of a drooping tip and convexity on profile view. (*A–C*) Preoperative nasal views. (*D–F*) Thirteen- year postoperative views demonstrating long-term tip support and stability of the result. (*G*) Operative schematic demonstrating CS, cephalic trim, conservative profile reduction, small radix graft, osteotomies, and a small tip graft (*H*) intraoperative photograph creating the pocket for CS graft. (*I*) Placement of the graft with cartilage forceps into narrow pocket.

projection and rotation combined with retrusive caudal septums.[6,7]

The design of the SEG has changed over the years and will depend on several factors: available septal cartilage and degree of projection/rotation needed. When not enough native septal cartilage is available other cartilage grafting options must be explored as is discussed in "If Septal Cartilage Is not Enough for Your Septal Extension Graft or Columellar Strut, What Other Cartilage Options do You Use and do You Have Any Special Techniques" section.

The big difficulty encountered over the years when using an SEG was defining the design and the amount of cartilage that was going to be invested in this type of graft. Many articles have been published on this topic and possibly the conclusion is that there is not an only design for this type of graft.[8–10] Today I routinely use a template fashioned from a piece of cardboard from the sutures that are used in surgery, a trick learned from Dr Brian Wong. The available harvested cartilage is painted on this cardboard and then a possible SEG is designed depending on the amount of available cartilage and the patient's needs (**Fig. 3**A). The template is then cut and tried on the patient's caudal septum in an overlapping manner (side to side; **Fig. 3**B). Once the template has been adjusted properly, the cartilage is cut

as a mirror image to the cardboard template (**Fig. 3**C). In this way, cartilage is used in an efficient manner and remaining cartilage is saved for other uses in the nose.

The design of the SEG today mimics an irregular pentagon shape where the superior portion has one side longer than the contralateral side (**Fig. 3**D). Several things must be taken into account when designing an SEG: (1) How much is it going to extend from the natural ASA; (2) Is it going to project, rotate, or both; (3) How much is it going to overlap the existing caudal edge of the patient's septal cartilage; and (4) Is the SEG going to extend all the way down to the nasal spine.

Design of the SEG is very important because it defines the shape of the nasal tip lobule, and establishes the degree of projection and rotation of the nasal tip. Even though dimensions will vary from patient to patient, the shape is essentially the same.

How do You Place Your Septal Extension Graft or Columellar Strut? End to End or Overlapping, Extended to the Nasal Spine? Why?

Wong

I perform both side-to-side and end-to-end SEGs. The indications are fairly straightforward for me.

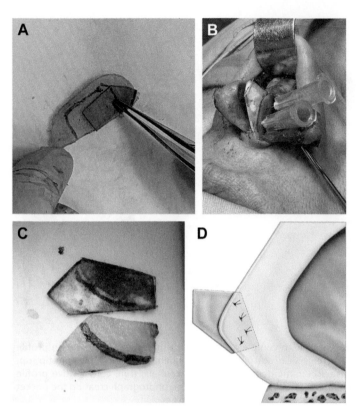

Fig. 3. Design of an SEG. (*A*) Graft is designed depending on available cartilage and the patient's needs. A piece of cardboard is used to draw the possible SEG. (*B*) The cardboard template is cut and placed overlapping the caudal edge of the patient's septum. (*C*) Available cartilage is cut using the cardboard template. (*D*) The design of the SEG usually has an irregular pentagon shape. The size is adapted depending on the patient's needs.

And that if there is a deviation of the ASA, then it is easy to put one in a side-to-side manner as it is less technically challenging, and it is very easy to suture into position. This is an effective strategy for most noses. However, if there is a significant caudal deformation that is beyond a minor ASA deviation, then it must be straightened. This would include maneuvers such as posterior septal angle (PSA) repositioning and septal batten placement. However, in cosmetic rhinoplasty, there are many noses where the ASA, PSA, and the midcaudal septum are aligned centrally. In those circumstances, I will use an end-to-end graft. The important take home point here is that the caudal septum should be resolutely straight. Apart from mild deformities of the ASA (on the order of the thickness of the septal cartilage), every effort should be made to create a central caudal septum. In general, the SEGs I placed do not extend to the nasal spine, the exception being where the caudal septum itself is relatively weak, again as in Asian patients where the cartilage is thinner and more flexible.

Williams/Urban

Once the graft is fashioned, a small vertical incision is made, typically on the right side, measuring only about 3 to 4 mm in length through the long axis of the right medial crura. Remember, the graft was designed with only 2 to 3 mm in width and thickness, and the incision and pocket are just large enough to accommodate the CS graft. A Stevens tenotomy scissor is used to dissect the pocket through the medial crura and down just past the nasal spine so it makes it easy to slide the strut in place. The Stevens scissors are then withdrawn and a dissection pocket is carried vertically between the medial crura up to the area of the nasal tip. By adhering to a pocket principle, the precise pocket is really made no larger than the graft itself other than the dissection off to one side of the nasal spine so that inserting the strut allows one to get the most anterior aspect into the incision before final placement and moving up between the medial curves toward the nasal tip. This is easily demonstrated with a video (Video 1). No sutures are necessary to secure the graft, and the vestibular mucosa is closed with interrupted 5-0 chromic sutures.

Notably, it is important to position the most posterior aspect of the CS graft a millimeter or two above the nasal spine, so it does not move from side to side or click. Placement is in between the medial crura from a millimeter or so above the nasal spine up toward the nasal tip, not to extend too far beyond the infratip, which would risk blunting the infratip break. It has been the senior author's experience that a very small amount of cartilage goes a long way in supporting the columella and nasal tip.

Cobo

Over the years, I have placed my SEG both overlapping and end to end. Today and for the past 4 to 5 years, I almost exclusively place an overlapping SEG that is stabilized on the contralateral side with a stabilizing or bolster graft. We call it the "reinforced overlapping septal extension graft" (ROSEG). The reason for this is that the main objective for me when placing the SEG is to gain projection and control rotation. In our patients, this increase in projection can be significant, and placing the graft overlapping the caudal edge of the septum will increase its stability.

The following sequential steps are performed when placing a ROSEG graft:

1. *Harvesting of septal cartilage (in primary rhinoplasty patients) leaving an L-Strut of at least 10 to 15 mm caudally and dorsally*. Correction of any septal deviations.
2. *Stabilizing caudal edge of septum in midline*. Ethnic and mestizo patients frequently have natural retrusive caudal septums with relatively short nasal spines and cartilage that is thin and weak.[3,4] It is imperative that this caudal edge be firmly positioned in the midline. For this reason, a 2 point fixation of the caudal edge of this cartilage is done. A first fixation point is performed at the nasal spine, and a second fixation point is performed 5 mm behind this first fixation point. Holes are drilled with a needle to the nasal spine and 5 mm behind this first fixation point, inferiorly to the maxillary bone. A 4-0 PDS suture is passed from the caudal edge of the septum to these 2 fixation points making sure the septum is stabilized in the midline (**Fig. 4**).
3. *Evaluation of stabilized caudal edge of septum*. The stabilized caudal edge is evaluated, and if there is any slight concavity or caudal weakness of the cartilage, the SEG is placed on this side. It is imperative that this caudal edge be in the midline.
4. *Placement of SEG*. This graft is placed on the side where there is a slight concavity of the caudal edge of the septum. If the septum is straight and is not weak, it can be placed on either side. This graft usually does not extend all the way down to the nasal spine (unless there is a specific need for this) and is placed angulated overlapping the ASA and projecting forward to increase projection. The graft is fixed with 5-0 running PDS sutures (**Fig. 5**).

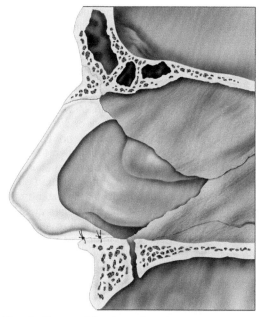

Fig. 4. The caudal edge of patients' native septal cartilage is fixed and stabilized in the midline with a 2 point fixation with 4-0 PDS. The first fixation suture is done at the nasal spine, and the second suture is placed 5 mm behind this first suture.

5. *Placement of contralateral bolster graft*. All of my SEG are stabilized on the contralateral side with a "bolster stabilizing graft." This is a trick I learned from Renato Sousa from Brazil

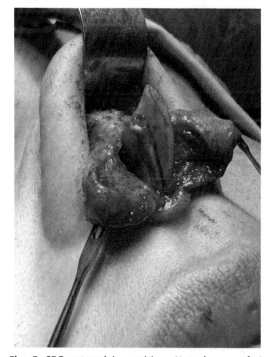

Fig. 5. SEG sutured in position. Note how graft is overlapping on left side of patient.

and adapted to my own particular needs. This bolster graft is placed depending on what I want to stabilize. It can be placed as a short extended spreader graft, an angulated graft or a mirror graft of the SEG. Everything is sutured in place with 5-0 PDS sutures (**Fig. 6**).

There is always the question of whether this contralateral graft will create bulk or will obstruct the nasal valve area. This is usually not the case because the septal cartilage of our patients is usually very thin, 1 to 2 mm, and if bulk is seen in the internal nasal valve area, the graft is thinned out.

The bolster stabilizing graft usually extends all the way up to the tip of the contralateral SEG and should be long enough to stabilize and give support to the leading edge of this SEG.

In cases of revision patients where the caudal septum is deficient, I usually place a mirror stabilizing graft on the contralateral side of the SEG (**Fig. 7**).

How do You Define Nasal Tip Position? How do You Measure It?

Wong

Tip position is absolutely critical, and I am of the school of thought that our eyes deceive us, particularly with regard to projection. I believe it is important to be quantitative and track tip position at multiple time points during surgery. For this, I use a projectometer device. The inventor of the original projectometer is unclear, but it may have been

Richard Webster, Jack Anderson, or Calvin Johnson (personal communication, Peter Hilger, MD March 2024), and at present, there are many commercially available devices that are all quite similar in design. The nasal projectometer is a surgical stereotaxis device that can track landmark movement during surgery. I think the singularly most important application is for tracking the position of the nasal tip and recording differential changes in projection and rotation. **Fig. 8A** illustrates the placement of the Davis projectometer (Marina Medical Instruments, Davie, FL) prior to surgery. This projectometer consists of a carriage that is placed midline over the nose with 2 registry markers. Inferiorly, there is a flange with a dental stop that registers to the maxillary incisors. Superiorly, a cradle embraces the forehead, and a surgical marker is used to trace its shape on the forehead. There are 4 metal pins. Three terminate in a rounded point while a central one ends in a "T" shape. One pin has an additional degree of freedom allowing precision placement along the columella. Collectively, these create fiducials at the glabella, over the rhinion, anterior tip defining point, and the nasal–labial junction. They are secured into place with set screws. The pins and carriage have millimeter scale bars that are recorded and provide micrometry information. They record data along a caudal-cephalic and

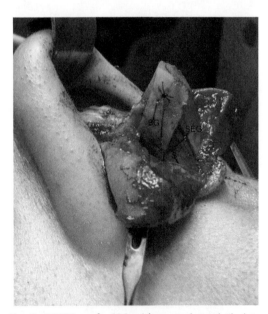

Fig. 6. ROSEG graft. SEG with contralateral "bolster graft" sutured in place. BG, bolster graft; S, septum; SEG, septal extension graft.

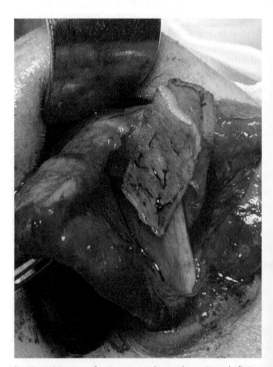

Fig. 7. Mirror graft. In cases where there is a deficient caudal septum, a contralateral graft is placed, which mirrors the SEG placed.

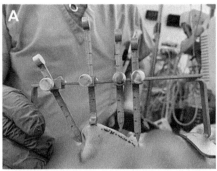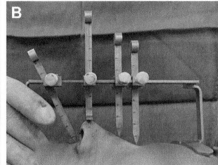

Fig. 8. (*A, B*) Projectometer placement before surgery and at the end of the operation.

anterior-posterior direction. They specify coordinates in 2 dimension. The device can be positioned just after sedation, sterilized, and then returned to the surgical field. Likewise, measurements may be first performed entirely on the sterile surgical field prior to local anesthetic injection thus avoiding resterilization. I repeat these measurements throughout surgery to link intraoperative changes with estimates made in preoperative computer simulations. After specific maneuvers (eg, hump reduction, SEG placement, and so forth), the 4 pins are readjusted, and the differential change is noted. Again as noted earlier, with regard to SEG use, I incorporate a template method to increase my precision in graft design. As noted, my SEG will specify the location of the tip defining point. Once the SEG is secure, I will replace the skin soft tissue envelope, and record tip position with the Davis projectometer. I tend to initially over project and counter rotate the tip defining point by 1 to 2 mm at this point, but this is transient. I then use a scalpel to refine and correct the contour until the precise shape I want is achieved. Projectometer measurements are repeated. One does have to compensate a bit for the impact of edema, and that will vary with skin type. It is generally well less than 1 mm over the tip. In contrast, if the SEG following initial suture fixation is deficient in projection or rotated in excess, then the only solution is removal and repositioning. You can easily trim an SEG, but you cannot make it larger readily. One of the challenges and intrinsic elements of imprecision is the measurement of the tip defining point with the projectometer. Generally, the T bar is placed tangent to the most anteriorly defining point, and in a broad, amorphous tip, a precise position is hard to ascertain. This matters most in gauging rotation. Further, following tip surgery, the shape generally becomes more refined. Hence, the rotation measure for the tip is less valuable for me compared to the projection measure. **Fig. 8B**

illustrates the placement of the Davis projectometer following skin closure. There is much published information on the use of projectometers in the literature, and there are many commercially available designs. I believe in the near future, these devices will be replaced with operative 3 dimensional imaging platforms that will provide real-time intraoperative micrometry in 3 dimensions and link to preoperative simulations.

Williams/Urban

The senior author's general approach in rhinoplasty is best described as structural endonasal rhinoplasty whereby very few reductive techniques are performed, and the nose is rebalanced through structural reorientation with suture techniques and cartridge grafting. This approach allows for the creation of harmonious nasal proportions without wide dissection and resection, thereby limiting the sequela associated with overly reductive rhinoplasty, such as delayed tip ptosis or loss of projection. The forces of scar contracture are relentless, and if surgeons truly follow their patients in the long term over multiple years, significant changes in the nasal tip position and shape are almost always evident.

While the CS is effective in buttressing the medial crura, providing strength to the nasal tip, and accentuating an esthetically appealing infratip break, the senior author's workhorse to maintain tip projection is the tongue-in-groove (TIG) maneuver. The TIG maneuver can fairly accurately give an optimal long-term tip support and rebalancing of the tip area when performed through an endonasal structural approach. The author's preference for the TIG maneuver is a 4-0 polydioxanone suture.

When there is a need for additional tip projection, the senior author often places small shaved flakes of septal cartilage via the pocket principle at the tip defining points. This will also help with tip refinement used with or without other techniques but also used in conjunction with a CS or TIG maneuver. It can be very powerful in maintaining and creating an esthetically pleasing tip and giving long-term tip support and balance. In cases with an extraordinary degree of tip ptosis, a lateral crural overlay flap may be performed to shorten the lateral limbs of the tripod and significantly rotate the tip, while also improving projection. This technique is best suited for individuals with thick skin to avoid palpable or visible irregularities.

The senior author has found that the aforementioned techniques reliably improve projection and support the tip while minimizing the deleterious effects of scar contracture over the course of multiple years. When these techniques are combined with rebalancing of the nasal length through a conservative dorsal reduction and radix grafting if necessary, this approach obviates an SEG in the vast majority of cases.

Cobo

Tip position and length is measured constantly during surgery. This is done not with a projectometer but with a ruler. Two distances are measured during consultation: the distance from the nasion to the nasal tip (N-T) and the distance from the alar groove to the existing nasal tip (A-T). When simulation is done, we calculate how much projection and or rotation is going to be needed, and this is documented. During surgery, measurements are verified once the patient is asleep and before infiltration (**Fig. 9**A, B). Measurements are repeated with the template in place and again measured once the ROSEG has been sutured in place. All of this is done with the skin redraped over the tip structure. These 2 measurements are documented before surgery and are taken again once the ROSEG is in place. These measurements are complemented with measurements of the angle of angulation of the ROSEG

with the dorsal line and the nasolabial angle and the distance in millimeters from the ASA to the position of the ROSEG.

Measurements vary from patient to patient and vary according to gender, but we try to achieve an N-T measurement of 45 to 50 mm, an A-T measurement of 31 to 34 mm, a dorsal angle of 130° to 140°, and a distance of the ASA to tip of graft of 5 to 10 mm. It is always easier to shorten or trim a long ROSEG graft. If it is too short, it becomes necessary to release it and suture it again in its proper position. As a surgeon, I know that unless something extraordinary happens, the nasal tip position will not vary significantly after surgery. Because of this, it becomes necessary not to overcorrect when placing these grafts.

If Septal Cartilage Is Not Enough for Your Septal Extension Graft or Columellar Strut, What Other Cartilage Options Do You Use and Do You Have Any Special Techniques

Wong

In every single patient that is undergoing primary rhinoplasty, I will also obtain informed consent for conchal cartilage as often septal cartilage alone is insufficient. While, costal cartilage is also readily available, I believe its use can be avoided in most primary cases with the exception of certain augmentation procedures. Structural grafts used in my operations generally include spreader, rim, and an SEG. The most important graft for me is the SEG as it will define the centrally and straightness of the nose. This is followed by rim grafts that I use approximately 30% of the time. Spreader grafts are strictly speaking non–load-bearing, and they mainly function as a space-occupying material. Hence, if cartilage is inadequate in a primary rhinoplasty, I will harvest auricular cartilage and most likely use it for a spreader graft. Of note, I do not cut any graft from the harvested

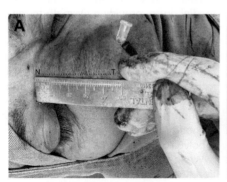
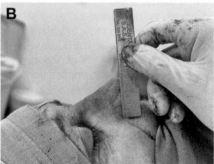

Fig. 9. (*A*) Distance from Nasion (N) to nasal tip (T). This distance is measured before surgery and after the placement of SEG to define necessary degree of projection and rotation. (*B*) Distance from alar groove (A) to nasal tip (T).

septal cartilage until I have traced with a surgical marker the shape every single graft I will use in the operation. This results in a very efficient use of available cartilage.

Williams/Urban

The key aspect for the successful implementation of the CS graft using the author's technique is to utilize a straight, thin, and strong piece of cartilage. Nasal septal cartilage is always the first choice for this. As mentioned earlier, the CS graft's dimensions through the endonasal pocket approach are significantly smaller than most SEG grafts, and thus septal cartilage may be adequate even in many revision cases.

If nasal cartilage is not available, rib cartilage is preferred because it retains strength even when thinly carved. Because rib cartilage is more rigid, additional care must be taken to avoid placement over the nasal spine. Fresh frozen and irradiated costal cartilage has garnered increased traction in recent years with a number of studies supporting its efficacy and safety. In our practice, autologous rib was the sole costal cartilage choice for over 2 decades; however, in recent years, we have transitioned to fresh frozen costal cartilage for many purposes including CS grafts. Autologous rib still remains the preference for more critical structural support grafts such as lateral wall reconstruction, particularly in younger patients. In years past, the senior author has utilized conchal cartilage for the CS graft, but because it tends to be thicker and softer with a lower tensile strength, it is a distance third option in the senior author's hands.

Cobo

If septal cartilage is not enough or not available for my ROSEG graft, I usually harvest ear cartilage or rib cartilage depending on individual patient needs. If the patient has had a previous rhinoplasty or a previous septoplasty and needs a rhinoplasty where projection is very important, I usually will speak to them on the need of harvesting rib cartilage. After septal cartilage, the ideal choice for grafting material for structural grafts is rib.

In the cases where there is available septal cartilage, but it will not be enough for the grafts needed for our patient, I will use ear cartilage. In these cases, I will use this ear cartilage either for spreader grafts or for the contralateral stabilizing bolster graft of the ROSEG graft. In some very specific cases, ear cartilage can be used to make the ROSEG graft. In these cases, the contralateral stabilizing graft is usually a mirror image of the SEG. Since the conchal cartilage tends to be concave, both concave sides are placed facing each other

and sutured in place overlapping the natural caudal edge of the patient's septum. ROSEG grafts fashioned from ear cartilage can be useful in those patients where the need for projection is not too important and where the skin-soft tissue (S-STE) is not overly thick.

When using SEG carved from rib cartilage, attention must be placed in making sure the graft is completely straight. If there is any slight concavity to the graft, it is better to place a thin contralateral mirror graft on the opposite side suturing them together to make sure the graft is straight and in the midline. ROSEG grafts fashioned from rib are usually placed overlapping the patients existing caudal septum and stabilized either with a mirror graft or with a contralateral bolster graft.

What Are the Complications of Using Septal Extension Graft or a Columellar Strut?

Wong

I think the biggest complication of septal extension use is in central placement. There is a tendency for these grafts to shift either to the left or right, and this may occur weeks postoperatively. They need to be secure and stabilized, and any forces acting on the SEG needs to be stabilized and balanced. This is particularly true when using lateral crural tensioning. This is less an issue with a side-to-side graft, but in one that is placed end-to-end, it is important that you have bridge grafts on both the right and left side to prevent any flexure of the graft. Grafts or the tip can shift to the right or left at the apex. This can occur as a consequence of asymmetric forces that act on the graft when the right and left domes were reattached. First and foremost, it is important to secure those grafts with the lateral forces balanced; second, you need to relieve the strain by placing a number of midline sutures securing the medial crura to the SEG, and then along the mucosal surface, through and through at the level of the PSA, midcaudal septum, and ASA. Each suture provides a small degree of strain release. I would say that midline shift (tip deviation) would be the biggest issue related to end-to-end SEG placement.

With side-to-side or overlapping grafts, I believe the biggest concern is airway obstruction. These grafts may encroach on the internal nasal valve and narrowing the air space. This is particularly true in narrow noses. One has to be very attentive to graft design to avoid this. The challenge is that graft is often used to provide additional structural stability to the septum or functions as a batten for several caudal deformities. Here graft placement is often focused on mechanical stability rather than on airflow. In some patients, the airway can be widely patent, but because of narrowing in the internal nasal valve, the patient may have perception or symptoms nasal airway obstruction due to pressure drops at a narrowed inlet.

Williams/Urban

Complications from CS are rare. In the early years, the most common mistake was fashioning a CS that was simply too large for the endonasal approach. This could result in clicking at the nasal spine or more rarely deformity of the infratip. If clicking of the nasal spine is encountered, the graft is easily trimmed through a stab incision in clinic. As mentioned earlier, the amount of cartilage required for the CS is much less when employed via the endonasal approach when the surrounding soft tissue support is undissected.

The senior author believes rhinoplasty surgeons have strayed from CS in the open approach because it can result in a wide columella and a very unnatural look to the base view, particularly if auricular cartilage is employed. While we are using the CS a little less frequently in recent years, the authors do feel it is a very powerful surgical maneuver.

Cobo

The biggest complications using an SEG is its placement and making sure it is completely in the midline, making sure that with the projection that is gained with this graft, it will not tilt to one side once the new domes are fixed to the ROSEG graft, and making sure there will be no compromise of the internal nasal valve.

If the existing caudal septum of the patient is exactly in the midline, placing an SEG with a contralateral bolster graft (ROSEG Graft) will align the whole pedestal structure in the midline. Care, of course, must be taken to thin out the portion of the graft that is in the internal nasal valve area. It becomes important to tension the domes to the ROSEG graft and the tissue of the internal nasal valve must also be meticulously sutured to the ROSEG graft to make sure it is aligned and tensioned properly.

There is a limit to how much projection is gained without having the graft tilting to one side, and this must be evaluated by the surgeon. In my experience, an increase in projection of more than 10 to 11 mm when measured from the ASA becomes very difficult to control.

Over the years, in many articles, surgeons have mentioned that stiffness of the nasal tip can be a complication. I have not found this to be the case in my patient population. It does become important to be able to carve grafts that are not overly thick and create too much bulk as this will definitely have an impact on nasal tip stiffness and in nasal obstruction. Grafts must be thinned out in the area of the internal nasal valve and thoughtful carving must be performed to avoid columellas that look overly thick and bulky.

How Have Your Techniques in This Area Changed over the Last 2 Years?

Wong

One technique that I have been using, which is a lot of fun, is to split cartilage in the central sagittal plane partially bivalving it. It is slipped over the ASA and sutured into place. I have been referring to this approach as a (Caudal Septal Extension Graft "Split CSEG"). It is a simplified approach that is a modification of the boomerang graft I described earlier. **Fig. 10** illustrates the use. **Fig. 10**A is a view of the graft from the side, and it is rectangular. **Fig. 10**B shows the graft rotated and on the left, one can appreciate how this edge is slightly displaced outward. **Fig. 10**C shows this partially bivalved graft placed over the ASA. **Fig. 10**D shows the graft reversed, and the 2 flanges of the graft are clearly visible. **Fig. 10**E shows placement of the graft over the ASA. In **Fig. 10**F and 27 G needles secure the graft over the ASA prior to suture fixation. It is very nice, it is midline, but it requires a fair amount of precision in order to make the sagittal cut. I generally alternate between #11 and #15 blades, and the process is slow and meticulous. Ideally, the cartilage should be at least 2 mm thick. This approach is not particularly consumptive of cartilage, it eliminates the need for a bridge graft and provides a significant amount of biomechanical stability. It also does not widen appreciably the septum at the ASA. The downside of course is that if one is not prudent in graft designed, you may end up with a degree of overrotation.

Williams/Urban

In the past 2 to 5 years, the senior author has progressively employed the TIG maneuver more frequently than a CS. As discussed earlier, the combination of TIG maneuver and very fine tip grafting with or without CS graft allows for an adequate projection and long-term tip support in the majority of cases. That being said, the senior author has recently begun experimenting with SEG placement as part of the structural endonasal approach. This requires an extended inferior marginal incision with wider dissection and lower lateral cartilage delivery in order to adequately fixate the SEG to the caudal nasal septum. This is only required in a small minority of cases with severe tip deformity. The senior author does not have sufficient experience with this technique as

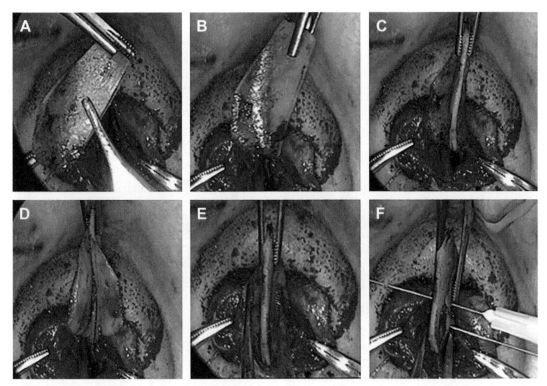

Fig. 10. (*A–F*) Split SEG.

of yet to form an opinion, and the workhorse still remains the TIG suture technique.

Cobo

My techniques have changed over the last 4 years, and the reason for this has been a loss of projection of the nasal tips over the years when using CSs. Studies have shown that there can be a loss of tip projection and rotation when using CSs.[11–14] With our patient population that has weak caudal septums and limited amounts of septal cartilage for grafting, tip support has always been a challenge. Initially, I started using SEG end to end but found that in my hands the stability of this graft with our very flimsy cartilage was not ideal. The changes I have made in my technique can be summarized as follows:

1. For this reason in the past 4 years, I have been using an overlapping SEG, and in the past 3 years, I have been using the ROSEG graft with very good long-term results. I have found that this graft gives me additional stability in the pedestal and serves as a very nice foundation for all the additional tip work that is performed.
2. In patients with platyrrhine noses (Asian patients, African descent patients among others) where we know available septal cartilage is

going to be very limited and thin, I routinely try to use rib cartilage. In these cases, we usually use ROSEG grafts where the bolster graft is a mirror image of the contralateral SEG.
3. In revision patients and patients that have had previous functional septal surgery, I routinely use rib cartilage to fashion my ROSEG grafts.
4. In all cases, the ROSEG graft that is fashioned is measured meticulously and thinned out in the areas that are overlapping the nasal valve area.
5. In all cases, the patient's natural caudal septum is first stabilized in the midline with 2 important stabilizing sutures: the first suture is placed on the nasal spine, and the second suture is placed a few millimeters posteriorly stabilizing the posterior edge of the caudal L-Strut to the maxillary bone. These sutures are done with 4-0 PDS. Once the pedestal is fixed in the midline, the ROSEG graft is carved and sutured in place depending on patients' individual needs.
6. The long-term follow-up of these patients has been quite good. Projection and rotation are preserved, and there is no real loss of tip support over the years. This has proven to be a reliable technique for patients with retrusive caudal septums and problems with projection and rotation of the nasal tip (**Fig. 11A–H**).

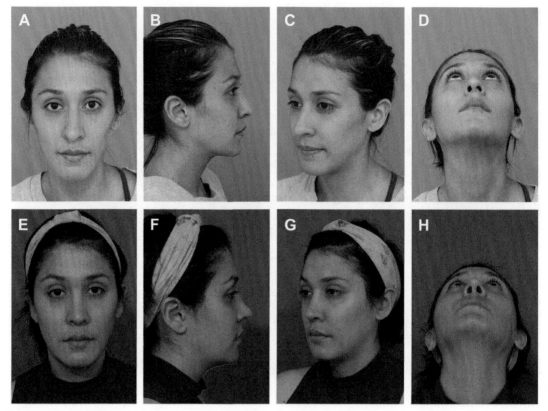

Fig. 11. A 2 year follow-up of a patient with a ROSEG graft where the objective in the tip surgery was to increase projection and rotation of the nasal tip. (*A–D*) Presurgical images. (*E–H*) A 2 year postsurgical images with placement of a ROSEG graft.

SUMMARY

SEGs and CSs have been used over the years to help control tip rotation and projection. In the past years, articles have been published showing that there could be a decrease over time in projection and rotation when a CS is used. This will depend on the underlying strength of the patient's caudal septum and medial crura. Because of this, there has been a shift in surgical techniques, and many surgeons today are using different variations of an SEG. The big downside to these techniques is that more cartilage has to be available for grafting.

Today, again we have new changes in rhinoplasty. With the use of the new preservation rhinoplasty approaches, there is a big discussion on trying to preserve or reconstruct the intercrural and interdomal ligaments (Pitanguy Ligament) and using it as additional support in the nasal tip. If this philosophy is used, this could mean using the SEG less frequently and focusing on reorienting ligament structures with smaller amounts of cartilage grafts to control projection and rotation. Only time will tell us if these new techniques will produce reliable long-term results.

SUPPLEMENTARY DATA

Supplementary data to this article can be found online at https://doi.org/10.1016/j.fsc.2024.06.005.

REFERENCES

1. Toriumi DM. New concepts in nasal tip contouring. Arch Facial Plast Surg 2006;8(3):156–85. PMID: 16702528.
2. Kridel RW, Scott BA, Foda HM. The tongue-in-groove technique in septorhinoplasty. A 10-year experience. Arch Facial Plast Surg 1999;1(4):246–56. discussion 257-8: PMID: 10937111.
3. Byrd HS, Andochick S, Copit S, et al. Septal extension grafts: a method of controlling tip projection shape. Plast Reconstr Surg 1997;100(4):999–1010. PMID: 9290671.
4. Peters RD, Vasudev M, Hakimi AA, et al. Boomerang Modification of the Septal Extension Graft: Graft Design and Functional Outcomes. Facial Plast Surg Aesthet Med 2024. https://doi.org/10.1089/fpsam.2023.0152. Epub ahead of print. PMID: 38215259.
5. Toriumi DM. Caudal septal extension graft for correction of the retracted columella. Operat Tech Otolaryngol Head Neck Surg 1995;6:311–8.

6. Cobo R. Management of the mestizo nose. Otolaryngol Clin North Am 2020;53:267–82.

7. Cobo R. Rhinoplasty in latino patients. Clin Plast Surg 2016;43:237–54.

8. Kim MH, Choi J, Kim MS, et al. An Introduction to the Septal Extension Graft. Arch Plast Surg 2014;41: 29–34.

9. Brandstetter M, Bhatt M, Pham M, et al. Comparative Analysis and Long-Term Results of Various Septal Extension Graft Types. Facial Plast Surg 2020;36:263–7.

10. Neves JC, Tagle DA. Lateral Crura Control in Nasal Tip Plasty: Cephalic Oblique Domal Suture, 7X Suture and ANSA Banner. Adv Plast Reconstr Surg 2020;4(3):1059.

11. Akkus AM, Eryilmaz E, Guneren E. Comparison of the Effects of Columellar Strut and Septal Extension Grafts for Tip Support in Rhinoplasty. Aesthetic Plast Surg 2013;37:666–73.

12. Sawh-Martinez R, Perkins K, Madari S, et al. Control of nasal tip position: quantitative assessment of columellar strut versus caudal septal extension graft. Plast Reconstr Surg 2019;144:772e–80e.

13. Toriumi DM. Discussion: control of nasal tip position: quantitative assessment of columellar strut versus caudal septal extension graft. Plast Reconstr Surg 2019;144:781e–3e.

14. Bellamy J, Rohrich R. Superiority of the Septal Extension Graft over the Columellar Strut Graft in Primary Rhinoplasty: Improved Long-Term Tip Stability. Plast Reconstr Surg 2023;152(2):332–9.

The Use of Costal Cartilage in Rhinoplasty

Fred G. Fedok, MD[a,b],*, Grace Lee Peng, MD[c], Eren Tastan, MD[d], Enrico Robotti, MD[e,f]

KEYWORDS

- Rib cartilage • Autologous rib • Cartilage grafting • Revision rhinoplasty reconstruction
- Carving rib cartilage

KEY POINTS

- Autologous rib cartilage can be safely harvested in both male and female patients.
- Rib cartilage harvest is integral to cartilage grafting in revision rhinoplasty cases as it provides adequate quantity of cartilage.
- Rib cartilage can be easily created into grafts for nasal reconstruction.

 Video content accompanies this article at http://www.facialplastic.theclinics.com.

PANEL DISCUSSION

Harvest Site/Technique?
Do you perform partial harvest of rib cartilage?
Which are your indications in Primary Rhinoplasty?
What Instruments do you use?
What Cartilage Carving techniques do you use and why?
How have your techniques in this area changed over the last 2 y?

QUESTION 1. HARVEST SITE/TECHNIQUE
Fedok

I have been harvesting costal cartilage for grafting material since the early 90s. Initially, I was doing larger harvests for microtia reconstructions. In those cases, a sizable amount of rib was removed from several ribs. Not infrequently this harvest caused a relative deformity in the area and the harvest was made through a larger incision.

My harvest of rib cartilage for rhinoplasty started out in the same time frame. This was relatively easier than the harvest for microtia. It could be done through a significantly smaller incision. It caused less pain and less of a resultant chest wall deformity. In my practice, the harvesting of costal cartilage for rhinoplasty was frequently for the management of post-traumatic deformity, after severe infection, or post-cancer surgery situations. The rhinoplasty patients were primarily being treated for saddle nose deformity, and those with a significant absence of midline septal support. In these situations, large dorsal grafts were placed to manage those rhinoplasty reconstructive challenges. The noses that were engaged in this fashion were largely those with severe deformity. Thus, most the time the complete cross section of rib was removed to create sizable midline dorsal grafts and central nasal support.

Initially, there was little finesse in these procedures. Larger incisions were made, and the harvest was performed using more traditional rib instruments, such as the Doyen elevator and Matson-Alexander elevators. Typically, the cartilaginous

[a] Department of Surgery, University of South Alabama, Foley, AL, USA; [b] Fedok Plastic Surgery, Foley; [c] Facial Plastic and Reconstructive Surgery, Beverly Hills, CA, USA; [d] ENT, Private Practice, Ankara, Turkey; [e] Private Practice, Bergamo, Italy; [f] Rhinoplasty Society of Europe, Italian Society of Plastic Surgery, Ospedale Papa Giovanni XXIII, Bergamo, Italy
* Corresponding author. Fedok Plastic Surgery, 113 East Fern Avenue, Foley, AL 36535.
E-mail address: drfredfedok@me.com

Facial Plast Surg Clin N Am 32 (2024) 565–583
https://doi.org/10.1016/j.fsc.2024.06.009
1064-7406/24/© 2024 Elsevier Inc. All rights are reserved, including those for text and data mining, AI training, and similar technologies.

rib was removed in its entirety, sometimes going beyond the bony-cartilaginous junction of the rib to harvest a composite graft. The majority of time the perichondrium was stripped on the deep side to limit the potential for violation of the chest cavity. Patients were frequently admitted to the hospital and placed on patient-administered pain pumps to manage the chest wall discomfort after removing the costal cartilage in this manner.

Over time, my harvest technique for obtaining costal cartilage for rhinoplasty has become a more limited endeavor. In general, because I am a right-handed surgeon, I harvest rib from the patient's right side of the chest. The goal is always to obtain an adequate amount of rib cartilage to obtain a sufficient quantity of cartilage grafting material while maintaining the esthetics of the patient's chest wall, whether or not the patient is male or a female.

I design the chest incision at a level and direction that is consistent with the patients relaxed skin tension lines on the chest wall and to take advantage of the inframammary crease where possible. The goal is usually to harvest portions of the sixth rib. The length of the incision depends on the patient's size and amount of subcutaneous fat over the chest wall where the graft harvest is anticipated. In a young thin female where there is less than 1 to 2 cm of overlying of soft tissue between the surface of the skin and the rib, a very small incision is possible that is, 2 cm or less. In the larger, heavier patient where literally one may have to dissect through 5 or 6 cm of adipose to get to the level of the rib, a larger incision is necessary. The incision may even extend to 4 cm or more in length. Skin retraction will be necessary, and some modification of the incision placement may be necessary in larger patients.

Modifications of technique I now use for the rib harvest is a compilation of advice I have received from colleagues over the years. Through their advice, I have learned the utility of retracting the incision and moving its location over several positions on the chest wall. Even a very small incision can be retracted back and forth over the chest wall to get access to different portions of the target rib.[1]

Another adaptation that I have utilized in harvesting rib cartilage was obtained through observation and discussion with thoracic surgeon colleagues. By performing the rib harvest via a "muscle sparing" technique, the patient experiences less incisional harvest pain.[1]

I make my skin incision with either 10 or 15 scalpels. The length of the incision depends on patient characteristics as I mentioned earlier. I will use the bovie electrocautery and blunt dissection to progress through the subcutaneous adipose. I will proceed through Scarpa's fascia in the same manner. At the level of the deep fascia, over the rectus abdominis or external oblique muscles, I will bluntly spread through the fascia and the muscle with a hemostat. Dissection proceeds in the direction of the muscle fibers to minimize trauma to the muscle until the rib periosteum is encountered. Utilizing retractors, one is able to keep the soft tissue out of the way and visualize the perichondrium over the rib. With careful retraction with the use of army-navy and/or Senne retractors, we are able to visualize the whole area of the rib and perichondrium we want to harvest while maintaining the smaller incision.

The instruments I use currently are smaller instruments than what I used in the past. The instruments I commonly use include a 10 or 5 scalpel, an Army-and-Navy retractor, Senne retractor, Freer elevator, and Adson and Cobb elevators. Rarely will I use a Doyen retractor.

My harvest technique continues in the answer to question #2.

Peng

I like to make a very small 1 cm, well placed and hidden incision for rib cartilage harvest. In the preoperative area, with the patient sitting up and facing me, I mark out the inframammary or infrapectoral crease as well as the xiphoid notch (**Fig. 1**). If the patient has larger breasts or pectoralis muscle, I have them hold up the breast/muscle so that I can see the crease. The incision lies within this marked crease, but the placement is finalized once the patient is supine on the operating room table.

With the patient supine, the crease can be easily seen and the incision is marked so that it is medial to the nipple line and approximately 6 to 10 cm from the midline xiphoid marking. I like to prep out the entire chest so that both sides are showing. Many of my female patients have breast implants it allows me to have constant comparison between the 2 sides. The small incision will become a small mobile incision. The goal is to shift the incision so that the small incision can cover a larger area underneath. Younger patients will have tighter skin. The concept of rib cartilage harvest can be likened to that of an inverse funnel (**Fig. 2**).

To get oriented, you have the skin at the top. The second layer is the subcutaneous and fatty tissue. The third layer is Scarpa's fascia which often looks as if it could be the fascia overlying the muscle but in many patients, there is additional, fatty tissue under this layer. The next layer is the true rectus or pectoralis fascia, underneath

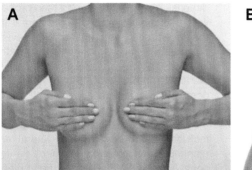
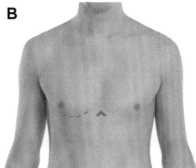

Fig. 1. Marking the inframammary crease and the xiphoid notch with the patient sitting up for the (*A*) female patient and (*B*) male patient. The *blue line* depicts where the inframmary crease is typically located.

which is the muscle. Immediately under the muscle is the rib with the anterior surface of the perichondrium (**Fig. 3**).

I usually make a 1 cm incision and dissect wider at each layer. I then shift the upper layers to allow for maximal exposure at the rib. The 2 landmarks I always look for are the synchondrosis and the bony cartilaginous junction. The incision is placed so that at the extent of the widest dissection the lateral edge is at the bony cartilaginous junction. Usually I am harvesting the sixth rib.

Once I am down to the rib, instead of the traditional H cuts in the perichondrium, I first incise a rectangle, and then make perpendicular cuts to the superior and inferior edge (**Fig. 4**). This way the piece of perichondrium can be used later at the tip or along the dorsum. I dissect the perichondrium off to expose the rib cartilage so that it can be removed en bloc.

Once I have identified the bony cartilaginous junction, I cut through it on the cartilage side with

a 15-blade. Then, the focus becomes at the synchondrosis where I elevate with the cottle slightly beneath the rib cartilage and cut through with the 15-blade until I make it through the entire synchondrosis. Once I reach the medial end of the dissection, a cut is made similar to the cut at the bony cartilaginous junction. The superior edge of the rib is dissected free from the posterior perichondrium as is the inferior aspect. The rib is then able to be gently lifted from the posterior aspect.

Once the rib is removed, I always check for any tears and confirm that there are neither leaks nor tears by doing 3 valsava maneuvers to 40 mm Hg.

Finally, it is important to close with maximal eversion at all the layers. I first close the muscle and the fascia together so that the sutures do not rip through the muscle using a 3-0 PDS running locking suture. I close Scarpa's with a 3-0 monocryl. I then close the deep dermal layer with a 4-0 monocryl and a running subcuticular with a 4-0 monocryl.

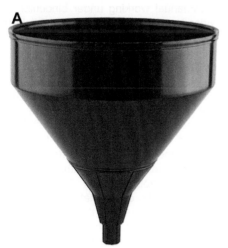
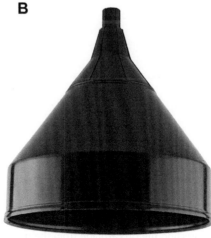

Fig. 2. The concept of rib cartilage harvest through a tiny incision is like that of an inverse funnel. A funnel has a larger opening on top with a small opening on bottom (*A*). An inverse funnel as a small opening on top and a larger, wider opening on the bottom (*B*).

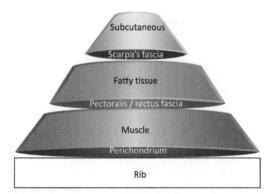

Fig. 3. The schematic of layers when you approach the "inverse funnel" for rib cartilage harvest.

At this time of this writing, I have personally performed over 1100 cases in the last 9 years. The average time is about 36 minutes. The rib lengths range from 2.5 to 6.8 cm and on average is about 4.5 cm.

Overall, rib cartilage can be easily and safely harvested as a reliable source of cartilage in rhinoplasty.

Tastan

Rib cartilage is frequently used by rhinoplasty surgeons in secondary rhinoplasties. Surgeons may be hesitant to harvest and carve rib cartilage because of the risks like pneumothorax, warping problems, scar, and postoperative pain. Surgeons need to be familiar with harvesting and carving of rib cartilage using the appropriate surgical tools and technique.

I always start the surgery with rhinoplasty dissection. I determine the required cartilage graft

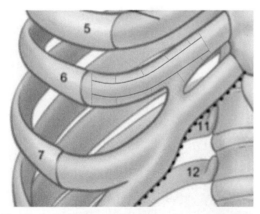

Fig. 4. Anterior rib perichondrium preserving technique while dissecting the rib cartilage from the posterior perichiondrium. Instead of the traditional H cuts, a rectangle is first incised into the perichondrium.

dimensions and volume, and then proceed to harvest the cartilage graft. Costosternal junction of the seventh rib and costal arch of seventh rib are palpated and marked. Between the sixth and seventh ribs, a 1.5 to 2 cm incision line is located, starting approximately 9 cm laterally from the costosternal junction and extending from lateral to medial. Since medial retraction of tissues is typically easier than lateral retraction at this region, the incision is started from the lateral end of the planned rib harvesting segment. In female patients, it is aesthetically preferred to place the incision along the inframammary crease as much as possible. If inframammarian approach is preferred, as it is relatively far from the target, 25% longer incision is advised. The lateral edge of the incision line which is 5 mm superior to the inframammary crease should align vertically with the lateral end of the planned incision line between the sixth and seventh ribs.

Incision size is often a matter of debate; from the surgeon's point of view, we need enough exposure to the surgical field and enough opening for to take the rib out, from the patient's point of view smaller and even invisible scar. When planning the length of the incision, it is critical to use the smallest incision feasible to ensure surgical exposure, permit rib harvesting, and minimum trauma to the wound edges. To have a better scar, it is necessary to avoid trauma to the wound edges. As the length of incision decreases, the amount of trauma increases. A full rib segment cannot be removed through an incision less than 1 cm. Tissue trauma increases with an incision less than 1.5 cm. If the incision is placed correctly, an incision longer than 3 cm seems unnecessary and usually does not provide additional exposure.

Bimanual working under binocular vision provides best control at the surgical field for to prevent complications. Endoscope is useful only for educational purposes.

The area is infiltrated with 4 cc of local anesthesia (1% lidocaine with 1:100,000 epinephrine), 10 to 15 minutes prior to the incision. After making the incision with a number 15 blade, dissection is carried down to the muscle fascia with a blunt tip scissor. Anterior surface of the fascia is exposed widely, and fascia incision is made with monopolar cautery between the sixth and seventh ribs extending approximately 6 to 8 cm medially. Then, blunt dissection that is parallel to the muscle fibers is performed at the lateral edge of the rib segment, so the anterior surface of the rib is exposed through a window between the intact muscle fibers. Another window opened 3 to 4 cm medially to the first one and the muscle layer is elevated from the anterior surface of the seventh rib like a muscle bridge. The preservation of muscle fibers is important as it will be helpful to lessen postoperative pain. A wide dissection plane is performed just anterior to the rib perichondrium so the whole rib segment surface is exposed and examined for the cartilage quality and dimensions. If the dimensions are not satisfactory, the neighboring sixth rib can easily be exposed and checked for an available segment.

I usually prefer to harvest the seventh rib, and if it is not suitable, then I harvest the sixth rib. The main differences between the sixth and seventh ribs are based on their anatomic features. The seventh rib has a narrower anteroposterior diameter but a longer, straighter segment. Posteriorly, it is mostly in relation to the abdomen, which makes it safer to harvest and allows for easier dissection since it is relatively mobile. On the other hand, the sixth rib is comparatively shorter but still offers enough length and has a thicker section. The sixth rib is adjacent to the pleura at its posterior border, requiring meticulous dissection.

I plan the perichondrial incision based on whether we need a perichondrial graft or not. If perichondrium is needed as a graft material, it is dissected from the whole anterior surface of the rib segment and the remaining perichondrium is carefully dissected from the inferior and superior borders of the rib without forcing to dissect the posterior surface of the perichondrium. If perichondrium resection is not planned as a graft material, then a longitudinal incision is performed that is 1 cm longer than the medial and lateral edges of the required rib segment.

I am using the "Oblique Split Method" (OSM) as a carving method, so the lateral incision is placed obliquely to provide a longer cross-sectional surface.[2] The rib segment needs to be taken as long as possible because ossification areas or other problems decreasing the cartilage quality can be present. The segment that includes the synchondrosis region has a narrow anteroposterior diameter, which is more appropriate for lateral crural reconstruction and produces more predictable results when modifying the straight OSM graft into a slightly curved one for alar wall support.

The segment to be harvested as a graft is precisely cut using an angled saw at the medial and lateral ends. I use "Tastan saw" that was designed specifically for rib harvesting. The purpose of this specially manufactured tool is to enable controlled incisions using the sensory feedback and pressure sensation in our fingertips, similar to the other saws I designed for use in nasal osteotomies (medial, transverse, and lateral nasal osteotomy microsaws) (**Fig. 5**A–D). Additionally, it is particularly helpful when separating the synchondrosis

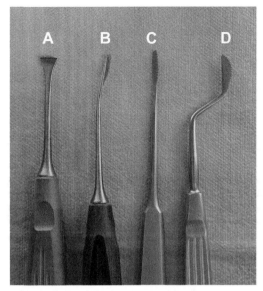

Fig. 5. Tastan saws used for (*A*) Transverse osteotomy, (*B*) Lateral osteotomy, (*C*) Medial osteotomy, and (*D*) Rib harvesting.

regions or when there are ossifications that are hard to cut with a scalpel. Starting rib incision with gentle pressure will allow the teeth to bury themselves in the cartilage tissue, and the incision will be made using back and forth movements. Once the cut is about halfway done, proceed with greater caution and progress in parallel movements with the anterior rib surface until you reach the posterior perichondrium. After both ends are released, the cartilage graft becomes relatively more mobile, making the elevation of the posterior perichondrium easier and safer due to the absence of rib cartilage stability. A blunt tipped, specially designed elevator made of harder steel, which does not bend, is used for the elevation of the posterior perichondrium. In order to reduce the risk of pneumothorax, the aim is therefore to perform posterior perichondrial dissection with less resistance.

The surgical field is filled with saline solution and positive pressure is applied to check pneumothorax (Video 1). Since I do not use a drain, hemostasis should be done carefully. The proper suturing technique is used to repair the perichondrium (4/0 Polydioxanone), muscular fascia (4/0 Polydioxanone), subcutaneous layer (4/0 Polydioxanone), and skin (subcuticular running, 5/0 poliglecaprone 25). The area of the wound is covered with pressure dressing for 3 days. In postoperative follow-up, if you notice any seroma collection, aspirate with an 18-G needle and continue pressure dressing for a few more days.

Robotti

In women, I invariably use an inframammary incision for harvesting rib. Since several years, I moved from the initial concept of looking for the best rib to the decision of always going exactly along the inframammary fold (IMF), then adapting rib selection and exposure to this prerequisite: a least visible access.[3–5] (**Fig. 6**) My technique has essentially been progressively modified from that described by Jack Gunter in 2008.[6] Preliminary palpation will allow the choice of the rib best suited for harvest, corresponding, superior, or inferior to such incision. From personal observation and repeated experience in about 110 to 120 cases per year, I developed and use the following parameters for marking: a vertical line tangential to the medial edge of the areola and carried to the IMF will correspond to the junction between bony and cartilaginous portion of the rib. From that point, the incision is marked extending medially for 2.5 to 3 cm exactly on the fold (**Fig. 7**). It doesn't matter to me which rib that will be: usually it is 5 or 6, depending on the specific anatomy of the rib cage. When a breast implant has been previously placed through the IMF, I will use the same incision, although I usually must extend it a little more medially. My scar will be around 3 cm or even 4 cm on some occasions in heavier patients, but it will hardly be noticeable, especially if 1 or 2 mm of skin at the edges is taken out with a serrated fine scissor at skin closure. This is in fact the portion of skin subject to traction and contusion, and thus more prone to scarring. I understand the benefit of an alternative minimal incision to harvest the seventh rib lower on the chest wall with the additional advantage of preventing the risk of pleural injury, as championed by Toriumi,[7] but, in my perspective, (a) pleural injury should not be a problem if one uses careful technique in harvesting under direct vision, and (b) using such a small access incision will mean considerable traction with retractors as well as a less predictable harvest of the rib segment in continuity with its perichondrium. Such traction may translate in a whitish and wide scar patch, albeit short. The essence is that I want my scar exactly in the IMF. In men, I will look for a native fold in approximately the same position as the IMF in women. In many male patients, especially when you ask them to stand in front of you and relax their posture, you will identify a useable skin crease, and this is where I will place my incision.

Regarding any analysis or diagnostic tool that could address my choice of which rib to take, I do not really find much reason to use any of the multiple described methods, such as walking the needle through the skin to assess calcifications (I actually find this maneuver somewhat perilous) or assessing the correct rib by ultrasound or even by a computed tomography scan. I find these methods unnecessary since I will still go on whatever appropriate rib I find at a reasonable distance from the incision at the fold. Sometimes, this rib will be relatively straight and other times more curved, but I will still use it and then, obviously, laminate it differently. Of course, the rationale of a pre-op analysis is to detect calcifications, but if there are calcifications, they will usually be multiple and essentially unavoidable. My current thinking, stemming from experience, is that they are not necessarily related to the patient's age, at least to a certain degree, while possibly they could be related to the individual's metabolic and nutritional status. If I find calcifications, I will section the rib differently and, in some rare cases, even use a thin-bladed Piezo insert.[8] Calcifications may even become an asset if I want an adequate structure for my L-strut segments. The opposite will hold if I need rib for thin lateral crura struts in rebuilding my lower lateral cartilages. Then, I will try to avoid obviously calcified areas. In those instances, I will also often use composite techniques, in which that part of tip reconstruction is done by the limited quantity of available septum left.

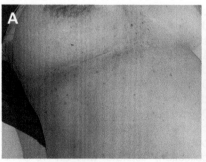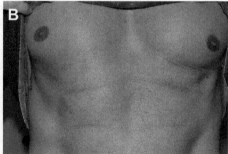

Fig. 6. (*A, B*) The scar following rib harvest at the inframammary fold is usually hardly visible.

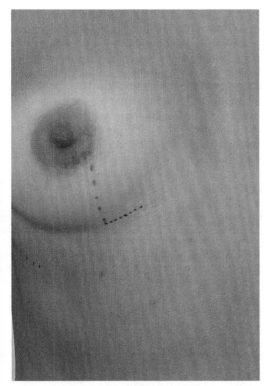

Fig. 7. The markings for where to place the incision for rib harvesting are demonstrated.

Technique

After incising dermis and fat, the superficial fascia becomes visible, and I mark it with methylene blue so as to facilitate its later suturing as a separate layer (Video 2). The fat below is readily visualized, and then, with a sweeping motion of a wide, sharp-edged elevator, the rectus fascia is exposed. This dissection is limited to the planned portion of rectus fascia harvest, as described by Cerkes,[9] in the frequent scenario when rectus fascia is needed later for the sandwich of perichondrium and fascia (SPF)-sandwich of perichondrium, rib lamination, and fascia (SPLF) construct. Usually, a 3 × 3 cm segment of rectus fascia is carefully elevated off the underlying rectus muscle by the use of a fine Bovie tip (**Fig. 8**). The fascia is then cleaned of residual muscle fibers, pinned to a silicone block, set aside for later use, and moistened under wet sponges. At this point, bipolar cautery is used to pre-cauterize some rectus muscle fibers along their direction (thus, almost perpendicularly to the skin incision). A gentle spreading motion then allows separation of the muscle without transecting its fibers, and easy subsequent exposure of the chosen rib segment. A full-thickness segment of rib, usually measuring between 3 and 4 cm, is harvested. The anterior perichondrium is left attached, while the

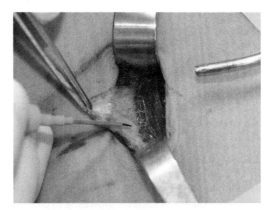

Fig. 8. The rectus muscle is separated along the direction of its fibers to allow rib harvesting, and it is not transected. This essentially respects its integrity.

posterior perichondrium remains on the chest wall. Specific, small right and left rib elevators, personally developed for this purpose (Marina Medical Instruments, West State Road 84 Davie, Florida, US), are used to carefully separate the harvested rib segment from its posterior perichondrium, while the previously used wide sharp-edged elevator or a thin, straight osteotome usually allows division of the rib medially, just away from the bony junction, as well as laterally. The same instrument will allow transection of synchondroses with adjacent ribs. As described by Gerbault,[8] Piezo can find an indication in the infrequent presence of voluminous calcifications that resist transection by the aforesaid instruments. Residual, sharp, palpable, edges at the periphery of the harvested rib segment are then softened by the use of a double-action rongeur. Then, the wound is filled with saline and a Valsalva maneuver performed by the anesthesiologist so as to confirm pleural integrity. Finally, closure is done in independent layers. A total of 7 to 8 mg of ropivacaine (Naropine) is instilled in the wound through a large-bore IV cannula which had been previously positioned in the residual cavity below the muscle repair, the needle is withdrawn, and the catheter is taped to the skin.[3] The excised rib segment is placed over a soft cutting block on a side table, and its anterior perichondrium is peeled off by a large elevator. Then, lamination begins by the use of a hair transplant blade, as will be described later.

As a final note, I find it interesting that patients invariably have quite little pain following rib harvest. I believe that this occurs because, when employing the technique described earlier, the rectus muscle is not split transversally or cauterized, but is essentially gently separated along its fibers, and then simply resutured (see **Fig. 8**). I find no reason to use pain pumps or other strong analgesics. We use an IV catheter which is placed at the end of surgery with around 7 or 8 mL of Naropine instilled, with the same dosage repeated the following morning before the catheter is removed at discharge.

QUESTION 2: DO YOU PERFORM A FULL CROSS SECTION OR PARTIAL HARVEST OF RIB CARTILAGE?
Fedok

I usually perform a partial harvest of the rib. To further clarify, I usually allow a portion of the rib, usually along the inferior medial segment to remain in continuity. I do this because it allows me to procure a sufficient amount of rib cartilage to create the appropriate number of grafts, I need to complete a successful rhinoplasty. In addition, because it limits movement of the chest wall, and coupled with the muscle sparing technique, it eliminates much of the chest wall pain for the patient. In fact, in cases where I have had the need to harvest both ear cartilage and rib cartilage, the patient frequently has found the ear to be more painful than his chest wall. If I need a full thickness amount to be harvested to complete my rhinoplasty tasks, I will remove the rest of the cartilage. I leave the posterior perichondrium down. After retrieving the costal cartilage segment, the wound bed is flooded with saline, and the patient undergoes a Valsalva maneuver to confirm the integrity of the parietal pleura.

Occasionally, I will remove the whole cross section of the rib, particularly when I am preparing a large graft for a dorsal replacement of a severe saddle nose deformity, and loss of structural cartilage.

This technique is easier in the younger patient with softer cartilage, where I can actually harvest the graft after cutting through the rib cartilage, on an angle, with a Freer elevator.

Peng

I always perform a full, en bloc harvest of the rib cartilage. I make sure that the dissection down to the rib cartilage allows for adequate exposure and visualization of the bony cartilaginous junction as well as the synchondrosis. With careful dissection of the superior and inferior edges of the perichondrium, I am able to remove the rib without any issues. I always perform 3 Valsalva maneuvers up to 40 mm Hg to confirm that there are no leaks and no violation of the posterior perichondrium.

Tastan

I perform a full cross-section harvest of rib segment because I am using the OSM for carving the rib grafts. As stated in the OSM, the graft obtained

from the cross-sectional surface of the rib is in balance in terms of the effecting forces. During partial harvesting of a layer from the anterior surface of the rib, there may be microfractures in the cartilage tissue and may damage the equilibrium of forces. I use the peripheral layer of the rib in onlay tip grafting to support the external nasal valve, for alar rim grafting, or for diced cartilage grafts.

It is better to keep in mind that the structural characteristics of rib cartilage may vary from patient to patient. For example, if there are gaps in the cartilage, the details of carving have to change accordingly (Video 3).

Robotti

The answer to this is never. I don't really understand why this should be done. If the decision is taken to harvest the rib, one should gain the maximum advantage. This means taking a full-thickness portion of rib from which (a) multiple laminations can be derived of different thickness length so as to provide an ample manual of choice, (b) perichondrium can be harvested along the anterior surface, usually for my SPF-SPLF construct[10] (c) the white peripheral portion can be used for deriving a plaster-like substance which we denominated "rib plaster" and which is, once one tries it clinically, immediately, and evidently superior to diced cartilage.[11]

The prerequisite thus becomes having enough material to do what is needed, regarding rebuilding the L-strut in its vertical and horizontal components as well as fashioning lateral crura struts for the tip, using perichondrium for dorsal camouflage or as an ingredient of the SPF-SPLF graft and, not least, having further substance from which to derive "rib plaster". If one performs a partial harvest, be it in a wedge shape or by bisecting the rib anteriorly, one may feel that the approach is safer regarding a possible pneumothorax, but this carries a substantial limitation since one will end up with a few segments which may not be optimal or may not be enough. Specifically regarding the risk of pneumothorax, I think it can be avoided entirely (no instances in all my experience so far) by careful technique, as I detailed earlier. Finally, if one would do a partial rib harvest, the initial steps needed for exposure and the donor site closure would be essentially the same. Not much to be gained, and quite a lot to be lost for a little extra security.

QUESTION 3: WHAT ARE YOUR INDICATIONS IN PRIMARY RHINOPLASTY
Fedok

My indications for the use of rib grafting in primary rhinoplasty are quite limited. The patients where I would decide to use rib cartilage as the source of donor material are those patients who will require a large amount of cartilage grafting. In addition, it is anticipated that the amount necessary will be beyond what is reasonable to be able to be harvested from their septum and ears. These situations include patients who have suffered a loss in the amount of septal cartilage available because of previous septoplasty, septal perforation, and infection. They may present with saddle nose deformity. If patients have had previous trauma or a severely deviated septum, the septal deformity may preclude the use of septal cartilage, so that another source is necessary. Patients with variations of Binder syndrome or other growth disturbance may prevent there to be an adequate amount of septal cartilage. In some patients of Asian derivation or with markedly platyrrhine noses, there may be insufficient donor sources except for the rib.

In summary, patient who presents with nasal anatomy that requires a large amount of cartilage grafting to be performed, and presentswithout a sufficient amount of septal or ear donor material, I will go immediately to the chess wall. In this way, I prevent harvesting inadequate amounts of grafting materials from the septum and ears and then encountering problems during the procedure.

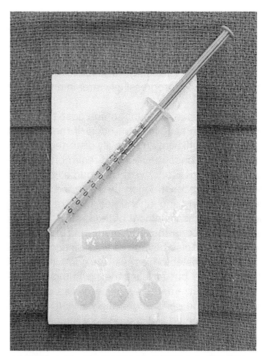

Fig. 9. Dorsal onlay graft made with ultra-finely diced cartilage with droplets of fibrin glue.

Peng

I will often use rib cartilage during a primary rhinoplasty when there is insufficient cartilage from the septum itself such as.

- Smaller native septal cartilage as often is the case in Asian, Black, or Hispanic noses
- Need for dorsal augmentation during which I will dice the cartilage very finely and use fibrin glue in order to make a dorsal onlay graft **(Fig. 9)**
- Need to multiple grafts for nasal reconstruction such as internal and external nasal valve collapse or need for a strong caudal septal extension graft

Tastan

The primary reason for using rib cartilage in primary rhinoplasty is the depletion of cartilage. The following patient groups are candidates for rib cartilage grafting: septoplasty or severe trauma history, caudal septum depleted patients, severely crooked nose, short nose, saddle nose, ethnic nose, patients having thick skin and weak cartilage, etc. Also, patients having dynamic alar collapse are prone to have graft material that is inadequate in dimension and resistance.

Even though there may be certain indications for rib cartilage harvesting, sometimes predicting this can be challenging. When in doubt, informing the patient about it will help you feel more comfortable during the surgery if you need rib cartilage.

Robotti

Currently, practically none. I touched briefly on this when answering some questions in the other section of this Clinics issue regarding the management of the middle vault in primary rhinoplasty. The reason is my progressive adoption, however, with several modifications, of preservation techniques in managing the dorsum. Even in asymmetric midvaults I can still "play" by preserving the dorsal keystone area (DKA) by my modified dorsal-split cartilaginous pushdown or full letdown approach.[12] If I still need grafting at that point, it would be for very small spreader/s to even out asymmetries between the 2 sides, which will be placed in a pedestal fashion between the upper laterals and the septal border of the septal T. Most patients have far enough cartilage for this. Another important fact is that, since I have adopted the use of long Piezo inserts for harvesting a single piece of septum, usually in a composite fashion, including a portion of the quadrangular plate and perpendicular plate of ethmoid, while leaving a proper L-strut, I use my harvested septum productively, without waste or piecemeal combination of scarcely useable segments. This makes taking rib usually unnecessary.

Of course, there may still be exceptions, although they are progressively rarer in my current practice.

A different situation is that of the post-traumatic nose, in which saddling can occur if the residual septum is insufficient and heavily distorted. I place these cases conceptually in the realm of secondary rhinoplasties and yes, of course, they will need dorsal reconstruction by extended or staggered spreaders and, oftentimes, need reconstitution of the vertical element of the L-strut. Rib may well be needed in these cases (**Fig. 10**). Usually, bone work will also be required, consisting in osteoplasty and osteotomies, with a combination of Piezo or burr, but at least the tip, although distorted and asymmetric because of the deviated septum, will be per se consisting of native lateral crura to be treated like in a primary rhinoplasty.

QUESTION 4: WHAT INSTRUMENTS DO YOU USE?
Fedok

As stated in the previous section, I use a paucity of instruments to accomplish harvesting of rib cartilage for rhinoplasty. The instruments I commonly use include a 10 or 5 scalpel, an Army-and-Navy retractor, a Senne retractor, a Freer elevator, and Adson and Cobb elevators. Rarely will I use a Doyen retractor.

Peng

I have curated rib tray set that I put together in conjunction with Black and Black surgical (**Fig. 11**). which contain very small instruments to facilitate with a tiny incision. The Senn retractors are 5 mm wide and 22 mm in length. I use a small cottle with round sharp edges. The larger side is 5 mm in diameter and the smaller side is 2.5 mm in diameter. The smaller end can be used to cut through calcifications. I also do all of my dissections with a mosquito to decrease the instrument footprint and allow for a smaller incision.

Tastan

The surgical instruments I use for harvesting rib cartilage and carving cartilage grafts are as follows: specially designed saws, elevators, dermatome blade, No: 15 and 11 blade, forceps, needle holder, retractors, scissors, and monopolar cautery.

The instruments worth discussing are specially designed saws, elevators, and dermatome blade that I have been using for more than 10 years. The purpose of specially designed saws is to harvest rib cartilage with minimal damage to the tissues. Tastan rib harvesting saw enables controlled incisions using the touch and pressure sensation in our fingers similar to the other saws I designed for use in nasal osteotomies. It is easy and safe to cut the rib segment from medial and lateral ends as well as synchondrosis region with this saw under binocular vision, bimanual work. Also, in certain cases where rib cartilage is

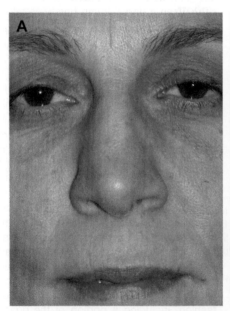
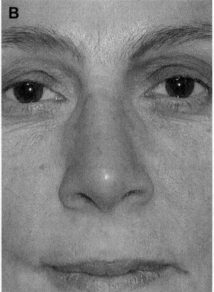

Fig. 10. (*A, B*) Pre-zoomed and post-zoomed frontal view demonstrating reconstitution of the dorsum and aesthetic dorsal lines by L-strut reconstruction by rib grafting in a post-traumatic nose. An SPF graft has reestablished the contour.

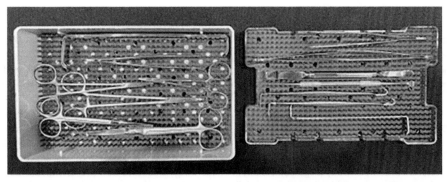

Fig. 11. Peng Rib Tray by Black and Black contains very small sens retractors as well as a small Peng elevator which is a double-sided elevator with 1 tiny oval side and 1 small round side. Both have very sharp edges to help with elevation and cutting through rib cartilage itself.

ossified, it is difficult to incise the cartilage and it would be better to use the saw in these circumstances. After all attachments of the segment are released, it becomes relatively more mobile, making the elevation of the posterior perichondrium safer in order to reduce the risk of pneumothorax.

For the elevators, any kind of blunt tip perichondrium elevator is suitable for anterior surface perichondrium dissection. However, it is necessary to use a blunt-tipped curved elevator to dissect the perichondrium from the posterior surface of the rib segment. In order to prevent unwanted damage to the posterior perichondrium, this elevator needs to be sufficiently strong and rigid (**Fig. 12**A–C).

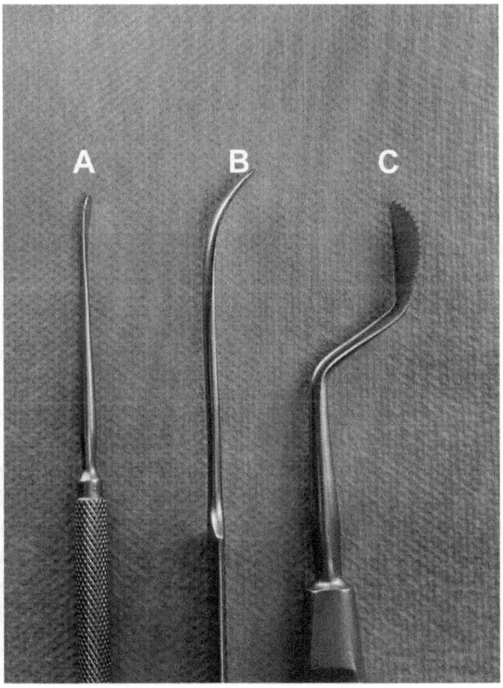

I recommend using a dermatome blade when preparing cartilage grafts from rib cartilage (Video 4). It is crucial to achieve a smooth graft surface to ensure equilibrium between inner and outer zone forces. Thus, it would be more suitable to use a sharp dermatome blade rather than a scalpel. Grafts prepared with a scalpel often exhibit surface irregularities, affecting the balance of forces and can lead to bending. When using a dermatome blade, it is important to pay attention to the sharp edge and alignment. Specialized handles can be used if necessary.

If there are areas of ossification within the rib cartilage, it may be difficult to use the dermatome blade. In such cases, manual straight micro saw for medial osteotomy, or electric powered saws can be used. If the rib is ossified, shaping the OSM graft with a diamond burr is preferable for dorsal onlay graft preparation.

Robotti

Let us go back to the technique to answer this question. I will highlight the instruments I use in italics:

After skin incision, delineation of the superficial fascia (marked with methylene blue for later re-suturing to avoid contour depression), and its transection, the correct plane on the rectus fascia is easily visualized. A wide sharp-edged elevator is used in a sweeping motion to expose the fascia and some perforators are treated by bipolar before they can retract. The rectus fascia is then harvested by a Valleylab Bovie tip. The rectus muscle is exposed and muscle fibers are first pretreated by a nonstick bipolar tip and then gently splayed in a longitudinal direction which follows their anatomy. Once the fibers are split without transecting them, 2 army-navy retractors are used to gain

Fig. 12. Surgical instruments for dissection of perichondrium. (*A*) Perichondrium elevator, (*B*) specially designed posterior surface perichondrium elevator, (*C*) Tastan rib harvesting saw.

exposure to the readily seen rib. Then, a sharp-edged wide elevator is used to define the edges of the perichondrium on the anterior surface of the rib and the same elevator is worked laterally on both sides to gain access to the posterior surface of the rib, with the posterior perichondrium is left attached to the chest wall. Customized small right and left rib elevators, personally developed for this purpose (Marina Medical Instruments, West State Road 84 Davie, Florida, US), are then used to dissect the harvested segment from its posterior perichondrium carefully (**Fig. 13**). Finally, the rib will need transection of both ends, usually done by a straight 4-mm osteotome. Only in the occasional cases in which a sizable calcification is encountered, Piezo is used for the same purpose.

QUESTION 5: WHAT CARTILAGE CARVING TECHNIQUES DO YOU USE?
Fedok

I harvest the rib cartilage early in the rhinoplasty procedure so that the rib can be observed for up to 20 to 30 minutes for warping after the initial harvest. In that way, I can be preparing the nose and gain my exposure while the rib is already harvested. I do not wait and watch the rib. I am doing something else while the rib is on the back table. My technique is relatively simple. I use a paucity of instruments for carving. After the rib cartilage is harvested, I place it in saline on the back table. I remove the perichondrium from the entire harvest most of the time since most of the time I will not be using a large thick graft. For the next 10 or 15 minutes, I allow the graft to be subject to some of its internal stresses so I can ascertain in what plane or vector the harvest will warp. I do additional

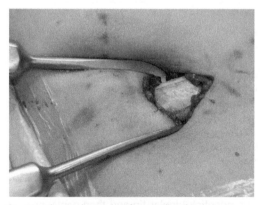

Fig. 13. The Right and Left specific rib elevators are shown. Their curvature serves well to dissect the posterior surface of the rib from its perichondrium, which will be left attached to the chest wall.

exposure tasks or prepare the recipient sites while the rib is processed.

I carve the cartilage either on a plastic carving block or on a small stack of blue towels depending on the facility. The cartilage is carved using a sharp, frequently changed #10 scalpel. The cartilage is held with a Kocher clamp and forceps. The cartilage is carved in the plane that takes advantage of the plane the graft is warping in. I usually carve my grafts in stages, so I will first carve the cut the block of cartilage in half along its long axis and let the 2 halves demonstrate how they will warp. I might do that several times. Eventually, I will carve the larger cartilage harvest into the number and dimensions of cartilage grafts that are useful for the procedure. Typically, the grafts are thin, usually no thicker than 1.5 mm to 2 mm. As this is done in stages, I can usually obtain grafts that are suitable and that do not warp in the patient's nose (**Figs. 14** and **15**).

Most the time I am in need of several types of "grafts": spreader grafts, extended spreader grafts, septal extension grafts, septal replacement grafts, dorsal grafts, among others. Even with significant saddles, it is rare for me to use thick grafts anymore. Most of the grafts are the thicknesses described.

Peng

I like to carve cartilage in accordance with the lie of the cartilage using straight blades on a chopping board. There is usually 1 side, either anterior or posterior where the cartilage lies flatter and with less movement on the cutting board (**Fig. 16**). Then, depending on the size of the grafts needed, I will angle my eccentric cuts. The outer portions of cut rib cartilage will always have a higher chance of warping compared to the ones more in the center. The center pieces I always save for caudal septal extension grafts and leave the outer pieces for other grafts.

Tastan

Rhinoplasty is the process of disrupting the current balance of forces and establishing a new balance. To reconstruct a new balance, it is essential to understand the cartilage behavior and equilibrium of effecting forces. Since rib cartilage is a unique tissue by nature, each patient's cartilage is of a distinctive quality; ossification, internal structure, texture, homogeneity, dimension, shape, and other characteristics may vary from patient to patient. In rhinoplasty, straight cartilage grafts of various thicknesses are required. The equilibrium of forces is altered when a rib segment is carved to obtain cartilage grafts.

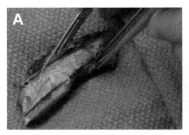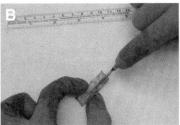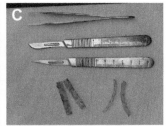

Fig. 14. (*A, B*) Carving of the harvested costal cartilage into large segments devoid of perichondrium. (*C*) Prospective grafts showing tendency to warp, thus noting magnitude and direction. (*From* Fedok FG. Costal Cartilage Grafts in Rhinoplasty. Clin Plast Surg. Jan 2016;43(1):201-212, Figure 11.)

Gibson and Davis reported that the warping of the cartilage is caused by a difference in tension between the outermost layers of cartilage and the inner zone.[13] An intact rib segment has these forces nicely balanced to preserve a stable shape. The matrix tends to expand when cut or carved, whereas the outer stretched layer contracts; therefore, warping occurs.

We can section the rib in 3 different planes; one is parallel to longitudinal axis along superior-inferior direction (SID), other one is parallel to longitudinal axis along anterior-posterior direction (APD), and the last one is crossing the longitudinal axis for to utilize cross section of the rib which is called "Oblique Split Method (OSM)."

The OSM provides a complete rib segment with an intact surface layer in which the diametrically opposed forces are equal and can easily be carved according to the principle of the balanced cross section also.

The cross section of the rib will result in a graft with equal circumferential forces of contracture, and we can also speculate that the cell groups at one cross-sectional surface are in continuous at the other surface, so the forces are balancing each other. Carving the rib at narrower angles to

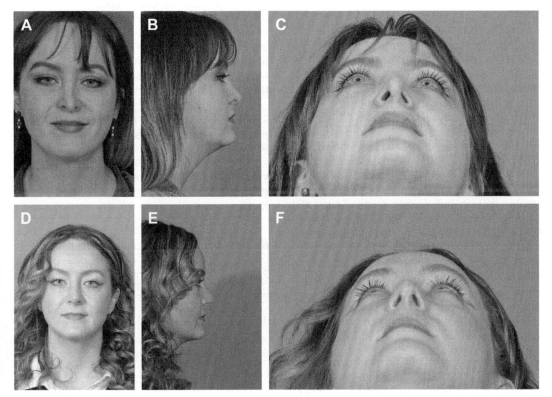

Fig. 15. (*A–C*) Preoperative images of a patient seen for revision rhinoplasty with insufficient septal cartilage. (*D–F*) Postoperative images of the patient after revision rhinoplasty via open approach and use of sixth rib costal cartilage to place a caudal septal extension graft, bilateral extended spreader grafts, and the placement of bilateral alar contour grafts.

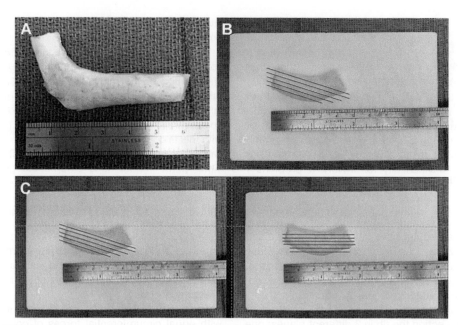

Fig. 16. (*A*) Orientation of rib cartilage. It is either anterior on top and posterior on bottom or anterior on bottom and posterior on top. This depends on how well it lies on the cutting board and the orientation, which will allow less movement while cutting. The goal is for it to lie as flat as possible so that cutting will be more precise. (*B*) Orientation of the cuts depends on the lengths of the grafts you need. (*C*) Other possible orientation.

obtain longer cartilage grafts does not effect the equilibrium of forces.

The elliptical OSM grafts maintain their straight shape even after being transformed into rectangular grafts because the contracting forces are in balance. By considering the equilibrium of forces, it may be possible to carve the grafts asymmetrically or bevel the edges meticulously.

All the frequently used grafts in rhinoplasty (spreader, columellar strut, caudal extension, alar batten, shield and cap grafts, to name a few) can be obtained from a single OSM graft. It is necessary to reconstruct the L-strut segmentally, using both the dorsal and caudal struts. Segmental reconstruction enables fine adjustment of height of the reconstructed septum and provides consistent results.

A dorsal onlay graft can be carved from a single OSM graft in almost all cases. If needed, 2 cartilage grafts can be sutured end to end, side by side, or by overlapping manner after the edges have been modified. Costal perichondrium may be sutured over the dorsal onlay graft to camouflage and for soft tissue padding.

Cartilage grafts used in rhinoplasty are typically straight in shape. If necessary, curved grafts for lateral crural reconstruction can be prepared from a straight OSM graft by beveling the edges.

It presents a challenge to the surgeon to deliver thin, straight grafts in patients with depleted septal cartilage. The OSM is unique in that it provides straight grafts as thin as septal cartilage or even in paper thickness. Additionally, because the OSM graft contains both the central and peripheral rib zones, a significant amount of graft material can be obtained from a given volume of costal cartilage.

I have been using this innovative method for costal cartilage graft carving for the past 17 years, and the OSM consistently produces reliable long-term outcomes.

Costal cartilage grafts carved with the OSM provide grafts that are at the intended thickness, even less than 1 mm, and they preserve their straight form.

Robotti

My concept essentially is that of deriving multiple laminations from a specific full-thickness rib segment, usually measuring 3 to 4 cm in length so that I can have an extensive "rib menu" from which to derive the segments I need for specific applications. Those applications consist of (a) extended or staggered rib spreaders for the horizontal portion of the L-strut, (b) smaller segments which can be used as bilateral splints, for instance, for a septal extension graft or to strengthen the vertical segment of the L-strut, (c) a segment to be used as vertical L-strut in combination with the residual septum, if available, and, lastly, (d) thin rib laminations to be used as lateral crura struts to splint residual lateral crura segments, or to replace them in toto.

It stands to reason that I need multiple choices and an array of options to derive the best segments for a specific purpose. This is why I never do a segmental rib harvest, as I explained earlier, but I always use a single whole piece. After harvesting, I first remove the perichondrium from the anterior surface, which I will often use as an ingredient of my SPF-SPLF graft, and then lamination begins. As well as making longitudinal segments, I also laminate a few segments perpendicular to the long axis of the rib: those will measure around 1 to 5 cm and can often be used as small splinting elements, for instance, bilateral support for a septal extension graft. For laminating the rib, I use a hair transplant disposable knife, which allows me the benefit of a solid handle and ideal width of the cutting portion of the blade (**Fig. 17**). Notably, a non-slippery rubber or silicone board should be used.

Regarding the direction of subsequent lamination, I have no absolute preference regarding concentric carving or other options.[14,15] What I essentially do is to observe the rib. It may be more or less straight, or curved, or wider on 1 side. After evaluating it, I form the impression of where the straightest segment would lie, and then I proceed with the first cuts. Those will be longitudinal or often obliquely oriented. Cutting obliquely, as described by Tastan,[16] is definitely beneficial in avoiding warping. I deliberately take some thicker and thinner pieces and mark them differently. In the past, I constantly used to try and achieve long rib segments, measuring up to 4 cm, but over the recent years I have often turned to using shorter segments which I will then employ in a staggered fashion for my horizontal L-strut reconstruction (**Fig. 18**). As I said previously, I will also derive some short, transverse laminations, prevalently perpendicular to the axis of the rib (**Fig. 19**). I mark the segments as I cut them with

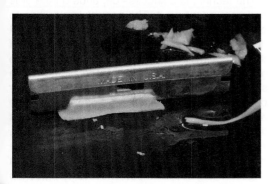

Fig. 17. A hair transplant knife is well-suited for laminating rib.

different symbols so as to identify later which options I have for spreaders (which obviously will be wider and more robust, and here calcifications may actually be of help) or, for instance, for lateral crura struts. Obviously, there is a learning curve. There is also a kind personal feel, which will come in time together with experience.

QUESTION 6: HAVE YOUR TECHNIQUES CHANGED IN THE LAST 2 YEARS?
Fedok

In the last 2 years, my technique has not changed at all. What have changed over the 10 years are the modifications to lessen pain and minimize dissection.

Peng

Have not had any changes over the last 2 years.

Tastan

OSM is a reliable technique we have been using confidently with our colleagues for years.

In the past 2 years, I have not made any changes to my technique for harvesting and carving the rib and preparing cartilage grafts. OSM provides straight grafts in varying thicknesses and the OSM grafts preserve their straight form at long postoperative period (Video 5).

Among the technical details that have changed in the last 5 to 10 years, I can mention that I use intact cartilage grafts instead of diced cartilage to provide more defined dorsal aesthetic lines. Additionally, due to variations in absorption rates, diced cartilage might not provide consistent results. I also prefer the cortex portion of the rib segment as a onlay tip graft due to higher suture security and flexibility.

Robotti

My techniques regarding using rib in secondary rhinoplasty have changed both concerning principles and practice. Also, because of several specific modifications, the premise is that I use rib in over 80% of my secondary cases, which constitute about more than 50% of my exclusively rhinoplasty practice.

Regarding principles, I could say that the major change has been to try and apply finesse concepts in a rib harvesting and application. This means that I take my time in laminating the segment of full-thickness rib, which I have harvested and pre-plan segments for the applications I will need, considering that I want multiple choices available. In practical terms, it means deriving the thinnest segment which will do its job, meaning that will

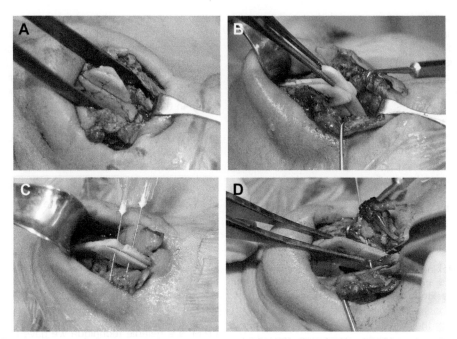

Fig. 18. (*A–D*) Different configurations of L strut reconstruction with rib Laminas of different length and thickness are shown. These are just a few examples of the many combinations possible.

be sturdy enough for the application it should serve. I learned this the hard way over the last years, since initially I was overgrafting and my grafts were essentially rather big. I changed this in time, now striking a proper balance between the function of support and the aesthetics of refined shape that patients desire.

Regarding techniques, I must again go beyond the 2 years stated in the question. The game-changer for me has been the SPF-SPLF graft for dorsal reconstruction graft for dorsal reconstruction. After first progressively tailoring and customizing the DCF (diced cartilage fascia) construct,[4,5] we then abandoned the DCF entirely and started,

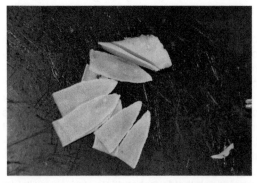

Fig. 19. Short transverse segments are derived by cutting the rib perpendicularly (or with some obliquity) to its axis.

since 2017, using varying combinations of Perichondrium, Fascia, and rib Laminations.[10]

The acronym SPF means "Sandwich of Perichondrium and Fascia," and consists of a layer of perichondrium at the bottom (which will be placed on the dorsal plateau in the same orientation as it originally had on the rib) together with a layer rectus fascia at the top, again oriented in the same way as it originally was in the rectus muscle (**Fig. 20**). Precise measurements are again essential.

The acronym SPL F means "Sandwich of Perichondrium, (rib) Lamina and Fascia" and consists of the addition, between the layers of an SPF as described earlier, of a straight or mildly convex, thin, and precisely constructed rib lamina gently beveled at is sides (**Fig. 21**).

The technique's success depends on the time and care spent on it. The correct lamina has to be chosen and it has to be reshaped to exact desired measurements of length and width. If there is a mild convexity to the shape of the graft, the convexity will be placed facing up. In some instances, its width will be slightly greater between the upper third and distal thirds of the nose, so as to allow a mild trapezoid shape of the dorsum such as desirable in male patients. The lamina has to precisely fit between the perichondrium and fascia juxtaposed layers, like a finger in a glove, without excess. The overlap at each side, where the perichondrium edge meets the rectus fascia's edge, must be stitched

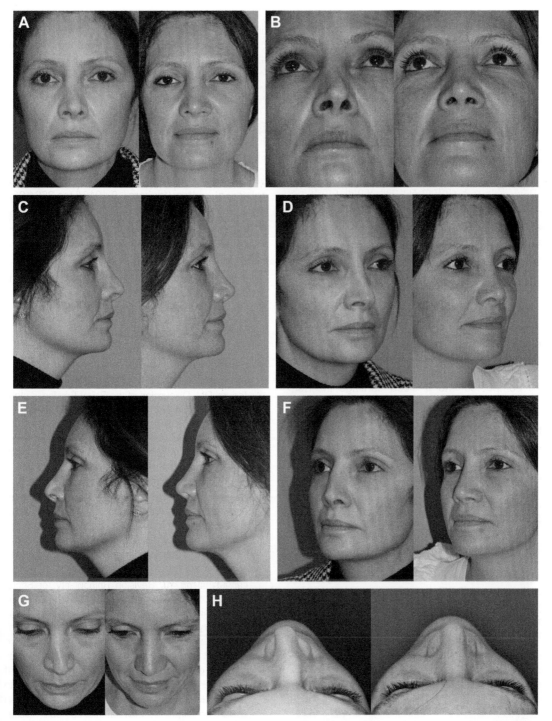

Fig. 20. (*A–H*) An example of aesthetic dorsal reconstruction with an SPLF graft in a secondary rhinoplasty patient.

precisely (Video 6). This tissue fringe will then serve for fixation to the residual edge of the upper lateral cartilages on either side. A transosseous bony cerclage suture, will then be placed proximally and override the construct without undue compression so as to avoid any lateral shift at the radix. This is the same "transcutaneous transosseous cerclage (TTC) suture" as described by Gubisch and Haack,[17] that I invariably use for solid fixation between rib spreaders

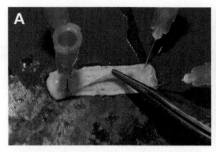
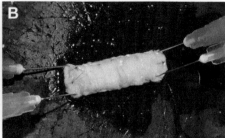

Fig. 21. (*A, B*) The SPLF construct consists of a Sandwich of Perichondrium, rib Lamina, and Fascia.

and proximal bone after custom slots have been configurated by Piezo. Should it be necessary, another lamination can be added, although it is best sutured to the previous one separately on the table. Alternatively, some finely diced cartilage can also be carefully inserted, via the distal edge of the construct left open until final assessment of the augmentation required.

Over the last 2 years, we have, however, substituted diced cartilage with "Rib Plaster" specifically derived by scraping the wide peripheral portion of the remaining rib after the perichondrium is removed and laminations done.[11] This is a putty-like substance with unique properties and can be well compacted into a diced cartilage inserter, smoothly injected, and is easily moldable (Video 7).

However, over the last couple of years, we have also implemented other variations, since we originally in the SPF-SPLF technique. Those consist in a lateral fringe from the fascia to adapt to the lower upper lateral cartilages, in double laminations, when necessary, in addition of rib cartilage plaster, in a fascial extension for the radix to avoid any step off (**Fig. 22**).

I now believe that the SPLF-SPF construct has allowed me to achieve the really natural-looking dorsum, which we had sought for so many years, and which is not equally unachievable by diced cartilage fascia (DCF) construct or, in my opinion, by solid rib. This construct will attach solidly to the underlying dorsal structure by virtue of its perichondrium, and it will resemble a native dorsum if

well-crafted and precisely sutured (see **Fig. 20**). On this topic, we are now completing a paper summarizing the possible modifications, but the striking element is that we have observed no warping whatsoever in over 300 cases done at the time of this writing.

SUPPLEMENTARY DATA

Supplementary data related to this article can be found online at https://doi.org/10.1016/j.fsc.2024.06.009.

REFERENCES

1. Fedok FG. Costal cartilage grafts in rhinoplasty. Clin Plast Surg 2016;43(1):201–12.
2. Taştan E, Yücel ÖT, Aydin E, et al. The oblique split method: a novel technique for carving costal cartilage grafts. JAMA Facial Plast Surg 2013 May; 15(3):198–203.
3. Robotti E, Penna WB. Current practical concepts for using rib in secondary rhinoplasty facial. Plast Surg 2019 Feb;35(1):31–46.
4. Robotti E. Rhinoplasty. In: Cohen M, Thaller S, editors. The unfavorable result in plastic surgery: avoidance and treatment. 4th edition. New York: Thieme; 2018. Chapter 23.
5. Robotti E. The role of preoperative planning in secondary rhinoplasty. In: Rohrich R, Ahmad J, editors. Secondary rhinoplasty by the global masters. Boca Raton, FL: Thieme CRC Press; 2016. p. 1–1816.
6. Marin VP, Landecker A, Gunter JP. Harvesting rib cartilage grafts for secondary rhinoplasty. Plast Reconstr Surg 2008;121(04):1442–8.
7. Toriumi DM. Dorsal augmentation using autologous costal cartilage or Microfat-infused soft tissue augmentation. Facial Plast Surg 2017;33(02):162–78.
8. Gerbault O, Daniel RK, Kosins AM. The role of piezoelectric instrumentation in rhinoplasty surgery. Aesthet Surg J 2016 Jan;36(1):21–34.
9. Cerkes N, Basaran K. Diced cartilage grafts wrapped in rectus abdominis fascia for nasal dorsum augmentation. Plast Reconstr Surg 2016;137(01): 43–51.

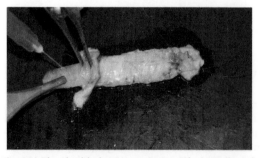

Fig. 22. The double lamina variation of an SPLF graft is shown.

10. Robotti E, Leone F. The SPF-SPLF Graft: building the ideal dorsum in revision rhinoplasty. Plast Reconstr Surg 2020 Jun;145(6):1420–4.

11. Robotti E, Leone F, Malfussi V, et al. RIB plaster: a versatile, moldable derivative from scraping the periphery of the rib. Plast Reconstr Surg 2024;154(1):85e–9e.

12. Robotti E, Cottone G, Leone F. Modified dorsal split preservation hybrid rhinoplasty for cartilaginous pushdown and full letdown applications: A PROM-Based Review of 100 Consecutive Cases. Facial Plast Surg 2023 Aug;39(4):441–51.

13. Gibson T, Davis WB. The distortion of autogenous cartilage grafts: Its cause and prevention. Br J Plast Surg 1958;10:257–73.

14. Rosenberger ES, Toriumi DM. Controversies in revision rhinoplasty. Facial Plast Surg Clin North Am 2016;24(03):337–45.

15. Farkas JP, Lee MR, Lakianhi C, et al. Effects of carving plane, level of harvest, and oppositional suturing techniques on costal cartilage warping. Plast Reconstr Surg 2013;132(02):319–25.

16. Taştan E, Yücel ÖT, Aydin E, et al. The oblique split method: a novel technique for carving costal cartilage grafts. JAMA Facial Plast Surg 2013;15(03):198–203.

17. Rezaeian F, GubischW Janku D, Haack S. New suturing techniques to reconstruct the keystone area in extracorporeal septoplasty. Plast Reconstr Surg 2016;138(02):374–82.

Dorsal Preservation Rhinoplasty

Jose Carlos Neves, MD[a,b,c],*, Dean M. Toriumi, MD[a,d], Abdülkadir Göksel, MD[a,e]

KEYWORDS

- Dorsal preservation rhinoplasty • Surface dorsal techniques • Preservation impaction techniques
- Subdorsal flap techniques • Low strip technique

KEY POINTS

- Preservation rhinoplasty effectiveness can be enhanced with techniques like the Ballerina maneuver and the Dorsal Aesthtetic Lines split maneuver.
- Potential drawbacks like residual humps, radix drop, supra-tip saddling, and post-surgical nasal deviation can be addressed by choosing patients carefully and having a clear knowledge of the nasal and septal anatomy.
- Dorsal preservation techniques preserve the integrity of the middle cartilaginous vault leaving more available septal cartilage for structural grafting in the nasal tip.

PANEL DISCUSSION

In what patients is preservation rhinoplasty indicated, when is it not indicated?
How to decide on the proper technique?
How can I safely introduce dorsal preservation techniques in my surgical armamentarium?
Do I need any special surgical instruments?
How can I prevent complications?
How have your techniques in this area changed over the last 2 years?

QUESTION 1. IN WHAT PATIENTS IS PRESERVATION RHINOPLASTY INDICATED, WHEN IS IT NOT INDICATED?
Neves

At the outset of my career, I was fortunate to receive a fellowship under Wilson Dewes in 2007, who predominantly employed conservative approaches to the dorsum. He meticulously tailored his techniques to maintain the dorsal anatomy across various nasal types, utilizing push/let down concepts for the lateral wall and SPAR A (high strip) and SPAR B (low strip) techniques for the septal wall.[1] This methodology supports the assertion that nearly all patients are candidates for preservation rhinoplasty (PR).

Transitioning back to my own practice, I experienced varying degrees of success with dorsal PR. During certain periods, I predominantly performed PR, while at other times I focused on structural rhinoplasty, influenced by the challenges and limitations encountered in both approaches. As the principles of PR evolved, the introduction of new tools and techniques has facilitated more precise and detailed outcomes. Consequently, some conditions that were once considered absolute contraindications for PR are no longer viewed as such in light of these advancements.

However, there continue to be optimal indications for the preservation of the nasal dorsum, as well as situations that we still consider best avoided in this approach, clearly depending on the strategy and surgical experience with PR.

[a] Toriumi Facial Plastics, 60 East Delaware Place, Suite 1425, Chicago, IL 60611, USA; [b] International and European Board Certified in Facial Plastic and Reconstructive Surgery (IBCFPRS - EBCFPRS); [c] Facial Plastic Surgery, MYFACE, Clinic and Academy, Lisbon, Portugal; [d] Department of Otolaryngology–Head & Neck Surgery, Rush University Medical School, Chicago, IL, USA; [e] Rino Istanbul Facial Plastic Clinic, Istanbul, Turkey
* Corresponding author. Facial Plastic Surgery, MYFACE, Clinic and Academy, Lisbon, Portugal; Toriumi Facial Plastics, 60 East Delaware Place, Suite 1425, Chicago, IL 60611.
E-mail address: jcneves@myface.pt

Facial Plast Surg Clin N Am 32 (2024) 585–602
https://doi.org/10.1016/j.fsc.2024.06.010
1064-7406/24/© 2024 Elsevier Inc. All rights are reserved, including those for text and data mining, AI training, and similar technologies.

For optimal indications, I would say that these include noses with a projected dorsum requiring deprojection but with little curvature, minimal angulation at the rhinion; without a low radix; without a low supratip; with well-defined dorsal aesthetic lines (DAL), ideally of proper width; and tension noses. Noses exhibiting lateralization are considered ideal for this approach since it involves mobilizing the entire structure to center it along the midline. In techniques that disarticulate the cartilaginous septum from the perpendicular ethmoidal plate (such as the Low-Strip approach or Tetris 3), this maneuver is particularly powerful. However, in the initial stages of the learning curve, the greater complexity of this approach may be a reason for hesitancy, as is often expressed by some colleagues. Therefore, a straight nose would be an excellent indication for PR, particularly in the early stages of learning.

Indications that require greater expertise include, beyond greater lateralization of the pyramid, a nose with more than 1 axis of deviation (S shape deviations); a wide nose in which DAL need to be redefined; a nose with a low radix or low supratip; and a nose with a highly angled rhinion.

Today, I categorize as a potential contraindication the presence of a traumatic nose that exhibits numerous surface irregularities or depressions in the bone or cartilage, as well as a septum with multiple fracture lines. In such cases, re-establishing a new central structure over which the lateral nasal wall reconstruction is to be conducted might be considered a preferable option. Certainly, in circumstances where there has been previous surgical intervention, such as septoplasty or rhinoplasty, we often find conditions that contraindicate a preservation approach.

Toriumi

I started using dorsal preservation in June of 2019. In the beginning, I was very selective in the patients that I chose for dorsal preservation.[2] I selected patients with a V-shaped dorsal hump and straight nose. These are ideal patients for starting dorsal preservation. After performing my first 20 dorsal preservation cases, I used the high strip, subdorsal Z-flap, and low strip (Cottle or SPQR). My comfort level increased significantly in the first 20 cases. I eventually incorporated the Tetris as introduced by Jose Carlos Neves and other techniques such as the spare roof type B.[3,4] As I gained more experience, my indications for using dorsal preservation expanded to most all primaries including; crooked noses and patients with S-shaped dorsal humps.

The deviated nose is an ideal indication for dorsal preservation. Preservation techniques are particularly helpful in patients with an axis deviation of their nasal dorsum (**Fig. 1**).

I started using a subdorsal grafting technique to correct the saddle nose deformity and also to augment the low nasal dorsum. Initially, I used

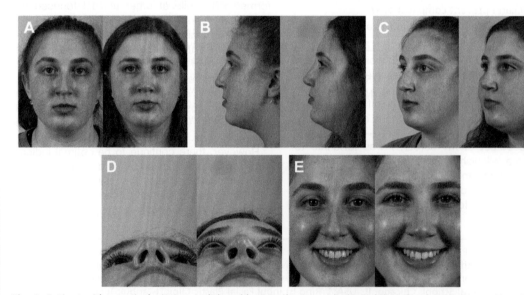

Fig. 1. Patient with an axis deviation and dorsal hump. She is an ideal candidate for dorsal preservation. In this case an overlapping subdorsal Z-flap was used to straighten her nose and reduce her dorsal hump. (*A*) Preoperative frontal view showing deviated nose (*left*). 1 year postoperative frontal view showing straight nose (*right*). (*B*) Preoperative lateral view (*left*). Postoperative lateral view showing straight dorsum (*right*). (*C*) Preoperative oblique view (*left*). Postoperative oblique view (*right*). (*D*) Preoperative base view (*left*). Postoperative base view (*right*). (*E*) Preoperative smiling frontal view (*left*). Postoperative smiling frontal view (*right*).

subdorsal spreader grafts and then progressed to using a subdorsal cantilever graft to augment the dorsum in the ethnic rhinoplasty patient.[5] This expanded the use of dorsal preservationin patients who otherwise would require dorsal grafting.

I also expanded the use of dorsal preservation for revision rhinoplasty patients who had residual dorsal humps. If the patient underwent prior rhinoplasty and had rasping of the dorsum without component hump reduction, a letdown with a subdorsal Z-flap or low strip could be used to straighten the dorsum. In these cases, care must be taken to carefully assess the status of the nasal septum to ensure there is adequate septal cartilage to permit a subdorsal Z-flap, Tetris, or low strip.

At this point, I use dorsal preservation on almost all primary rhinoplasties with a dorsal hump or those needing dorsal augmentation. I also use dorsal preservation in a small number of revision rhinoplasty patients requiring dorsal augmentation. I perform a good number of Asian rhinoplasty surgeries where patients need dorsal augmentation or need their implant removed with immediate dorsal elevation to reestablish proper dorsal height.

I believe dorsal preservation is not indicated in patients who have a complex deformity of their nasal bones or middle vault. In these cases, there is little to preserve, and a structured approach with spreader grafts will be needed to reconstruct the middle nasal vault.

Göksel

The main indications for PR are primary cases in which hump elimination is desired. PR is particularly beneficial for patients who own the following features.

- A primarily cartilaginous, dorsal hump.
- Short V-shaped nasal bones.
- An elevated or normal radix height.
- Straight linear DAL, even if they deviate from the midline axis.
- Narrow tension noses.

The surgeon's expertise is crucial in expanding the indications for PR to include more prominent noses and scoliotic nasal pyramids. This can be achieved by applying techniques such as dorsum-plasty, ostectomies, and asymmetric lateral osteotomies.[6,7]

However, even if the patient falls under the criteria mentioned above, some relative contraindications still exist for PR.

- Septal pathologies such as trauma with multiple fractures, large septal perforations, and severe deviations.

- A partial or complete septum reconstruction is necessary due to a previous aggressive septoplasty.
- Severe S-shaped dorsal axis deviations.
- Revision cases, particularly if open roof deformity is present.
- Less than 150 degrees angle between nasal bones and upper lateral cartilages (ULCs) (the angle between the internasal suture and the midline fusion of the ULC on a sagittal view)

QUESTION 2. HOW TO DECIDE ON THE PROPER TECHNIQUE
Neves

The field of PR has witnessed an explosion of new ideas and concepts, making it challenging to delineate its conceptual boundaries today. In my 17 years of endeavoring to understand the optimal path that aligns with my surgical skills and objectives, I have come to focus on preserving what lies between the 2 DAL, which I refer to as the dorsal platform. This approach aims to maintain continuity between the bone and cartilage in the rhinion region, where the skin is thinnest and surgical vestiges are most readily apparent. Additionally, it helps to preserve the integrity of the nasal septum and ULCs as a unit. Consequently, the entire surgical strategy is centered on the preservation of this platform. Following this line of reasoning sequentially, I explore the following options.

Surface approach
The dorsum is slightly projected (up to 2 mm): In these cases, surface maneuvers such as rhinosculpture are almost always sufficient. I begin with shaving of the nasal dorsum, typically using burrs, although piezo and rasps are also effective. After achieving the desired height of the bony dorsum, I adjust the cartilage projection. Burrs can also be used, but performing a shaving with a cold blade scalpel is another possibility. I have employed electrosculpture (using the cut of the monopolar electrocautery) which provides great precision in cartilaginous sculpting, without completely separating the septum/ULC unit.

Cartilaginous impaction
The bony dorsum is slightly elevated, with a predominantly cartilaginous hump: The dorsum is addressed with rhinosculpture, and the cartilage is deprojected using the Tetris concept. I perform a cartilagineous sub-dorsal flap (Tetris flap) to define the height of the cartilaginous dorsum.

Full pyramid impaction
This is my most frequent approach, which involves impacting the entire nasal pyramid, necessitating

work on the nasal septum and the sidewalls. Regarding the septal wall, the position of the ethmoidal plate primarily guides the choice of the impaction technique.

1. If the ethmoidal plate shows no significant deviations, the technique of choice is the Tetris Concept[8] (**Fig. 2**), a sub-dorsal flap that guides and stabilizes the new position of the nasal dorsum. After resecting the excess nasal septum beneath the flap, board-to-board sutures are applied. There is the option of Tetris 1 (the original description, where the flap is defined cephalically at the highest point of the nasal hump and caudally at the caudal border of the ULCs) and Tetris 2 (cephalically the same but caudally the cut is made below the ULCs halfway between the rhinion and W point, thus providing a support point to the caudal cartilaginous vault above the nasal septum).
2. In minor deviations of the nasal pyramid and ethmoidal plate, we use the same concept but consider the possibility of overlapping the flap with the basal septum to compensate for the deviation, it is the lateral Tetris.[8]
3. In cases of marked deviations of the ethmoidal plate, where continuity with the septal cartilage is maintained, both the nasal pyramid and the caudal septum persistently exhibit deviations. In these cases, I always opt for a basal and posterior disarticulation of the septal cartilage. We then have 2 options: the Low Strip approach (popularized by Cottle and later Wilson Dewes, SPAR B) or Tetris 3. This Tetris option is based on a sequence that assesses the need for the extent of disarticulation, whether partial or total. After centering the caudal septum at the anterior nasal spine (ANS) and reducing the projection of

the nasal dorsum with the Tetris flap, I assess the degree of deviation of the ethmoidal plate, its location, and its impact on the deviation of the anterior nasal pyramid and septum. Sometimes this ethmoidal plate deviation is more basal, and I disarticulate the septum from the entire pavement and from the basal portion of the plate; I then reevaluate the impact of this maneuver. If it is not sufficient, I perform a complete disarticulation, leaving the septal cartilage detached from the ethmoidal plate, now able to freely perform a swinging door maneuver. It is important to note that this technique completely frees the septal cartilage from its surroundings, thus it is imperative to define a stable sequence. This actually represents a high strip with a subdorsal Tetris flap combined with a Low Strip approach release, thus integrating the advantages of each: better control of the final position of the nasal dorsum and the release of the septal cartilage to correct septal and pyramidal deviations.

Regarding the sidewall, I primarily use the let-down maneuver, not only in the basal portion of the osteotomy but also in the transverse to avoid blocking points. The sidewall is seen more as a facilitator of movement, leaving to the nasal septum the task of defining the position of the nasal profile. An exception to this concept is the "lateral-push", described by Wilson Dewes, for deviated pyramids. This involves performing a let-down on the longer sidewall and a push-down on the shorter side, to facilitate centering of the nasal pyramid.

Toriumi

Choosing the proper dorsal preservation technique can be somewhat confusing as the indications can

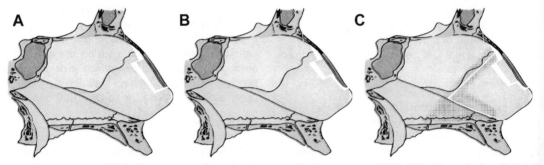

Fig. 2. The Tetris Concept. (*A*) *Tetris 1*: Original description of the subdorsal Tetris flap; the caudal incision is placed at the level of the caudal border of the upper lateral cartilages (ULCs); the cephalic incision at the highest point of the nasal hump; (*B*) *Tetris 2*: The caudal incision was shifted cephalically to preserve some of the quadrangular cartilage below the cartilaginous vault, increasing support to the supratip area; (*C*) *Tetris 3*: After the subdorsal flap is stabilized and the posterior septal angle is fixed in the mid-line, the pyramid is analyzed to detect any residual deviation that may be caused by a deviation of the ethmoidal perpendicular plate. If this is the case, we free the quadrangular cartilage from the ethmoidal plate and perform a swinging door movement. This procedure results in a *Full Release* of the quadrangular cartilage.

vary or overlap. For example, many primaries with a V-shaped dorsal hump can be treated with a high strip, intermediate level strip (subdorsal Z-flap, Tetris, Ishida) or low strip. I chose to use the subdorsal Z-flap, Tetris or low stripin most primaries that have a V-shaped dorsal hump with a normal radix and good supratip position. I will use a Tetris in patients that require more precise control of the supratip position due to a lower or higher supratip position. In the deviated nose, the low strip, subdorsal Z-flap and Tetris work well if there is an axis deviation with a moderately deviated septum with a midline ethmoid bone. If I use an intermediate level technique, I will overlap the subdorsal Z-flap or Tetris to the side opposite the deviation to shift the dorsum to the midline. I also prefer a letdown and in cases with an axis deviation, I will take out a bone strip on the side opposite the deviation and a conventional lateral osteotomy on the side of the deviation.

I prefer to use a low strip in patients with a deviated nose and deviated septum that involves a quadrangular cartilage that is too large for the space it occupies or in the case with a high ethmoid deviation. In these cases, the quadrangular cartilage can be freed from the nasal spine, maxillary crest, vomer, and ethmoid and then resized to fit into the space and resuture the septal flap to the nasal spine. The low strip (Cottle, SPQR) is a very powerful technique and can correct severe septal deformities without performing a subtotal septal reconstruction or extracorporeal septoplasty (**Fig. 3**).[9]

I will use the subdorsal cantilever graft to perform dorsal augmentation in most patients requiring augmentation to avoid using larger dorsal grafts. I do not use diced cartilage and fascia grafts as I believe they are problematic and can leave deformity and can be difficult to revise.

In many situations, the dorsal preservation techniques are interchangeable or can be combined. For example, the subdorsal Z-flap and Tetris are almost interchangeable. In some cases, a Tetris or Z-flap can be combined with a low strip using the low strip to correct the septal deformity and to straighten the nose and the subdorsal Z-flap or Tetris to lower the dorsal hump (Jose Carlos Neves, personal communication, 2022).

Göksel

After a patient's suitability for dorsal preservation is elected, the surgeon must then make critical decisions regarding the surgical approach (open or closed), the conservation of ligaments, the dissection extent of the skin-soft tissue envelope (SSTE), septal management, dorsal work, and the potential need for adjunctive tricks such as the Göksel's Ballerina maneuver or bony cap removal.[6,7]

This preoperative analysis is immensely significant in determining the extent of SSTE dissection in PR because the degree of ligamentous preservation directly influences the redraping of SSTE and the resolution of edema, in my anecdote.[6,7,10]

To ease this process, we recently introduced a classification system for patients, grouping them into 3 classes based on the presence of dorsal deformities. This categorization assesses the suitability of the case for ligamentous conservation, which allows for an individually tailored and practical application of preservation techniques.[6,7]

1. Patients with a straight dorsal aesthetic line necessitating solely reduction of the cartilaginous hump: This group can be managed through limited SSTE dissection along the nasofacial groove, which allows the lateral osteotomies while preserving the SSTE attachment to the dorsum. The dissection should be minimally invasive to achieve the anticipated results (**Fig. 4**A).
2. Patients with straight DAL with a bony hump that requires minor adjustments. Here, a dorsal SSTE elevation and partial ligament dissection are needed. This technique allows access to the central dorsal and symmetric lateral nasal bony compartments. By carefully managing the dorsal skin and selectively dissecting ligaments, surgeons can address the raised bony hump while preserving the overall dorsal aesthetics (**Fig. 4**B).
3. Patients with dorsal irregularities and asymmetries: Those cases may still undergo a PR employing dorsum-plasty and classical preservation techniques. Here a complete dorsal SSTE dissection for restructuring without preserving ligaments. Following the necessary adjustments, the Pitanguy and Scroll ligaments are reattached before the surgery is finished. This allows for the correction of dorsal irregularities and asymmetries (**Fig. 4**C).

The next step is to decide on the best way to manage the septum. If the hump height is less than 4 mm with straight DAL, the high septal strip/subdorsal resection that has been popularized by Saban and colleagues[11] or Mid-Septal Strip/Subdorsal flaps of various configurations that have been described by Most and colleagues,[12] Neves and colleagues,[8] and Kovacevic and colleagues.[13] However, if we deal with a crooked nose with no pathology at the lower septum, the low septal strip (by Cottle.[14] or SPQR by Finocchi and colleagues[15]) works best for me as I need to change direction of the nose, and this is possible only through the separation of the attachment between the quadrangular cartilage and the perpendicular plate, which

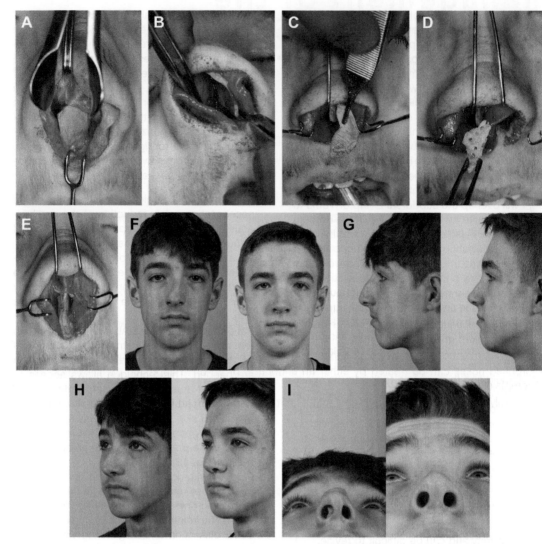

Fig. 3. Patient with a severely deviated nose and deviated caudal septum. (*A*) Severe septal deviation noted. (*B*) After release of the septal flap it was trimmed and rotated caudally. (*C*) Caudal septal extension graft used to reestablish proper length. (*D*) Ethmoid bone used to stabilize the extension graft. (*E*) Septal extension graft in place. (*F*) Preoperative frontal view showing severe deviation (*left*). 3 years postoperative frontal view showing a straight nose (*right*). (*G*) Preoperative lateral view showing dorsal hump (*left*). Postoperative lateral view showing straight dorsum (*right*). (*H*) Preoperative oblique view (*left*). Postoperative oblique view (*right*). (*I*) Preoperative base view showing severe caudal septal deviation (*left*). Postoperative base view showing symmetric nasal base and open airway (*right*).

is hard to achieve in the high-septal strip technique. The specific indications for each PR technique are illustrated in (**Fig. 5**).[6]

QUESTION 3. HOW CAN I SAFELY INTRODUCE DORSAL PRESERVATION TECHNIQUES IN MY SURGICAL ARMAMENTARIUM?
Neves

As previously mentioned, the variety of PR techniques is so vast that it is difficult to outline a single guidance path for beginning this journey. For

example, surface techniques, which today are also considered part of PR, have always been in the armamentarium of nose surgeons, regardless of their school of thought, since in various situations it would be necessary to refine the nasal dorsum, using rasps or motorized devices. Today, perhaps we take it a bit further, and thus include it in the PR repertoire.

Regarding impaction techniques, they rely on a 3-dimensional mastery of the entire nasal structure and the ability to predict how movement will occur in each segment, which undoubtedly requires a

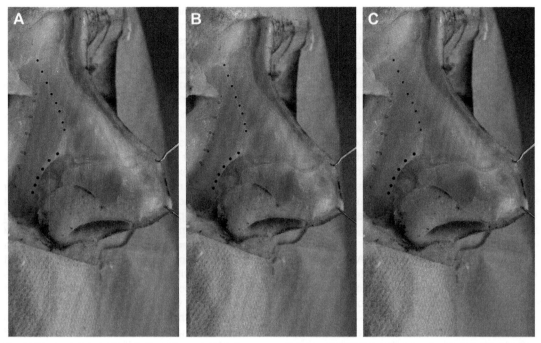

Fig. 4. The red dotted line defines the nasofacial groove, the blue dotted line refers to the site of the nasomaxillary ligament attachment, and the dotted black line delimitates the pyriform aperture. (*A*) Limited dissection with ligament preservation. There is no dissection on the dorsum. (*B*) Limited dissection with ligament preservation; the dorsum is dissected. (*C*) Extended dissection with no preservation of the ligaments.

learning curve and improvement of skills. It is important to note that several surgical actions are performed without observing a change in the pyramid until impaction is executed. This may be the significant difference from structured rhinoplasty, which plans each step sequentially, with each producing a visible modification. Therefore, mastery and control of nasal anatomy are absolutely crucial.

Beyond the obvious anatomy study, I believe it is very important to undertake hands-on cadaver

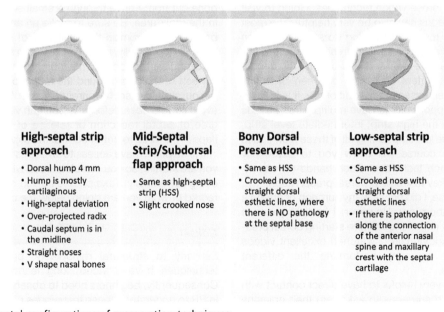

High-septal strip approach	**Mid-Septal Strip/Subdorsal flap approach**	**Bony Dorsal Preservation**	**Low-septal strip approach**
• Dorsal hump 4 mm • Hump is mostly cartilaginous • High-septal deviation • Over-projected radix • Caudal septum is in the midline • Straight noses • V shape nasal bones	• Same as high-septal strip (HSS) • Slight crooked nose	• Same as HSS • Crooked nose with straight dorsal esthetic lines, where there is NO pathology at the septal base	• Same as HSS • Crooked nose with straight dorsal esthetic lines • If there is pathology along the connection of the anterior nasal spine and maxillary crest with the septal cartilage

Fig. 5. Septal configurations of preservation techniques.

courses to understand structure and movements. It is also crucial to identify the surgeons whose concepts are most appealing and visit them to see these procedures in real time and clarify any doubts. Then, choose the ideal candidates. As mentioned, today we cannot say there are absolute contraindications in PR, but there are certainly optimal indications. To start, I would recommend a nose with a projected dorsum with a slightly kyphotic hump, without low radix or supratip, without deviations, and with well-defined aesthetic lines. It may also be helpful to include in this initial group of candidates male patients, who, in the event of ending up with a residual hump or a recurrence, generally accept this appearance as a characteristic perceived as masculine, even adding some naturalness.

Although I initially learned the SPAR B[1] (low strip approach) early in my career, this technique is, in my opinion, the most demanding of all and can present significant difficulties in controlling the nasal pyramid and septum. Therefore, in relation to impaction techniques, I would start with those that rely on a stable cartilaginous septum, where there has been no disarticulation with the ethmoidal perpendicular plate, such as the high strip (SPAR A[1], Saban[11]) or techniques similar to high strip with a sub-dorsal flap, also seen as an intermediate strip (Tetris,[8] Most,[12] Z-Flap[13]).

Toriumi

When incorporating dorsal preservation techniques into your practice, it is important to study the publications of different surgeons who have introduced preservation techniques. Going to visit these surgeons can also be very helpful. The most productive means of learning dorsal preservation is to attend a comprehensive fresh cadaver laboratory course. The ideal setting would be to attend a course that offers split time between didactics and cadaver dissections. Additionally, it is ideal to have the opportunity to have multiple fresh heads to practice the high strip, intermediate level strip, and then the low strip. Doing all of these techniques during the course will allow you to personally perform each technique. Such hands-on experiences are key to learning dorsal preservation.

In my case, I did not visit any surgeon or attend a cadaver laboratory. However, I had 30 years of rhinoplasty experience before starting dorsal preservation. Additionally, I watched excellent videos of master surgeons performing the different techniques.

It is also very helpful to have direct contact with experienced surgeons to ask them their opinions on choosing the proper cases. I was able to contact Yves Saban, Milos Kovacevic, Baris Cakir, and Aaron Kosins to ask for their opinion on case selection and the best techniques for each case.

There are many good references to gain information about dorsal preservation including the PR series as well as informative papers on the topic (Jose Carlos Neves, personal communication).[16]

I believe it is very important to learn structure before embarking on dorsal preservation as structure techniques may be needed as a "bailout" if dorsal support is lost.[5,17] Additionally, it is very helpful to be experienced in performing osteotomies as this is needed if performing pushdown or letdown techniques. Because I had over 30 years of experience performing osteotomies, it was an easier transition to performing foundational dorsal preservation techniques. If you have access to a piezotome, bone cuts can be made under direct visualization with great precision. This simplifies the execution of the foundational techniques but does require a wider field of dissection.

There are 2 major types of dorsal preservation methods. These include surface techniques and foundational techniques.[18] In some patients with a V-shaped dorsal hump, the hump can be managed simply by rasping the bony cap. This works with smaller V-shaped humps.

For a safe transition you should start with surface techniques involving modification of the bony cap with or without a Saban style high strip.[16] This approach allows you to convert to a structure approach with spreader grafts if you wish. A natural progression is then to transition to the push down with lateral and transverse bone cuts and radix bone cut. You should start making your radix bone cut from above through a small stab incision in the radix area. Be sure to make an angled radix bone cut to minimize the likelihood of radix drop (**Fig. 6**). Additionally, it is helpful to keep the periosteum and skin attached to the radix area to keep the support of the bone around the radix bone cut.

You should also be careful at the W point to avoid saddle nose deformity. You can vary the degree of septal resection or release of the septal flaps in this area to better control the supratip area.

It is helpful to have access to an endoscope when you are starting so you can clearly see what you are doing subdorsally. Take photos so you can keep a record of what you are doing below the dorsum.

Göksel

Similarly to structural rhinoplasty, preservation techniques have a steep, long learning curve. Consequently, beginners need to observe masters in PR to understand these techniques comprehensively. Moreover, finding an individual mentor with

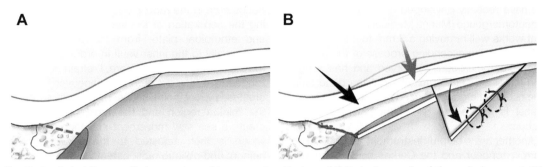

Fig. 6. Angled oblique radix bone cut used to prevent radix drop. (*A*) Note the angle of the radix bone cut. (*B*) The bone slides and does not drop to prevent descent of the radix.

good expertise in PR who can guide the surgeon's learning curve would be very beneficial.

It is also important to understand that PR has limitations and cannot be applied to all cases, so the wise selection of the optimal cases for those techniques is the most crucial safety measure. Here again, mentoring can be of great value in helping to choose the best patients for a PR technique. Furthermore, the supervisor can advise on the best techniques based on his/her mentee's familiarity with PR. For instance, starting with male patients with straight DAL is the best option, to begin with, as the most common complication in PR is a residual hump, which in turn could be desired in men to retain the masculine appearance of the face.

Regarding septal management techniques, starting with the high septal strip technique is advisable, as it allows easier revisions in case of postoperative complications.

QUESTION 4. DO I NEED ANY SPECIAL SURGICAL INSTRUMENTS?
Neves

If the answer were to be strictly a yes/no binary, it would be: No. Indeed, a conventional set of rhinoplasty instruments is sufficient to perform PR. It is noteworthy that this concept has been in existence for over a century. My mentor, Wilson Dewes, used a conventional, non-fancy set that included good quality osteotomes of 2 mm and 4 mm, both straight and curved, and a long scissors designed by him for addressing the nasal septum. In many of my surgeries, I continue to use the same osteotomes and a Heymann scissors for addressing the ethmoidal plate. However, power instruments have expanded our toolkit options.

The piezoelectric tool can enhance precision in performing osteotomies; it can be used in areas where impact might be more traumatic, such as

along the DAL; and can be safely used after the mobilization of the pyramid has been achieved. Similarly, burrs create smooth surfaces and are very effective in addressing the lateral wall and naso-facial groove.

In fact, these tools have made a positive addition to rhinoplasty in general, not specifically to PR.

Toriumi

There are a few instruments that can be helpful when performing dorsal preservation. If you can use a piezotome then this device can allow you to perform the bone cuts and also perform rhinosculpture. I have a piezotome but only use it rarely in cases where rhinosculpture is necessary or if I am planning on performing a spare roof type B. I use the piezotome most frequently in secondary rhinoplasty cases where the nasal bones are deformed and require sculpting. I will also use the piezotome in cases where costal cartilage is calcified and requires the piezotome to harvest the rib and sculpt the grafts.

In most primary rhinoplasty cases, I will use osteotomes to perform the bone cuts. If bony cap removal is needed, I will use a narrow rasp (Marina Medical Inc., Davie, Fla.) to take down the bony cap and to sculpt the bones. In most cases, I will use a 2 mm straight osteotome to perform the radix bone cut from below. This is an obliquely oriented radix bone cut to minimize the likelihood of radix drop. I use a 3 mm straight osteotome to perform a high and low bone cut on the ascending process of the maxilla to remove a banana-shaped bone strip. The transverse bone cut is performed through a 3 mm stab incision along the side of the nose near the medial canthus. I first use a Cerkes bone drill (Marina Medical Inc., Davie, Fla.) to make a trough along the path of the transverse bone cut then complete the cut using a 2 mm osteotome. This helps to prevent comminuted bone fractures.

I have recently developed a banana bone strip osteotome/gouge (Marina Medical Inc., Davie, Fla.) that works well removing a 3 mm to 4 mm strip of bone along the ascending process of the maxilla. The osteotome/gouge is curved and has a right and left-sided version to take out the bone strip. The osteotome/gouge is used after a subperiosteal tunnel is created to allow the passage of the instrument.

Another very helpful instrument is the Goksel narrow rongeur and the Cerkes narrow rongeur. The Goksel rongeur is longer and is helpful for taking out bone under the nasal bones. The Cerkes narrow rongeur is useful for taking out the lateral bone strips if you prefer not to use an osteotome making a high and low cut in the bones.

The specific instruments that you will need depend on your level of expertise as some instrumentation requires more skill to use them. This is where a cadaver laboratory will help tremendously so you can feel comfortable using such instrumentation.

Göksel

PR is possible with conventional and power instruments; experienced surgeons could achieve the anticipated results using either. Nonetheless, the Piezotome eases the osteotomy and offers extra safety margins, especially for beginners, as it is more predictable. For example, performing a sagittal orienting lateral osteotomy in a push-down might be challenging using an osteotome that usually follows the weakest point in the bone while it is manageable with the Piezotome. Surgeons should not hesitate to use the Piezotome because of its time-consuming nature.

QUESTION 5. HOW CAN I PREVENT COMPLICATIONS?
Neves

Complications or suboptimal outcomes may be observed from both the profile and frontal views.[19] In the profile view, potential issues include residual hump or recurrence of a hump; loss of control over the radix height; loss of control over the supratip; and loss of control over the entire nasal pyramid, which may result in an infantilized appearance of the nose. From the frontal view, potential complications can include deviation of the nasal axis; widening of the nasal pyramid; and loss of definition of the DAL.

The complication that most concerns surgeons, particularly those considering starting with PR, is the loss of control over the pyramid, especially in the radix region. My main strategies to avoid loss of control of the radix include: not detaching the

periosteum in the radix osteotomy area; performing the separation of the septum, both cartilage and ethmoidal plate, from the nasal pyramid tangentially to the inner vault in order to preserve the supporting pillar (therefore, I refrain from using rongeurs); the radix step-up maneuver[19] (which creates a pivot point between the split septal in the rhinion region and the radix osteotomy to create a see-saw movement elevating the radix, which is then adjusted to the desired dorsal height); and oblique radix osteotomy.

The most frequent complication in dorsal preservation (DP), which might rather be seen as a suboptimal outcome, is the persistence of a dorsal hump. This can be due to inadequate control of blocking points and poor execution of maneuvers that flatten the nasal dorsum. These maneuvers aim to allow the central (septal) and lateral walls to spread without resistance, promoting splitting movements.[3] In the nasal septum, at the highest point of the nasal hump, a vertical chondrotomy should be performed to enable forward splitting; on the sidewall, we have 2 options: disarticulation of the lateral K stone area (LKA), popularized by Goksel as the Ballerina maneuver, which promotes lateral splitting or the DAL split maneuver, which allows advancement of the bony sidewall along with the ULC, achieving the same effect of flattening the dorsum.

Distinguishing between a residual hump and the recurrence of a hump is not always straightforward. However, recurrence may be due to inadequate stabilization. Despite controlling all blocking points, the tissues' inherent elasticity can promote the recurrence of the nasal hump. Therefore, robust stabilization is important. The purpose of introducing a sub-dorsal flap (the Tetris flap), as also observed in the work of Most[12] and Kovacevic,[13] is precisely to stabilize the final position of the nasal dorsum more accurately. The traction suture of the flap downward to a stable septum has proven very effective. Similarly, when performing a low strip (SPAR B) or Tetris 3, an oblique suture is executed from the ANS toward the rhinion to stabilize the dorsal position. In these specific cases of Low Strip mobilization, proper stabilization of the posterior border of the nasal septum to the ANS is crucial. Here, I introduce another concept that offers enhanced stability: the sublaminar dissection of the septum[20] (**Fig. 7**). This dissection allows for the preservation of the nasal septum's perichondrium, being performed immediately below the lamina propria, which provides superior resistance to suture passage and avoids the cheese-wire effect, thus safeguarding the position of the quadrangular cartilage and, consequently, the entire nasal structure.

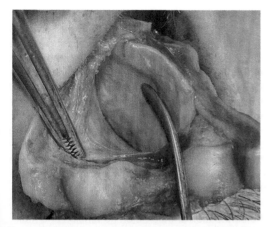

Fig. 7. Sub-laminar septal cartilage dissection allows for observation of the perichondrium overlying the cartilage. Simultaneously, the lamina propria can be observed within the dissected flap.

Another interesting point that should be addressed is the shape of the bony dorsum, which may require surface techniques to flatten the profile. This is especially true for an S-shaped bony dorsum. After achieving the ideal projection of the dorsum, I initiate the second phase of the surgery, which involves refining the profile line. The S-shaped or kyphotic dorsum is addressed using burrs, piezo, or rasps, as previously described in our surface strategies. The same issue can occur with the cartilaginous dorsum which, despite being well-positioned, may present a convexity that needs to be smoothed.

Regarding drawbacks observed from the frontal view, the widening of the nasal dorsum is a common complaint. Even if the width of the impacted nose remains unchanged, the perception that the nose appears wider is common due to the changed relationship between width and projection. However, actual widening of the cartilaginous pyramid can be observed if the cartilaginous blocking points are not controlled. This issue, though seldom discussed, particularly involves the posterior edge of the ULC, which may experience limited movement due to the presence of undissected soft tissues at the base of the sidewalls. For this reason, in most cases, I begin the dissection of the lateral wall at its most basal portion, leaving the dorsal platform undisturbed, which, if necessary, can be elevated later.

To correct a wide nasal dorsum, I follow a sequence of possible strategies. A bone shave can be performed, serving as a surface technique, to narrow the bony wall in cases requiring minor adjustments. If the dorsum is truly wide, I may then opt for DAL osteotomies to redefine the angle of the sidewalls and the width of the dorsal. If I

anticipate narrowing the dorsum or defining the DAL, and aim to flatten the nasal dorsum, then I perform the DAL split maneuver.[21] This technique allows to achieve all these objectives with a single maneuver. For an enlarged bony-cartilaginous dorsum, I may consider performing a continuous mattress suture with 5.0 polydioxanone (PDS) at the level of the T plate to control the angle and width of the wall.[22] The use of electrocautery may also be interesting to sculpt the cartilaginous wall.

Toriumi

The primary potential complications when performing dorsal preservation include; radix drop, saddle nose deformity, deviation, comminuted bone deformity, and collapsed nose. A residual dorsal hump or recurrent dorsal hump is not a complication but a suboptimal outcome.

Preventing a residual or recurrent dorsal hump requires proper execution of the technique, proper selection of the technique, and management of the potential blocking points. One of the primary blocking points includes leaving bone and or cartilage under the bony hump. In most instances, 4 mm to 5 mm of bone and or cartilage should be removed below the bony hump to make room for the hump to be reduced (**Fig. 8**). Cartilage can be removed using a 15-blade or rongeur. If there is bone under the dorsum this can be removed with a long narrow rongeur.

When performing the lateral bone cuts or bone strip removal and the transverse bone cuts, if the junction between the 2 is squared off, the corner of the bone can act to block the downward rotation of the dorsal hump. This can be avoided by taking out a banana-shaped bone strip as described by Sabastian Haack. Creating more of

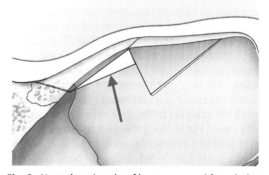

Fig. 8. Note the triangle of bone removed from below the bony hump to allow the hump to descend and not drop excessively. *Red arrow* points to the triangular segment of cartilage removed from under the dorsal hump to prevent blockage of hump reduction.

a continuous curvature from piriform aperture and the radix bone cut will allow a more uniform reduction of the dorsal hump.

The lateral keystone or connection between the caudal nasal bone and the upper lateral cartilage can act as a "tension band" that will prevent complete reduction of the dorsal hump and could result in a popping up of the hump. To prevent this tension effect, a lateral keystone release as described by Goksel will divide the connection and allow more freedom for the 2 zones to separate and allow the hump to "stretch" flat.

Another potential blocking point is Webster's triangle, where a segment of bone can block the full reduction of the dorsum hump. This blocking point can be removed by taking out a strip of bone along the ascending process of the maxilla. In this area, the periosteum can be elevated to free the bones to release.

When performing a Saban-style high strip, a strip of cartilage and bone is removed under the middle vault and nasal bones. When this strip is removed it is difficult to remove the cartilage flush to the undersurface of the ULCs. In this case, a strip of cartilage is left that runs continuously along the undersurface of the dorsum passing across the rhinion. This strip of cartilage can act as a tension band across the undersurface of the hump. To remove the tension band effect, a couple of vertical incisions can be made across the strip of cartilage to break up the tension band effect and allow the hump to stretch flat. Saban describes this tension band effect as the "clothes hanger effect."

To avoid complications, there are other maneuvers that can be executed. To avoid radix drop, the radix bone cut can be made in an oblique or beveled orientation. This is accomplished by angling the osteotome at a 30-degree to 40-degree angle off of the horizontal plane. This can be performed either from above or from below. I find it easier to accomplish this by performing the osteotomy from an angled orientation from below. In this case, a comminution of the bone of the radix may be created as opposed to a clean cut that is accomplished using the piezotome or saw. Even greater support of this area can be achieved by leaving the skin and periosteum attached to the bone. In this case, any comminuted bone segments are all left attached to the periosteum and keep the radix intact, not allowing the radix to drop. An additional way to avoid radix drop or the infantile radix, is more bone can be left under the bony hump as this will block the descent of the nasal bones and radix. However, enough bone should be removed to allow the hump to reduce.

Preventing the saddle nose deformity will depend on the specific technique used in the subdorsal septum. For example, if a high strip is used, the strips of cartilage can be removed sequentially to avoid excessive lowering of the supratip. If a subdorsal Z-flap is used, the caudal end of the Z-flap can be preserved leaving a continuity of support from the rhinion to the W-point. If a Tetris is used, the caudal cut of the flap can be adjusted anterior or posterior to set the position of the supratip. If a low strip is used, saddling can occur if too much cartilage is trimmed off of the undersurface of the quadrangular cartilage septal flap (QC flap). Saddling can also occur if the QC flap becomes dislodged from the attachment to the nasal spine. To prevent detachment, the connection should be on no tension and multiple sutures can be used to solidify the connection.

Deviation of the nose can be prevented by choosing the proper technique for the problem. For example, in cases with a severe septal deviation, the low strip is likely the best option for correction. It is important to avoid applying too much tension to the QC flap to prevent deformation of the septum and late deviating of the nose. In most low-strip cases, I will place a very thin plastic stent over the septum to aid in fixation and stabilization. This maneuver can also help prevent disruption of the connection between spine and the QC flap.

Deviation can result when an intermediate-level septal flap such as the subdorsal Z-flap or Tetris is used to correct a deviated nose that involves more than a pure axis deviation. In these cases, the overlapping of the intermediate-level septal flap can improve the deviation but could shift other parts of the dorsum to create a crooked nose. To prevent this problem, a low strip swinging door maneuver can be performed to straighten the septum. Then a Z-flap or Tetris can be used to reduce the dorsal hump. In these cases, most of the straightening is accomplished by overlapping the septal flap on the side opposite the deviation. Instead of this approach, the low strip swinging maneuvers are used to straighten the deformity, and then the independent Z-flap or Tetris are performed just to reduce the dorsal convexity.

When using osteotomes to make the bone cuts, inevitably some comminution of the bones can occur. If the periosteum is left attached to the bones, the bone fragments will remain in the proper orientation.

Fortunately, nasal collapse is uncommon. In most of these cases, the septum was left distorted, weak, or overly reduced. For example, if too much tension is applied to the septal remnant at the nasal spine, the attachment can be compromised resulting in loss of tip and or supratip support.

Göksel

Complications such as residual hump, radix step, and supra-tip saddling occur in PR. Besides the correct indication for PR, understanding the techniques' biodynamics is the key to avoiding those unpleasant results. Consequently, releasing all the anatomic blocking points described by Göksel and colleagues[23] These points can potentially create intrinsic resistant tensile forces, impeding intraoperative dorsal lowering or allowing the osseocartilaginous framework to revert to its original height.

Moreover, adopting a sequential intraoperative approach would significantly reduce the risk of complications.

QUESTION 6. HOW HAVE YOUR TECHNIQUES IN THIS AREA CHANGED OVER THE LAST 2 YEARS?
Neves

Over the past 2 years, there has been a focus on stabilizing concepts previously developed and acquired, closely observing and reinforcing the best options, and understanding the reasons behind certain drawbacks. However, 2 areas have particularly gained prominence in this period: the implementation of the DAL split maneuver[21] and Tetris 3.

The introduction of DAL osteotomies, refined with burrs or Piezo, has enabled the operation on patients with PR who were previously considered absolute contraindications. Following these osteotomies, a new concept of lateral wall splitting has evolved, which avoids the need for LKA disarticulation (Ballerina maneuver), thereby achieving the same effect of dorsum flattening. The DAL split maneuver (**Fig. 9**) results in a flat dorsum, a narrowed bony dorsum, and enhanced definition of the DAL. Furthermore, an interesting advantage is observed when compared to LKA disarticulation. When impacting the bony wall during LKA

disarticulation, it undergoes a posterior (deprojection) and cephalic movement. This cephalic movement creates the most significant blocking point in the bony wall at the region of the transverse osteotomy, necessitating an ostectomy at this level, commonly referred to as a banana ostectomy. By performing the DAL split maneuver, the movement of the sidewall follows the ULC to which it is still attached, resulting in posterior (deprojection) and caudal movements. This caudal movement effectively avoids the blocking points at the level of the transverse osteotomy.

Regarding Tetris 3, it defines itself as the amalgamation of 2 concepts that provide the best of both worlds: the precision of stabilizing the nasal dorsum with a subdorsal flap (Tetris flap) and the ability to correct nasal deviations with a low strip approach (SPAR B). SPAR B is a fantastic technique, with unique capabilities to correct deviations of the nasal pyramid and septum, which was the predominant technique I utilized at the beginning of my journey in PR. However, besides being a less forgiving technique—since loss of control can have more dramatic effects—it lacks precision in defining the new position of the nasal pyramid. Once the entire nasal septum and pyramid are mobilized, defining the new profile position heavily depends on the surgeon's experience, as the reference points are eliminated by this mobilization. Therefore, whenever possible, I prefer to perform the Tetris Concept, which, in contrast, maintains its reference points until the end, allowing me to control the degree of deprojection of the nasal dorsum meticulously. But, when there is a clear deviation of the perpendicular ethmoidal plate without its disarticulation from the nasal septum, I cannot achieve adequate mobilization for effective correction of the nasal pyramid and septum. Thus, Tetris 3 allows for the deprojection and precise aesthetic correction of the nasal dorsum and subsequently mobilizes the quadrangular cartilage freely after

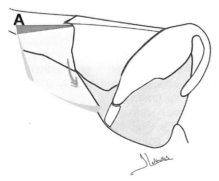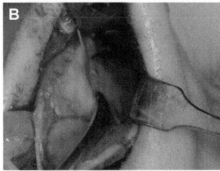

Fig. 9. (*A*) Dorsal Aesthetic Line (DAL) split maneuver. (*B*) A full-thickness DAL osteotomy is performed, enabling the sidewall to advance in conjunction with the ULCs. This maneuver flexes the dorsal profile and controls the width of the bony structure. (Image Courtesy: [*A*] Jose Carlos Neves.)

its disarticulation from the prependicular ethmoidal plate. This results in a *Full Release* of the quadrangular cartilage (see **Fig. 2**B).

A final note regarding my approach to the soft tissues and ligaments of the nose. I always perform a sub-areolar (supra-perichondrial) dissection across the entire extent of the nasal tip cartilages and the middle third of the nose, and a subperiosteal dissection of the upper third.[24] For septal dissection, I perform a sub-laminar (supra-perichondrial) dissection (see **Fig. 7**) on the quadrangular cartilage and a subperiosteal dissection on the bony septum.[20] Maintaining the perichondrium on all cartilages has proven to significantly increase the resistance and stability after suture placement. In the dissection of the midline at the nasal tip, I preserve the Fusion Sling (**Fig. 10**) connected with the cephalic margin of the lower lateral cartilages (LLCs) along their entire length, which will serve as the ultimate anchor for stabilizing the position of the nasal tip. The Fusion Sling, an embryologic structure that connects the cephalic border of the LLCs to their vicinity, consists of perichondrium-like material in the scroll and supra-tip regions and dense connective tissue fibers between the medial crura, intercrural fascia. This structure will be reconstructed in a hook shape over the Anterior Septal Angle, supporting and defining the position of the medial crura and consequently the nasal tip. Over the last 4 years, this has been my workhorse for stabilizing the nasal tip with exceptionally stable results. The vertical ligaments of the supra-tip (Pitanguy) and the scroll are re-sutured for enhanced definition of the supra-tip and supra-alar crease (**Fig. 11**).

Toriumi

Over the past 2 years, I have improved some of the existing techniques with relatively minor adjustments. One of the biggest changes was the change

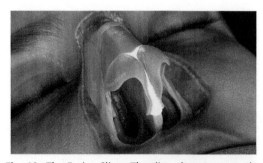

Fig. 10. The Fusion Sling. The sling that connects the cephalic border of the lower lateral cartilages to the adjacent structures. It is formed during the embryologic merging process of the lateral placodes. (Image credits: Kaminskyi team.)

I made in how I performed the lateral bone strip removal. When I started in June of 2019, I began using foundation techniques in the form of a push-down in combination with a push-down with bilateral lateral osteotomies. I then shifted to using a letdown using a 3 mm osteotome to make a high and low bone cut on the ascending process of the maxilla, then removing the banana-shaped bone strip (**Fig. 12**). I then shifted to using a Cerkes narrow rongeur (Marina Medical Inc., Davie, Fla.) to remove the lateral bone strips. Using the narrow rongeur, I tended to leave a narrower gap at the junction between the lateral bone strip and the transverse bone cut. This resulted in a corner at the junction between the 2 bone cuts and left a blocking point at that junction. This resulted in some residual dorsal humps. I then shifted back to using the 3 mm osteotome to make the high and low bone cuts and removing the intervening banana-shaped bone strip that removed the corner between the lateral bone strip removal and the transverse bone cut.

It can be difficult to pass a 3 mm osteotome high and low precisely and then remove the banana-shaped bone strip. This is why I developed the Toriumi banana bone strip osteotome/gouge. Using this right and left-sided instrument, I can easily remove the bone strips along the ascending process of the maxilla.

Another change in the past 3 years is the introduction of the "push-up" for management of the saddle nose deformity and also for dorsal augmentation.[5,17] Working with Milos Kovacevic, we developed a technique that we used to correct the saddle nose deformity by placing a costal cartilage graft under the middle vault after releasing the lateral keystone and piriform ligaments, then pushing up the middle vault to correct the saddle nose deformity. Initially, spreader grafts were used to push up the middle vault.[17] This was accomplished by performing a high strip release of the septum from the ULCs. The spreader grafts were sutured to the septum to push up the middle vault.

Then I further developed the push up concept to incorporate a subdorsal cantilever graft.[5] This costal cartilage graft was modified into the subdorsal cantilever graft type A and the subdorsal cantilever graft type B.[5] The subdorsal cantilever graft type A was used to raise the dorsum with little to no effect on the position of the radix. After completing the high subdorsal incision and extending this to a notch made in the bone under the bony dorsum, this graft is advanced into the notch made under the nasal bones that is then extended caudally to integrate with a caudal septal extension graft. This graft was ideal in patients

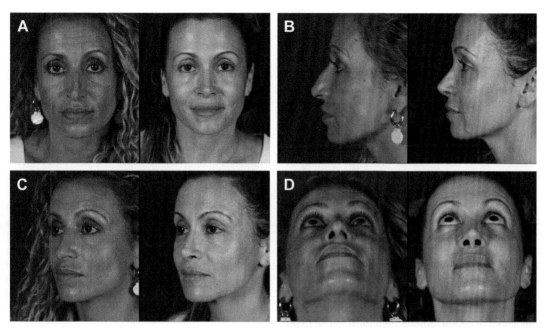

Fig. 11. Clinical case: 2.5-year follow-up. (*A–D*) The patient presented with a slight axis deviation, a dorsal hump, and a ptotic tip, making this a suitable case for dorsal preservation rhinoplasty. I performed a septoplasty and a subdorsal Tetris Flap to center the nose and flattened the dorsum; let down with rhinosculpting with cylindrical drill. The tip was stabilized using Fusion Sling fixation and an anterior nasal septal angle (ANSA) Banner.

who need primarily elevation of the middle vault and caudal nasal bones and worked well for the saddle nose deformity and Asian patients who do not desire to have their radix elevated.

The subdorsal cantilever graft type B, is a longer costal cartilage graft that extends through a radix bone cut after the entire bony vault is freed up by performing radix, transverse and lateral osteotomies with a lateral keystone release and division of the piriform ligaments (**Fig. 13**). This graft is more complex and has a tongue of cartilage that extends through the radix osteotomy site and integrates with the caudal septal extension graft

below. This graft must be very rigid and preferably partially calcified to hold up the entire dorsum. The graft has a convexity where it sits under the middle vault to adequately push up the ULCs. The graft is fixed to the nasal bones to prevent caudal migration of the graft.

Another change made in the past couple of years is the use of dorsal preservation in the acute nasal trauma patient. In this setting, dorsal preservation techniques such as the low strip, subdorsal Z-flap, or Tetris are used to treat deviations of the septum and nose early after nasal trauma. The advantages of this use of dorsal preservation are that

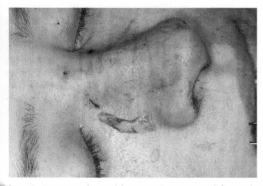

Fig. 12. Banana shaped bone strip removed from the ascending process of the maxilla to allow the bony hump to reduce.

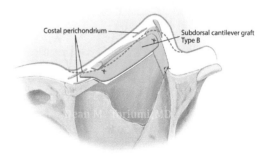

Fig. 13. Subdorsal cantilever graft type B extending through the radix bone cut to sit on the frontal bone and also fixated to the caudal septal extension graft caudally.

it is more effective in correcting the septal deviation and nasal deviation than using an open or closed reduction of the nasal fracture. Care must be taken when using dorsal preservation in the acute nasal fracture as it is possible to lose control of the septal support if a severe septal fracture is present. Therefore, the surgeon must be experienced in using structural techniques such as subtotal septal reconstruction and extracorporeal septoplasty. Additionally, the surgeon should be experienced in using costal cartilage grafting in rhinoplasty.

If the nasal support is lost at any time, a subdorsal cantilever graft can be used to complete the reconstruction and reestablish septal support. If complete nasal septal support is lost, a subdorsal cantilever graft type B can be used to set radix position and support the lower two-thirds of the nose as the L-strut support is reestablished with the subdorsal cantilever graft sitting on the frontal bone and the inferior edge of the graft is integrated with a caudal septal replacement graft that is fixed to the nasal spine.

Jose Carlos Neves has introduced the combination therapy using the low strip in combination with the Tetris to correct a deviated nose with a septal deviation (Jose Carlos Neves, personal communication). In this technique, the low strip swinging door is used to straighten the septum and straighten the nose. Then he used the Tetris to reduce the dorsal hump. The advantage of this approach is that there is no need to perform the overlapping of the Tetris flap as this can create some intrinsic deviations in the nose. As an extension of this Neves concept, I have started using the

subdorsal Z-flap in combination with the low strip swinging door for the same reasons.

I have also developed a "reverse" subdorsal Z-flap that is oriented with the vertical limb at the supratip area to reduce prominent supratip convexities.

The incorporation of dorsal preservation into my practice has evolved over the past 5 years and now is used in most of my primary rhinoplasties. The incorporation of dorsal preservation has resulted in shortening of the operation and having more cartilage for structural grafting of the nasal tip.

I have also recently starting performing PR via the endonasal approach. This approach involves using the polygon tip concepts of Baris Cakir with preservation of the Pitanguy ligament and scroll ligaments to better control tip projection and supratip contour.[25,26,27] These changes are dramatic shifts from the purely open structural approach that I have used for over 35 years.

Göksel

Over the past few years, I shifted from an open to a closed approach to PR in most cases. Conservation of the SSTE and its ligamentous attachments to the osseocartilaginous framework has gained paramount importance in my practice. The game changer for me was the Ballerina maneuver that I have previously described, as it solved the dorsal widening and the hump recurrence.

I mainly performed a high-septal strip at the beginning of my PR journey. However, I changed to a low-septal strip for a crooked nose. In this case, the direction of the nose needs to be changed,

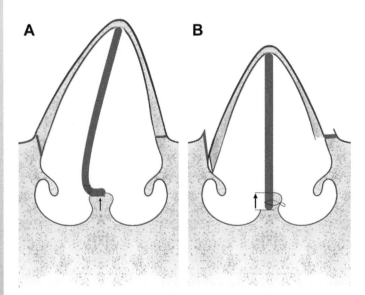

Fig. 14. The red arrow represents the height of the low septal excision, while the black arrow refers to the anterior nasal spine (ANS). The red lines represent the lateral osteotomies in different orientations (sagittal on the right nasal bone and horizontal on the left side) (A) It shows a deviated nasal axis with nasal bones of different lengths between the 2 sides besides basal septal pathology. (B) Shows how the septum overlaps with the ANS side by side, which is why we should count the height of the ANS in our excision.

and this is possible only through the separation of the attachment between the quadrangular cartilage and the perpendicular plate, which is hard to achieve in the high-septal strip technique.

Regarding the low septal strip excision, my resection measured the exact height I anticipated as a dorsal reduction and was timed just before closing the incision. Meanwhile, I am removing a thinner strip to avoid the supra-tip area depression. Moreover, I am considering the height of the ANS in my calculation of the magnitude of the strip excision as the septum would eventually need to be sited on the side of it in a side-to-side fashion to correct the nose deviation from the midline (**Fig. 14**).

I used the convex nasal bones only to rasp the bone; however, beneath the nasal bone, there is a corresponding upper lateral cartilage shoulder that I started to trim.

CLINICS CARE POINTS

- If an S-shaped dorsal hump is treated, typically the bony cap needs to be altered. Bony cap reduction can be performed using one of many techniques.
- An angled radix osteotomy can help to prevent radix drop and an infantile dorsum.
- Managing blocking points are important to prevent dorsal hump persistence or recurrence.

REFERENCES

1. Dewes W, Zappelini CEM, Ferraz MBJ, et al. Conservative surgery of the nasal dorsum: septal pyramidal adjustment and repositioning. Facial Plast Surg 2021;37(1):22–8.
2. Toriumi DM. My first twenty rhinoplasties using dorsal preservation techniquesfacial. Plast Surg Clin N Am 2023;31:73–106.
3. Neves JC, Arancibia G, Dewes W, et al. The split preservation rhinoplasty: The Vitruvian Man split maneuver. Eur J Plast Surg 2020;43(4).
4. Gonçalves FM, Ishida LC, Ishida LH, et al. Spare roof technique b. step-by-step guide to preserving the bony cap while dehumping. Plast Reconstr Surg 2022;149(5):901e–4e.
5. Toriumi DM. Subdorsal cantilever graft for elevating the dorsum in ethnic rhinoplasty. Facial Plast Surg Aesthet Med 2022;24(3):143–59.
6. Goksel A. Piezo assisted let down rhinoplasty. In: RK Daniel PP, Saban Y, Cakir B, editors. Preservation rhinoplasty. 3rd edition. Septum Publishing; 2020. chap 217-242.
7. Goksel A, Tran KN. Open preservation rhinoplasty using the piezo electric instrument. Facial Plast Surg Clin North Am 2023;31(1):59–71.
8. Neves JC, Arancibia D, Dewes W, et al. A Segmental approach in dorsal preservation rhinoplasty: the tetris concept. Facial Plast Surg Clin N Am 2021;29:85–99.
9. Finocchi V, Vellone V, Ramieri V, et al. Pisa tower concept: a new paradigm in crooked nose treatment. Plast Reconstr Surg 2021;148(1):66–70.
10. Saadoun R, Riedel F, D'Souza A, et al. Surgical and nonsurgical management of the nasal skin-soft tissue envelope. Facial Plast Surg 2021;37(06):790–800.
11. Saban Y, Daniel RK, Polselli R, et al. Dorsal preservation: the push down technique reassessed. Aesthetic Surg J 2018;38(2):117–31.
12. Patel PN, Abdelwahab M, Most SP. Dorsal preservation rhinoplasty: method and outcomes of the modified subdorsal strip method. Facial Plast Surg Clin North Am 2021;29(1):29–37.
13. Kovacevic M, Veit JA, Toriumi DM. Subdorsal Z-flap: a modification of the Cottle technique in dorsal preservation rhinoplasty. Curr Opin Otolaryngol Head Neck Surg 2021;29(4):244–51.
14. Cottle MH. Nasal roof repair and hump removal. AMA Arch Otolaryngol 1954;60(4):408–14.
15. Finocchi V, Vellone V, Mattioli RG, et al. A 3-level impaction technique for dorsal reshaping and reduction without dorsal soft tissue envelope dissection. Aesthetic Surg J 2022;42(2):151–65.
16. Daniel RK, Palhazi P, Saban Y, et al. Preservation rhinoplasty. 3rd edition. Istanbul (Turkey): Septum Publishing; 2020.
17. Toriumi DM, Kovacevic M. Subdorsal cantilever graft: Indications and technique. Fac Plast Cl N Amer 2023;31(1):119–21.
18. Ferreira MG, Toriumi DM. A practical classification system for dorsal preservation rhinoplasty techniques. Facial Plast Surg Aesthet Med 2021;23(3):153–5.
19. Neves JC, Arancibia-Tagle D. Avoiding aesthetic drawbacks and stigmata in dorsal line preservation rhinoplasty. Facial Plast Surg 2021;37(1):65–75.
20. Neves JC, Regalado P. Cable and mirror sutures and the nasal septum sublaminar dissection. Thieme Medical Publishers; 2023. https://doi.org/10.1055/a-2021-0280.
21. Neves JCM. Dorsal aesthetic line (DAL) split maneuver in dorsal preservation rhinoplasty. Facial Plast Surg 2024. https://doi.org/10.1055/s-0044-1780509.
22. Neves JC, Erol O, Arancibia-Tagle D, et al. Precision segmental preservation rhinoplasty: avoiding widening, defining new dorsal esthetic lines in dorsal preservation rhinoplasty. Facial Plast Surg Clin North Am 2023;31(1):155–70. PMID: 36396286.
23. Goksel A, Cason RW, Tran KN, et al. The blocking points: the keys to consistent success in preservation rhinoplasty. Plast Reconstr Surg 2023. https://doi.org/10.1097/prs.0000000000010851.

24. Neves JC, Zholtikov V, Cakir B, et al. Rhinoplasty dissection planes (Subcutaneous, Sub-SMAS, Supra-perichondral, and Sub-perichondral) and soft tissues management. Facial Plast Surg 2021;37(1): 2–11.

25. Cakir B. Aesthetic septorhinoplasty. 2nd edition. Budapest (Hungary): Springer; 2022.

26. Cakir B, Saban Y, Daniel RK, et al. Preservation rhinoplasty. Istanbul (Turkey): Septum Publications; 2020.

27. Cakir B, Oreroglu AR, Dogan T, et al. A complete sub-perichondrial dissection technique for rhinoplasty with management of the nasal ligaments. Aesthetic Surg J 2012;32(5):564–74.

Dorsal Preservation Versus Structural Techniques and Their Application

Dean M. Toriumi, MD[a],*, Russell W.H. Kridel, MD[b], Ira D. Papel, MD[c,d], Sam P. Most, MD[e], Priyesh N. Patel, MD[f]

KEYWORDS

- Structure rhinoplasty • Preservation rhinoplasty • Dorsal preservation • Cartilage grafting
- Dorsal hump • Structural grafting • Subdorsal Z-flap • Tetris

KEY POINTS

- Structure and preservation rhinoplasty can be used in a hybrid approach applying dorsal preservation in the upper two-thirds of the nose and structure techniques in the lower third of the nose.
- Dorsal preservation allows preservation of the integrity of the middle vault eliminating the need for spreader grafts. This leaves more cartilage for the structural grafting of the nasal tip.
- Dorsal preservation can be used in most primary rhinoplasties and also for augmentation rhinoplasty in ethnic patients.

PANEL DISCUSSION QUESTIONS

Discuss How They Differ
What is more effective?
How to decide on proper technique.
What is the optimal patient for preservation rhinoplasty?
What is the optimal patient for structural approaches?
How have your techniques in this area changed over the past 2 years?

INTRODUCTION

Structure rhinoplasty and preservation rhinoplasty are two important rhinoplasty philosophies that have been around for many years. Structure rhinoplasty was introduced in 1989 by Johnson and Toriumi and involved using structural grafts such as columellar struts and spreader grafts in rhinoplasty.[1] These grafts were applied using the external rhinoplasty approach. At that time, the use of cartilage grafts and the open approach were felt to be unnecessary. Over the years, many surgeons have adopted structure techniques into their surgical armamentarium. Additionally, the open approach has become a favored approach for performing rhinoplasty. Before structure rhinoplasty came to the forefront, endonasal rhinoplasty techniques were the primary approach for rhinoplasty. With the introduction of structure rhinoplasty, there was a movement away from endonasal rhinoplasty.

Thirty-five years later, we are in a time when there is a resurgence of endonasal rhinoplasty. However, the endonasal approach used these days is much different from that used pre-structure (before the

[a] Otolaryngology Head & Neck Surgery, Rush University Medical School, Chicago, IL, USA; [b] Department of Otolaryngology, University of Texas Medical Branch, Galveston Texas and Facial Plastic Surgery Associates, Houston, TX, USA; [c] Aesthetic Center at Woodholme, Baltimore, MD, USA; [d] Facial Plastic Surgicenter, Ltd, Baltimore, MD, USA; [e] Division of Facial Plastic and Reconstructive Surgery, Stanford University School of Medicine, Stanford, CA, USA; [f] Division of Facial Plastic and Reconstructive Surgery, Department of Otolaryngology, Vanderbilt University Medical Center, Nashville, TN, USA
* Corresponding author. Toriumi Facial Plastics, 60 East Delaware Place, Suite 1425, Chicago, IL 60611.
E-mail address: deantoriumi@toriumimd.com

Facial Plast Surg Clin N Am 32 (2024) 603–624
https://doi.org/10.1016/j.fsc.2024.06.011
1064-7406/24/© 2024 Elsevier Inc. All rights reserved, including those for text and data mining, AI training, and similar technologies.

early 1990s). Previously endonasal rhinoplasty was primarily a reductive operation with significant cephalic trim or division of the domes of the lateral crura and classic Joseph humpectomy using a rasp or Rubin osteotome.

The resurgence of endonasal rhinoplasty has coincided with the increased popularity of dorsal preservation. Dorsal preservation has been around since the early 1900s.[2–5] Yves Saban was a critical figure in the resurgence of dorsal preservation.[5] With the increased interest in dorsal preservation, there has been an improvement in nasal tip concepts that align with the concepts of dorsal preservation. Many of these concepts have been refined by Baris Cakir with his polygon tip concept.[6–8] Rollin Daniel has termed this new improved form of endonasal rhinoplasty as "preservation rhinoplasty."[9] Preservation rhinoplasty focuses on the preservation of the native anatomy of the nose including the cartilage, bones, ligaments, and soft tissues. The term "preservation" refers to the approach used to access the structures, preservation of the nasal dorsum, and preservation of the tip structures (lateral crura). Whether or not this is a true preservation technique is not the point. The primary point is to preserve ligaments and structures that can positively impact the outcomes and potentially simplify the operation. For example, dorsal preservation involves preserving the leading edge of the nasal dorsum (dorsal aesthetic lines) and therefore eliminating the need for camouflaging the edges of the cut nasal bones and the need for reconstruction of the middle vault using spreader grafts or spreader flaps.

The polygon tip surgery described by Cakir focuses on innovative delivery of the tip cartilages using an endonasal approach, preservation of the Pitanguy and scroll ligaments, and managing the nasal tip with a columellar strut, tip suturing, and tensioning of the lateral crura.[6–8] These tip concepts incorporate elegant preservation of important support structures coupled with minimally invasive maneuvers to alter tip contour.

With the resurgence of endonasal rhinoplasty, we have circled back to the "closed rhinoplasty," however, with a newfound respect for the nasal structures to increase the control of postoperative healing and improved command of important features such as the supratip break and facet contour.

HOW DO STRUCTURE AND PRESERVATION DIFFER?
Kridel

Both methods are used to reduce the dorsal bony and cartilaginous nasal bridge, commonly when there is an unwanted hump present.

Traditional structural methods are much simpler and have many fewer potential and easily remedied complications: a rasp, chisel, or drill (piezo or regular drill burr) directly remove the top layer of the bony dorsum and a knife is used to take down the cartilaginous contribution to the hump. A precise contour and smooth dorsum can easily be achieved. Personally, I prefer to use tungsten carbide rasps to take down the bone as any asymmetric irregularities (such as in a fractured or deviated nose) can be precisely contoured. With rasps or a drill, one does not have to worry about taking down too much bone as can occur with a chisel, which invariably can over shorten the lateral nasal bones, making an open roof more possible. If a large bony hump is removed, medial and lateral osteotomies are performed to maintain a narrow dorsum and prevent an open roof. The osteotomies must be complete with no green-sticking or else the nasal bones will later re-lateralize.

If a large component of cartilaginous dorsum is shaved down, the upper lateral cartilages will be separated from the septum and spreader grafts; either turn-in spreaders or spreader grafts are used to prevent a too narrow mid vault.

The area is irrigated out to prevent any bone particles from remaining. One can then palpate over the skin overlying the dorsum with a gloved wet finger to check for smoothness. If any irregularities are found, further rasping or excising can be done. If any small depressions are found, they can easily be filled in with finely crushed cartilage taken from the septum. If the individual has very thin dorsal skin as is seen in some revision patients, temporalis fascia or acellular dermis may be placed over the corrected dorsum.

One great advantage to this traditional technique is that one knows exactly what the dorsum will look like over time. No later changes occur to the dorsal profile except in rare instances. If a bony callus forms, it can be watched expectantly and if it is not resolved, an 18-gauge needle may be inserted through the skin in the office and the area scraped down. If this is not helpful or if true bony fullness exists, a simple rasping can be done in the office under local. In my practice, such an incidence is under 1%.

On the other hand, dorsal preservation rhinoplasty (DPR) techniques remove the support under the cartilaginous and bony dorsum, and the original dorsum is either "pushed-down" or "let-down" to a lower height. This "new" preservation technique is not new, but was first done about 100 years ago and then abandoned in the United States while it was still popular in Mexico, South America, and in parts of Europe. It has come back into fashion with the introduction of better tools such as piezo and is now being re-born in several arenas. Such maneuvers leave the cap of the dorsum intact and preserve its original contours except for the hump, which is pulled down and, in some cases, fixed by sutures.

However, to accomplish this, much has to be done to the underlying structures, which are not necessary in traditional structural reduction. The nasal septum must be entered, and various strips of septal cartilage are removed and/or sutured. There are no less than 4 major different septal cartilage excisions and suture techniques espoused by the various proponents of DPR with no current comparative studies analyzing which may be the best.

In the let-down technique, extensive lateral bone removal is accomplished bilaterally often with piezo instrumentation with the potential for uneven removal or excessive removal creating lateral step offs. In the push-down technique, the lateral nasal bones are dis-attached with piezo laterally, medialized, and pushed down into the nose, where they can create segments of bone that can be visible within the internal nose and can lead to nasal obstruction.

But what seems to be the most disruptive of normal dorsal support and contour is the transverse osteotomy across the nasion, which allows the superior portion of the dorsum to come in. The resulting step off created may not be visible in the immediate post operative period but when one looks at the x-ray of the area, one might be worried about the long-term result. Certainly, patients will be able to palpate this irregularity even if it is not initially visible and may be bothered by this. Carlos Neves MD, a proponent of the DPR, has published an article showing this step-off (**Fig. 1**)[10]

Neves also lists a table of "Drawbaks and Stigmata" with the DPR (**Box 1**).

It is notable that hump recurrence is number 1 on the list with DPR, which is in marked divergence with traditional hump removal. Another potential complication can occur when some surgeons add the Ballerina maneuver technique to this, which is a separation of the upper lateral cartilages from the undersurface of the nasal bones as espoused by Goksel to allow for a flatter push-down of the dorsum; an inverted V deformity can occur because of this dis-articulation.

Most/Patel

Fundamentally, while dorsal preservation and structural techniques, which the authors will hereafter describe as conventional hump resection (CHR) aim to lower a dorsal hump in an aesthetically pleasing fashion, the former aims at maintaining the complex relationship between the bony and cartilaginous dorsum/septum while the latter disrupts these relationships. Understanding the

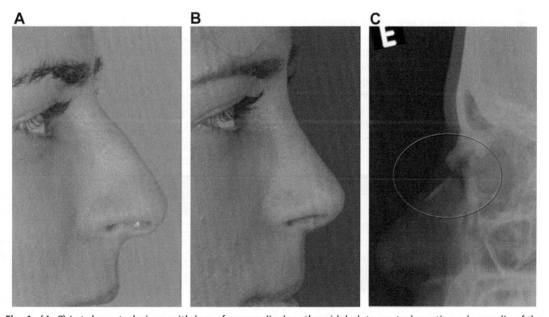

Fig. 1. (*A, B*) Let-down technique with loss of perpendicular ethmoidal plate control creating a low radix of the nose, that was partially compensated with grafts (*C*) The Rx image shows the loss of control of the patient's pyramid. *Circle* shows the drop in the radix position and bone step off. (*From* Neves JC, Arancibia-Tagle D. Avoiding Aesthetic Drawbacks and Stigmata in Dorsal Line Preservation Rhinoplasty. Facial Plast Surg. 2021 Feb;37(1):65-75. https://doi.org/10.1055/s-0041-1725101. Epub 2021 Mar 1. PMID: 33648013.)

Box 1
Drawbacks and stigmata

Profile view drawbacks and stigmata

Hump recurrence

Radix step

Low nasal radix and dorsum

Supratip saddling

Frontal view drawbacks

Pyramid lateralization

Pyramid broadening

Functional impairment

Blockage associated with push-down (bone impaction)

Blockage associated with LKA disarticulation

Abbreviation: LKA, lateral Keystone area.
From Neves JC, Arancibia-Tagle D. Avoiding Aesthetic Drawbacks and Stigmata in Dorsal Line Preservation Rhinoplasty. Facial Plast Surg. 2021 Feb;37(1):65-75. https://doi.org/10.1055/s-0041-1725101. Epub 2021 Mar 1. PMID: 33648013.

difference between these techniques requires an appreciation of the anatomic makeup of the dorsum.

The medial keystone of the nose consists of the intersection of the upper lateral cartilages with the bony and cartilaginous septum (**Fig. 2**). At this site, the septal cartilage extends under the nasal bones, and it has been found that the majority of the dorsal hump sits above the cartilaginous septum rather than the bony septum.[11] This has implications for both CHR and preservation techniques, albeit differently. When resecting a dorsal hump in CHR techniques, resection of bone will reveal a cartilaginous septum that commonly requires excision at its superficial component. In preservation techniques, excision of septal

cartilage lower in the nose (many times without bone) will allow for the lowering of both the bony and cartilaginous dorsum. In addition, at the dorsal bony-cartilaginous junction, there is a non-rigid fusion of the perichondrium of the cartilaginous vault with the periosteum of the nasal bones.[12] In preservation cases, this allows for at least partial flexion at this site in combination with the profile lowering necessary to reduce dorsal convexities. In CHR cases, direct excision of the convexity is instead performed to flatten the dorsum.

In preservation cases, the medial keystone is preserved. As such, the attachments of the upper lateral cartilage are maintained. Conversely, with CHR cases, there is separation of these attachments and potential additional manipulation of the upper lateral cartilage. As such, rebuilding of the midvault with spreader grafts or autospreader flaps are imperative, as are osteotomies to close an open roof. Since the external contour of the nose is not violated in preservation cases, these maneuvers are not required and there is a lower risk of superficial contour irregularities.

Importantly, preservation cases should not be differentiated from structural cases by a lack of resection. Both preservation and structural cases require excision and manipulation of the osseocartilaginous framework. In structural cases, direct excision of bone and cartilage at the dorsum achieves aesthetic goals. In preservation cases, the bony vault is separated from the attachments at the maxilla and frontal bone (with or without excision of bone at the lateral nasal sidewall) with additional septal resection to lower the dorsum. The osteotomies performed laterally in these cases mirror those performed in CHR cases. Ultimately, while preservation cases treat the osseocartilaginous vault as a single unit, CHR cases segmentalize these components.

It should also be noted that newer preservation techniques incorporate surface modifications

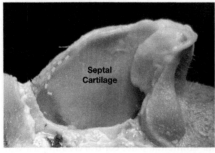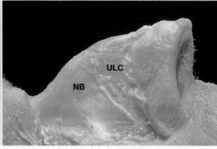

Fig. 2. The medial extension of the upper lateral cartilages under the nasal bones (NBs) and the bony-cartilaginous junction of the septum all contribute the medial/dorsal keystone (*dotted blue line*). This anatomic region contributes to the dorsal hump and is violated in conventional structural hump resection cases, whereas it is maintained in preservation cases.

with or without the need for osteotomies and some techniques separate the treatment of the bony dorsum from the cartilaginous midvault.[13] As such, there is a growing fusion between CHR and preservation ideologies for treatment of the dorsum. In addition, the combination of preservation techniques to the dorsum and open structural modifications to the nasal tip ("Structural Preservation") are similarly uniting these ideologies.

Papel

Structural rhinoplasty has been the dominant mode of nasal surgery for the past 30 to 35 years. The key intent is to preserve the key points of stability to not only provide good contour but resist the powerful factors of scar contraction and gravity for years after surgery. The most common techniques used include osseocartilaginous hump reduction, lateral and/or medial osteotomies, maintaining a septal L-strut, and tip techniques as indicated including grafts and sutures.

Preservation rhinoplasty, in its recent form, seeks to maintain the dorsal rhinion anatomic unit where the bone and cartilage come together. To accomplish this goal, techniques such as circumferential osteotomies, lateral bone excision, partial dissection of the lateral keystone area, and reduction of septal height with fixation are necessary. As in structural rhinoplasty, tip techniques can vary widely.

Toriumi

Structure rhinoplasty is primarily based on the open rhinoplasty approach and the use of structural grafting to stabilize the nasal structures after moderate degrees of reduction and division of the ligamentous support of the tip. Structure rhinoplasty incorporates compensatory maneuvers to account for what has been lost in the process of exposure and reduction of the nasal structures. The "tip split" approach to the nasal septum involves dissection between the medial crura to then perform septal work. This tip-split approach divides some of the critical support structures of the nasal tip. To compensate for this loss of tip support, most surgeons place a columellar strut or caudal septal extension graft.[1,14–16] The dorsal hump is lowered by removing the leading edge of the nasal dorsum, which necessitates reconstruction with spreader grafts or spreader flaps.

Preservation rhinoplasty, or specifically dorsal preservation, involves preservation of the leading edge of the nasal dorsum as the upper lateral cartilages meet the dorsal septum with some potential modification of the bony cap. The middle vault is not opened as the dorsal hump is lowered

by manipulating the nasal septum from below to align the profile. This can be accomplished by high, intermediate, or low septal manipulation.

The primary difference between structure and preservation lies in that the former resects and modifies necessitating structural grafting to stabilize the structure to withstand the forces of healing and reestablish proper contour. Preservation rhinoplasty preserves the favorable aspects of the nasal anatomy and limits the removal of tissues to minimize the need for restructuring the nose.

WHAT IS MORE EFFECTIVE?
Kridel

Both are just techniques to achieve the same results of a decreased dorsal profile while preserving dorsal aesthetic lines from the frontal view. Surgeons should use the techniques, which in their hands are the most reproducible with the best cosmetic result while preserving the nasal airway with the fewest possible potential complications. Most all surgeons agree, however, that the learning curve for the DPR method is indeed steep and more complex when compared to traditional hump reduction. For me, keeping it simple with bony reduction with a rasp and trimming the cartilaginous dorsum has stood the test of time in my practice for over 40 years and I see little need for DPR.

I have taken a strip of septal cartilage out over the maxillary crest when there is septal deviation and I have needed to go into the septum; this maneuver, when combined with freeing up the attachment of the cartilaginous septum from the bony perpendicular plate, allows a swinging door of the septum, and the caudal septum can then be sewn in the midline to the periosteum of the nasal spine. At those times, when I also wish to de-project the tip and a little bit of the dorsal cartilaginous septum, I have taken some extra septal cartilage in a strip leaving a small gap between the inferior portion of the septum and the maxillary crest, so that when I suture the caudal end of the septum to the spine, the Vicryl suture I use does de-project a certain amount depending on amount of gap created. However, when no septal work is needed when there is no septal deviation, not having to go into the septum at all reduces potential complications such as septal perforations and saves time.

Most/Patel

While preservation rhinoplasty can impart a negative connotation to excisional techniques, which have been labeled as "destructive," both structural and preservation techniques are effective in achieving universal goals in rhinoplasty: namely a functionally and aesthetically sound result that

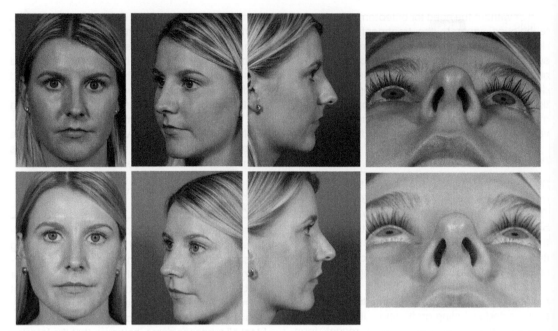

Fig. 3. Preoperative and 1 year postoperative images are shown here in a patient undergoing a structural preservation with a let-down and modified subdorsal strip method. Note that the preoperative dorsal aesthetic lines are preserved.

will stand the test of time (**Figs. 3–5**). For many years, the largely pervasive structural approach has resulted in high rates of patient satisfaction. Reported outcomes with preservation techniques are growing, but still more limited relative to the long-term data available for structural techniques.

Since preservation techniques maintain the external nasal contour on frontal view, in patients with ideal dorsal aesthetic lines preoperatively, preservation may be more effective in maintaining this appearance (see **Figs. 3** and **4**). Since CHR approaches require disruption of and recreation of the

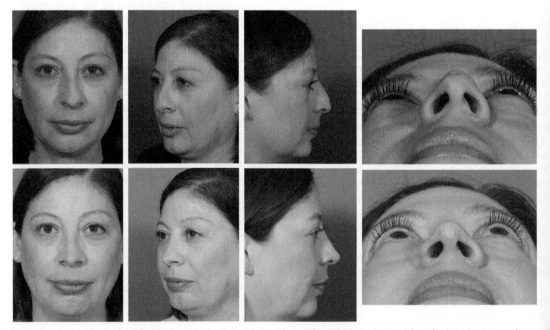

Fig. 4. Preoperative and 1 year postoperative images are shown here in a patient with a deviated nose undergoing a structural preservation with an asymmetric let-down, modified subdorsal strip method, and right septal extension graft.

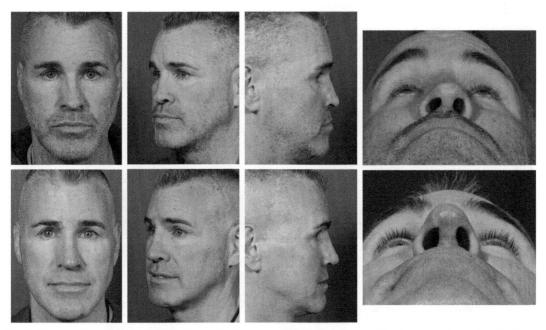

Fig. 5. Preoperative and 9-month postoperative images are shown here in a patient undergoing a structural revision rhinoplasty including anterior septal reconstruction, spreader grafting, and diced cartilage for camouflage. Note that in the interim, the patient was treated with a forehead flap (nasal tip only) by an outside Mohs surgeon.

dorsal aesthetic lines, there is a higher risk of having irregularities at the dorsum. Alternatively, CHR approaches will be more efficacious in correcting inherently deformed bones with irregularities or significant width of either the bones or midvault (as preservation techniques will not alter these deformities; see **Fig. 5**).[10,17] One concern with preservation techniques is the incomplete elimination of or recurrence of dorsal humps, with rates ranging between 3% and 12%.[18–23] This may be higher than CHR approaches in which a direct excision of the hump is performed.

Comparative studies between preservation and CHR techniques have shown varying results, but largely they have similar patient satisfaction outcomes. In a randomized prospective study comparing the modified preservation technique (spare roof technique) to component dorsal hump reduction (n = 250), functional and cosmetic visual analog scale (VAS) scores were superior in the former group.[24] However, in a cadaveric radiologic study, the internal nasal valve (INV) dimensions/angle did not change between the traditional letdown (LD) technique or Joseph hump resection with appropriate midvault reconstruction.[25] In a matched cohort study, Standardized Cosmesis and Health Nasal Outcomes Survey (SCHNOS) and VAS scores were no different between patients undergoing open approach LD preservation compared to open structural rhinoplasty.[26] A similar outcome

was noted in a comparison of Dorsal Preservation and Dorsal Reduction Rhinoplasty analyzing nasal patency and outcomes with Rhinomanometry, Nasal Obstruction Symptom Evaluation (NOSE) Scale, and SCHNOS outcomes.[27] These later studies suggest that while preservation rhinoplasty is a fundamentally sound methodology, well-executed CHR surgery with adequate midvault reconstruction yields similarly excellent results. It is important to note that some of our outcome measures may not be granular enough to elucidate some of the more subtle benefits (eg, quality of dorsal aesthetic lines) seen with preservation techniques.

Papel

The answer to this question will depend on the bias and experience of the surgeon. Comparison of both techniques' long-term results with scientific data is not available. Experienced surgeons will have long-term data on one technique or another, but this type of data are just beginning to build for the "preservation" techniques. It is important to point out that rhinoplasty with push-down and let-down techniques has been around for a very long time. I have found references in the literature about preservation type surgery as far back as 1932. Maurice Cottle taught these techniques extensively in the 1940s and 1950s in numerous courses and publications.

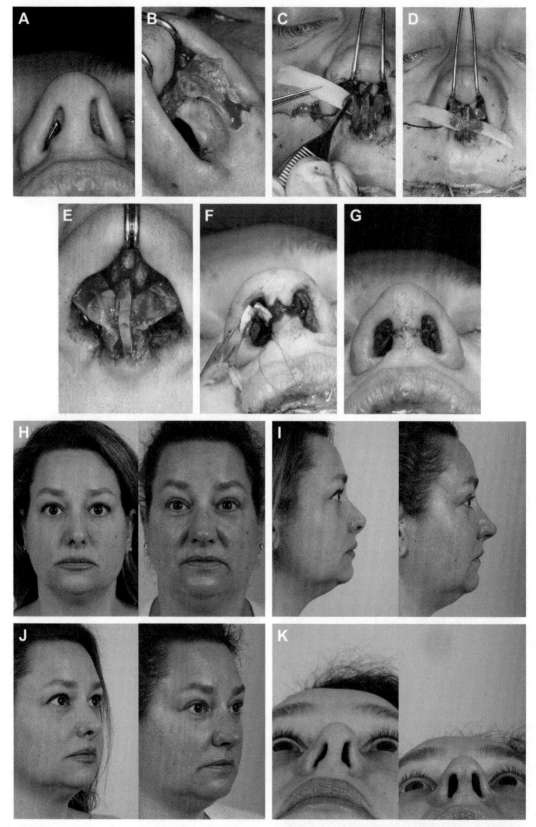

Fig. 6. This patient underwent prior rhinoplasties and required extensive structural grafting for reconstruction. (*A*) Preoperative base view showing nasal vestibular stenosis. The yellow arrow points to the right vestibular stenosis. (*B*) View of asymmetric and over-reduced tip cartilages. (*C*) Placement of lateral crural strut grafts. (*D*)

When I was a resident, we had several rhinoplastic surgeons in our community who were associated with the Cottle courses and routinely used push-down and let-down techniques in their surgery. My observation of these cases was that there was often persistent wideness of the dorsum, and hump recurrence was higher than expected. In addition, the lateral nasal bone excisions were difficult to judge and perform.

In summary, direct comparison is very difficult currently. With further experience by a wider number of surgeons, this should change.

Toriumi

Both structure rhinoplasty and preservation rhinoplasty are effective. Structure rhinoplasty is the most versatile of the philosophies as it can be used in almost all rhinoplasty cases. If a patient is not a candidate for preservation rhinoplasty, they would likely be a candidate for structure rhinoplasty. As to which is more effective, it depends on the application of the technique and the patient's specific anatomic findings and intended outcome.

In cases of revision rhinoplasty, structure rhinoplasty is far more effective as many of these cases require more of a reconstructive mode, and in many cases, there is little that can be preserved. In most revision cases, the nasal dorsum has been manipulated and the nasal tip likely has been altered. In these cases, structural cartilage grafting will be necessary to reconstruct the nasal dorsum and nasal tip. Costal cartilage or auricular cartilage may be needed for the cartilage graft stock. In many cases, I will use spreader grafts, caudal septal extension graft, and lateral crural strut grafts (**Fig. 6**). In these cases, there is little that is preserved and most of the major structures require some degree of reconstruction.

In some select revision cases, there may be a residual dorsal hump and the middle vault may be intact. In these rare cases, dorsal preservation can be used to reduce the dorsal hump and straighten the nose. I will use a subdorsal Z-flap, Tetris, or low strip to accomplish these tasks (**Fig. 7**). If the roof of the bony vault has been resected or the roof of the middle vault has been removed, dorsal preservation is not effective.

In revision rhinoplasty, a structural approach is very effective, and preservation is only rarely an option.

In primary rhinoplasty, preservation rhinoplasty is highly effective. I have shifted to using dorsal preservation in over 90% of my primary rhinoplasty cases. In most cases, I use a hybrid of structure and dorsal preservation (structural preservation rhinoplasty).[28] I will use dorsal preservation to manage the upper two-thirds of the nose to modulate the dorsal hump and structure in the nasal tip (caudal septal extension graft and lateral crural strut grafts). I find this hybrid approach to be very effective both aesthetically and functionally.

I also find the "push-up" using the subdorsal cantilever graft to be very effective in augmenting the nasal dorsum in the saddle nose deformity and in ethnic patients with a low dorsum.[29]

Both structure and preservation are effective approaches to rhinoplasty and in many cases, a combination of both provides the best outcomes.

HOW TO DECIDE ON THE PROPER TECHNIQUE?
Kridel

As stated earlier, there is no "proper" technique. It depends on the experience of the surgeon. There are many ways up the mountain. One should learn multiple techniques so that when one way is blocked due to the encountered physical anatomy, the armamentarium of the surgeon provides other approaches. For the novice surgeon, it is probably best to use the technique with the least chance for serious or multiple complications.

Most/Patel

Selecting the best technique in rhinoplasty is dependent on a number of pre-operative historic and examination findings. Despite the positive outcomes and patient satisfaction observed in both CHR and preservation techniques, we find that preservation minimizes the risks of dorsal irregularities requiring camouflaging and is superior at maintaining the dorsal aesthetic lines. Postoperatively, the dorsal contour appears smoother more immediately. Given these findings, preservation is a preferred technique where possible. Therefore, it is easiest to first determine if a patient is a candidate for preservation. If not, it is next determined if the patient's nasal morphology can be converted into a preservation case via surface techniques (eg, rasping/osteoplasty). If criteria are not met, then patients are treated with a CHR

Lateral crural strut grafts in place. (*E*) Tip after lateral crural strut grafts positioned. (*F*) Hinged auricular composite graft placed to open the right nasal valve. (*G*) Immediate postoperative base view. (*H*) Preoperative frontal view (*left*). Two-year postoperative frontal view (*right*) (*I*) Preoperative lateral view (*left*). Postoperative lateral view (*right*). (*J*) Preoperative oblique view (*left*). Postoperative oblique view (*right*). (*K*) Preoperative base (*left*). Postoperative base view showing open nasal vestibule (*right*).

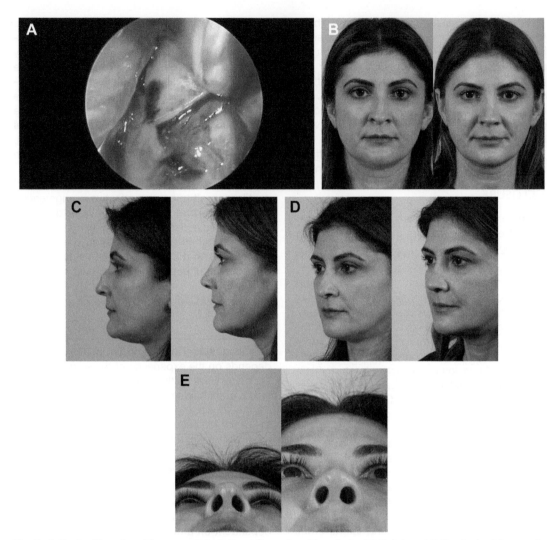

Fig. 7. Patient with a dorsal hump and deviation after prior rhinoplasty. (*A*) Subdorsal Z-flap incised for overlap to correct the deviation. (*B*) Preoperative frontal view (*left*). Two-year postoperative frontal view (*right*). (*C*) Preoperative lateral view (*left*). Postoperative lateral view showing straight dorsum (*right*). (*D*) Preoperative oblique view (*left*). Postoperative oblique view (*right*). (*E*) Preoperative base view (*left*). Postoperative base view (*right*).

approach. It is possible to convert from a preservation to CHR technique intraoperatively if needed.

Preservation cases ideally involve an aesthetically pleasing dorsum on frontal view (**Fig. 3**). If there is a break in the dorsal aesthetic lines and this is secondary to a small irregularity in the bone, many times this can be contoured. If there are straight axis deviations, this can also be corrected with preservation techniques incorporating asymmetric resection of bone (with more resected from the non-deviated size; see **Fig. 4**).[30–32] Significant deformities or S-shaped deviations will be difficult to correct with preservation strategies.

Significant violation and/or resection of the septum or dorsum from prior trauma or surgery may preclude preservation since integrity and structure in these areas are paramount to successful stabilization of the osseo-cartilaginous framework. Very significant septal deformities, for similar reasons, are better treated with CHR methods (see **Fig. 5**). Caudal septal deviations are not contraindications to preservation strategies. Preservation septal techniques such as the modified subdorsal strip method allow for complete anterior septal reconstruction and the cottle method allows for repositioning of the septum.[33–37]

Those patients with a significantly kyphotic hump (or S shaped nasal bones rather than V shaped) may not be appropriate candidates for preservation secondary to a risk of incomplete hump elimination/hump recurrence or a significant drop in the height of the radix while attempting to lower the dorsum.[10,13,17] Similarly, patients with deeper nasofrontal angles are at greater risk of a drop in the radix with DPR technqiues.[18] It should be noted that the use of bony contouring and radix grafts can be used to manage these issues and therefore these are not absolute contraindications to preservation rhinoplasty.

Papel

Most surgeons will decide to use techniques they are confident will provide good results. It is understandable that many are hesitant to change from structural rhinoplasty to preservation techniques when they have not seen a mass migration of surgeons move in that direction. American Academy of Facial Plastic and Reconstructive Surgery (AAFPRS) meetings, and other specialty societies, give much attention to preservation techniques, but I have not seen this playing out in the general community.

There has been much discussion about whether preservation of the dorsal osseocartilaginous subunit is really a "preservation" technique. To move the dorsum lower, or higher, aggressive mobilization of the entire bony structure, septal resection with designed flaps, and possible lateral separation of the keystone area (Ballerina Technique) are required. When this is accomplished, the entire dorsum is mobile, and the final position depends on accurate placement of septal sutures. Some see this as an aggressive (not preservative) technique with many moving parts. This possibly contributes to the hesitation of surgeons to switch from structural methods.

Toriumi

Many factors come into play when deciding on the proper technique in structure or preservation rhinoplasty. In structure rhinoplasty, the technique used depends on the type of grafting employed and the intended changes desired. You can choose between a columellar strut and a caudal septal extension graft to support the nasal base. My preference is a caudal septal extension graft if a tip-split approach to the septum is used.[14,15] I will use spreader grafts in most cases to reconstruct the middle vault if a component hump reduction was used to reduce the dorsal hump. I rarely do this anymore, so the spreader grafts are primarily used in revision rhinoplasty.

In preservation rhinoplasty, the technique used can vary depending on what the goals are and what type of deformity is noted in the patient. If the patient has a small dorsal hump that is primarily bony, it may be sufficient to use a surface technique with rhinosculpting of the bony cap and limited subdorsal work to lower the middle vault prominence. This could include a high strip, subdorsal Z-flap, or Tetris.[38,39] With larger dorsal humps, it will likely require foundational work such as a push-down of a letdown in combination with the subdorsal septal work (high strip, subdorsal Z-flap, or Tetris).

In patients with an axis deviation with a dorsal hump, a subdorsal Z-flap or Tetris can be used and overlapped on the side opposite the deviation and sutured in the overlapping orientation. If the patient has a deviated nose with moderate to severe septal deviation, a low strip (Cottle, SPQR) can be used to straighten the septum and reduce the dorsal hump.[4,40] The low strip can also be used in the deviated nose without a dorsal hump by performing a swinging door septoplasty where the quadrangular septal cartilage flap is reduced to fit properly in the space occupied by the septum and then fixed back to the nasal spine. In this case, the septal flap is not rotated to reduce a hump but just resized and shifted to the midline to fit into the subdorsal space.

An Ishida cartilaginous push down with or without bony cap preservation or spare roof type B can be useful in patients with a larger bony hump with some S-shaped characteristics. In this case, triangles of bone are removed along the sides of the dorsal hump and then the bony cap is collapsed on itself and sutured into a reduced position.[41] If the radix is low, it can be augmented with a small radix graft.

WHAT IS THE OPTIMAL PATIENT FOR PRESERVATION RHINOPLASTY?
Kridel

A patient who does not need tip work, in whom an endonasal rhinoplasty might alternatively be considered, and who has only a dorsal hump might be a candidate for DPR, especially if you do not like taking a dorsum down traditionally. But DPR is more disruptive and is a lot of extra work for something done much more easily via a rasp and a blade. If you do need to do tip work, you might as well do a traditional hump removal since you are already there. Additionally, with traditional rhinoplasty that requires middle vault trimming, spreader grafts are often needed which require cartilage for grafting. If a turn-in method is not used for spreaders, a patient who requires septal cartilage for other grafts might not have enough to do spreaders also and so might be considered for DPR.

Most/Patel

The optimal patient for preservation rhinoplasty has not had prior nasal surgery or significant

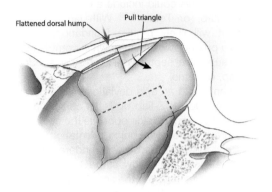

Fig. 8. Subdorsal Z-flap showing overlapping of the septal flap on the right side to correct axis deviation.

nasal trauma. Dorsal aesthetic lines are pleasing on frontal view. The profile view demonstrates a broad hump rather than significant kyphosis. Anatomically, this correlates with V-shaped and S-shaped bones, respectively. The latter group has a higher likelihood of an osseous residual hump without additional contouring maneuvers.[10,13,17] Ideally, the septum is either non-

deviated or has minor deviations lower and posteriorly. The dorsal hump in the ideal preservation patient has a greater cartilaginous contribution with a corresponding shorter nasal bone length.[18] Since the middle vault cannot be separated from its pyrifom attachments, it will flare as it descends. As such, the ideal preservation nose will not have wide or prominent upper lateral cartilage shoulders. The radix in the optimal patient should not be deep. Preservation has been reported to reduce revision rates in males compared with other surgical techniques, potentially due to less risk of feminization.[13] Higher revision rates may be observed in females due to the desire for greater dorsal height reduction.[13] However, both males and females with realistic expectations are great candidates for preservation techniques.

Papel

The ideal patient for let-down or push-down techniques would exhibit small to moderate humps, normal or high radix, have an intact septum, and a normal dorsal width.

Toriumi: The optimal patient for dorsal preservation will have a narrow dorsum with V-shaped dorsal hump with a normal radix and shorter nasal

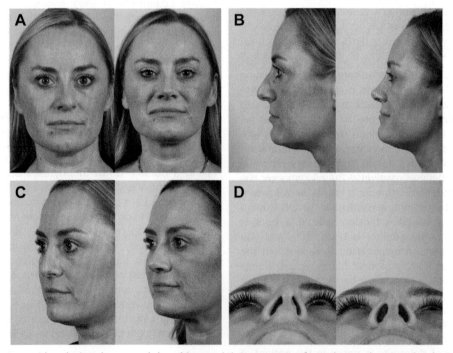

Fig. 9. Patient with a deviated nose and dorsal hump. (*A*) Preoperative frontal view showing the deviated nose (*left*). Two-year postoperative frontal view showing the straight nose (*right*). (*B*) Preoperative lateral view (*left*). Postoperative lateral view and the straight dorsum (*right*). (*C*) Preoperative oblique view (*left*). Postoperative oblique view (*right*). (*D*) Preoperative base view (*left*). Postoperative base view (*right*).

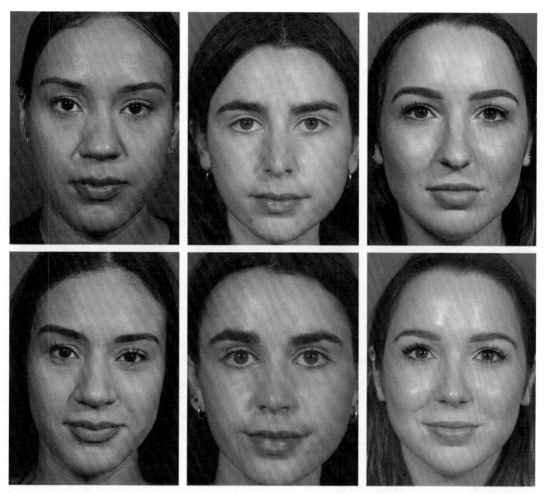

Fig. 10. Several before and after frontal views demonstrating patients treated with structural rhinoplasty techniques. In the first case, osteotomies as well as dorsal augmentation/camouflage with diced rib were performed. In the second and third cases, the dorsal aesthetic lines were narrowed using piezo osteotomy and osteotomy of the dorsum.

bones. It is more favorable to have shorter nasal bones as this equates to an easier dorsal reduction with the designated subdorsal manipulation. Depending on the technique chosen for the dorsal preservation, it may be more favorable to have a slight axis deviation that needs to be corrected. With the slight axis deviation, the subdorsal Z-flap can be overlapped on the side opposite the

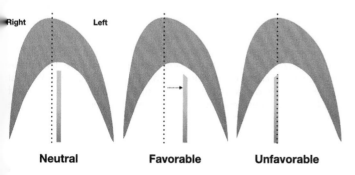

Neutral   Favorable   Unfavorable

Fig. 11. The relationship between the position of the high septum and the external nasal deviation may help identify patients that are better suited for preservation cases. As shown here, with an external deviation of the nasal pyramid to the right, a high septal deviation to the contralateral side will permit mobilization of the nasal framework to the left. The dorsal septal gap (DSG) is larger and therefore favorable for structural hump resections. If the septum has a high deviation to the ipsilateral side, there is a smaller DSG, which will limit the medialization of bone if doing a conventional hump resection. In this latter scenario, a preservation procedure may be more optimal.

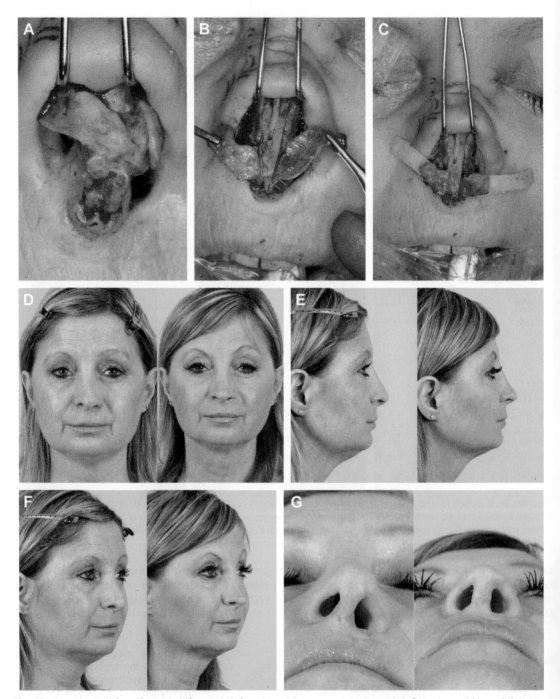

Fig. 12. A patient with unilateral cleft nasal deformity with asymmetric tip and deficient nasal base. (*A*) Intraoperative view of the asymmetric tip cartilages. (*B*) Lateral crural replacement grafts positioned. (*C*) Lateral crural strut grafts in place. (*D*) Preoperative frontal view (*left*). Two-year postoperative frontal view showing improved symmetry (*right*). (*E*) Preoperative lateral view (*left*). Postoperative lateral view (*right*). (*F*) Preoperative oblique view (*left*). Postoperative oblique view (*right*). (*G*) Preoperative base view showing asymmetries (*left*). Postoperative base view showing improved symmetry (*right*).

deviation providing a more stable fixation of the Z-flap to the remnant septal strut (**Fig. 8**; **Fig. 9**). On the other hand, with the high strip, it is better to have a straight nose with no axis deviation.

The optimal patient for a preservation rhinoplasty using an endonasal approach such as the polygon tip, will have a symmetric tip with more normally positioned lateral crura. It is also favorable to have longer stronger medial and lateral crura. Patients requiring shortening of their nose are also more favorable.

WHAT IS THE OPTIMAL PATIENT FOR STRUCTURAL APPROACHES?
Kridel

Structural approaches have stood the test of time for over 40 years, producing precise, long lasting, aesthetically pleasing, and functional noses with very minimal complications in the hands of a skilled surgeon in all patients. Those with such successful outcomes need not adopt a different approach DPR solely because those who are marketing this reborn old approach to the public as "the latest and greatest" are purporting it to be superior or the way to go. We need to be sure that those who advocate for DPR are inclusive in discussing the downsides of the procedure and that they present long-term results of at least 5 years in their presentations and that they benchmark their results with the traditional methods.

Most/Patel

Patients who are optimal candidates for preservation rhinoplasty will inherently also be great candidates for CHR rhinoplasty. This includes primary patients with realistic expectations and with good integrity of the septum and nasal framework. However, relative to preservation, CHR rhinoplasty will more optimally treat very deformed noses or wider noses on frontal view (**Fig. 10**). CHR techniques will also be more consistent in effectively treating very large dorsal humps. In a meta-analysis of 22 studies representing a cohort of 5660 patients undergoing a variety of DPR techniques, postoperative hump recurrence rates were 4.18%.[42] The rates in CHR rhinoplasty are likely lower, especially when considering large kyphotic humps, although this has not been definitively confirmed in long-term comparative studies. Regarding the dorsum, while patients with any skin quality are great candidates for preservation, the optimal patients for CHR rhinoplasty have medium to thicker skin. This is for the purposes of minimizing the visibility of any irregularity in the dorsum.

While the deviated nose and septum can be optimally managed with CHR methods, a caveat is worth noting. In the setting of high septal deviations, structural techniques work well if the side of the septal deviation is away from the side of the nasal deviation (**Fig. 11**). In this favorable scenario, after a hump takedown, there is a gap (the dorsal septal gap, DSG) for bone to medialize toward the deviated septum.[36] Alternatively, if the septum deviates to the same side as the deviated nasal vault, this will limit the medialization of bone and the ability to correct the deviation. (if doing a standard hump takedown). In this scenario, a preservation procedure may be more optimal.

Papel

This patient can have a hump of any size. The radix can also be variable. If the dorsum is wide, it can be managed easier with a structural plan. As always, an intact septum allows for more flexibility and potential grafts.

Toriumi

The optimal patients for structural approaches are patients who require reduction and reconstruction of the middle vault and tip. These patients are those with severe tip asymmetries and those with inherent middle vault cartilage deformity or extremes in projection. Patients who have undergone prior rhinoplasty and who require dorsal, or tip reconstruction are ideal candidates for the structure approach as long as cartilage is available for grafting. In most revision cases, costal cartilage will be needed if the septum has been operated in the previous operation.

Patients with cleft nasal deformity, nasomaxillary dysplasia/deficiency (Binders syndrome), and other nasal deformities are great candidates for structure rhinoplasty (**Fig. 12**).[5,43]

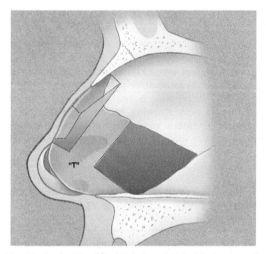

Fig. 13. In the Modified Subdorsal Strip Method, cartilage is resected from the intermediate portions of the septum (*blue*) with preservation of a subdorsal strut. Lower portions of septum can be resected (*red*) if there are deviations or for grafting needs. This leaves a "T" strut of cartilage that involves the caudal septum and an intact mid septal segment.

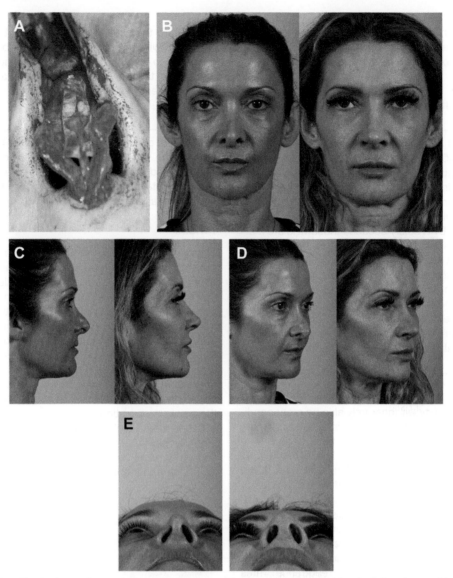

Fig. 14. A patient who underwent prior rhinoplasty with alar retraction, polybeak deformity, and inverted-V deformity with low dorsum. (*A*) Tall spreader grafts extending above the upper lateral cartilages for augmentation. (*B*) Preoperative frontal view showing inverted-V deformity (*left*). One year and 3-month postoperative frontal view showing improved dorsal aesthetic lines (*right*). (*C*) Preoperative lateral view (*left*). Postoperative lateral view showing augmented dorsum (*right*). (*D*) Preoperative oblique view (*left*). Postoperative oblique view (*right*). (*E*) Preoperative base view (*left*). Postoperative base view showing improved symmetry (*right*).

HOW HAVE YOUR TECHNIQUES IN THIS AREA CHANGED OVER THE PAST 2 YEARS?
Most/Patel

Until approximately 5 years ago, the most common technique used in our practice was a CHR method. This mirrors the rhinoplasty climate globally.[44] However, with time, and particularly over the past 5 years, preservation rhinoplasty has made up a larger majority of primary rhinoplasty cases. Importantly, as our practice includes a high number of revision or traumatic cases, structural techniques remain prevalent. It is important to recognize that these 2 techniques are not mutually exclusive and rather we feel together they contribute to the versatility of our rhinoplasty armamentarium.

As noted earlier, there are a number of techniques and modifications that have emerged within preservation rhinoplasty. Our preferred method is the modified subdorsal strip method, which affords the ability to address septal deviations (including

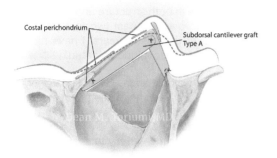

Fig. 15. Subdorsal cantilever graft type A showing extension under NBs to elevate the middle vault. Note the fixation to the caudal septal extension graft caudally.

caudal) and harvest cartilage for grafting purposes (**Fig. 13**).[36] This technique has allowed for the treatment of functional complaints in addition to aesthetic concerns, allowing for its expanded use in our practice. Additionally, we find that we are increasingly converting patients to preservation candidates through surface modifications (eg, osteoplasty) where possible. Again, as part of our algorithm, the goal is to perform preservation where feasible. The fusion of conventional open structural techniques for the nasal tip and preservation

methods for the dorsum ("structural preservation") has additionally allowed for us to increasingly incorporate preservation into practice.[45] This may be especially important for rhinoplasty surgeons who are starting to utilize preservation. As with any method in rhinoplasty, preservation techniques certainly have a learning curve and we continue to learn about the nuances and remain critical of our results as time progresses.

Papel

I have been observing push-down and let-down techniques for many years. While rare in the United States until recently, these operations have been common in parts of Europe, the Middle East, and South America. I have had the good fortune to have visited these areas frequently and directly observed surgical procedures on a regular basis. Therefore, I have had a long exposure to these procedures.

> I have often observed how the midportion of the nose is so mobile and the final position dependent on a single polydioxanone (PDS) suture pulling the dorsum down to the septal strut. This is not always an easy task but is critical to the success of dorsal preservation rhinoplasty.

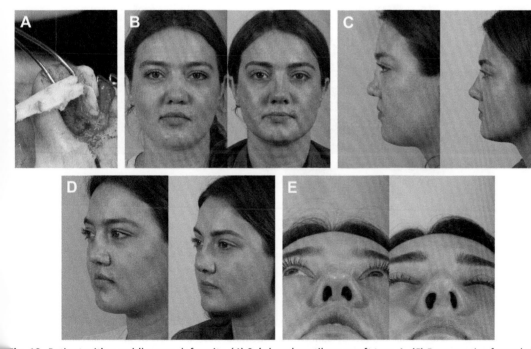

Fig. 16. Patient with a saddle nose deformity. (*A*) Subdorsal cantilever graft type A. (*B*) Preoperative frontal view (*left*). Fifteen-month postoperative frontal view showing improved dorsal aesthetic lines (*right*). (*C*) Preoperative lateral view showing saddle nose deformity (*left*). Postoperative lateral view showing improved profile (*right*). (*D*) Preoperative oblique view (*left*). Postoperative oblique view (*right*). (*E*) Preoperative base view (*left*). Postoperative base view (*right*).

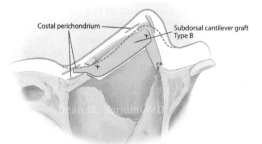

Fig. 17. Subdorsal cantilever graft type B showing cranial extension through the radix osteotomy site to raise the radix and fixation caudally to the caudal septal extension graft.

I have performed thousands of rhinoplasty procedures using a large variety of techniques. It is apparent that the modern preservation techniques are more subtle and better planned than what I saw more than 35 years ago. At this point, I feel I can control the rhinoplasty better with structural methods and depend on long-term stable results. With this said, I will continue to study and observe all new techniques, including modifications to the "dorsal preservation" methods, which have been described for more than 90 years.

Toriumi

My techniques in both structure and preservation have changed over the past two to 4 years. For structure, over the past 4 years, I have made 4 major changes in technique as noted.

1. One of the major changes is that I no longer use onlay dorsal grafts when I need to augment the nasal dorsum. I either use "tall spreader grafts" or the subdorsal cantilever graft. Tall spreader grafts are spreader grafts that extend higher than the existing dorsum to increase dorsal height.[16] The tall spreader grafts will reconstruct the middle vault and increase dorsal height. I use them in revision rhinoplasty cases. I do not need spreader grafts in primary cases as I do not open the middle vault. The tall spreader grafts can also create narrowing of the dorsum and provide symmetric dorsal aesthetic lines (**Fig. 14**). With tall spreader grafts, I can raise the dorsum up to 4 mm in height.

   For major dorsal augmentation, I will use the subdorsal cantilever graft to raise the dorsum in primary ethnic augmentation cases.[29] With the subdorsal cantilever graft, I perform a complete release of the nasal bones and lateral keystone, then

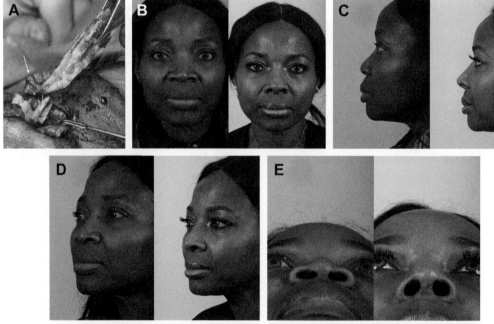

Fig. 18. Patient with a low radix and low dorsum with a wide nasal base. (A) View of subdorsal cantilever graft type B with attached perichondrium (*yellow arrow*). (B) Preoperative frontal view showing flat dorsum and wide base (*left*). Two-year postoperative frontal view showing improved dorsal aesthetic lines and narrower base (*right*). (C) Preoperative lateral view showing low radix (*left*). Postoperative lateral view showing higher radix and projected nasal tip (*right*). (D) Preoperative oblique view (*left*). Postoperative oblique view (*right*). (E) Preoperative base view showing wide base (*left*). Postoperative base view showing narrow nasal base (*right*).

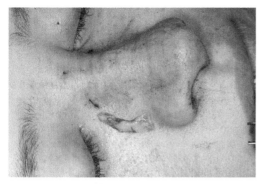

Fig. 19. Banana-shaped bone strip removal for letdown foundational reduction of the dorsal hump.

raise the dorsum (push-up) and hold it in an augmented position using a graft placed under the dorsum. The subdorsal cantilever graft type A raises the dorsum with minimal radix augmentation and is ideal for saddle nose repair (**Figs. 15** and **16**). The subdorsal cantilever graft type B raises the radix as well as the dorsum of the nose (**Figs. 17** and **18**). I find the subdorsal cantilever graft to be very effective for ethnic augmentation cases requiring dorsal augmentation.

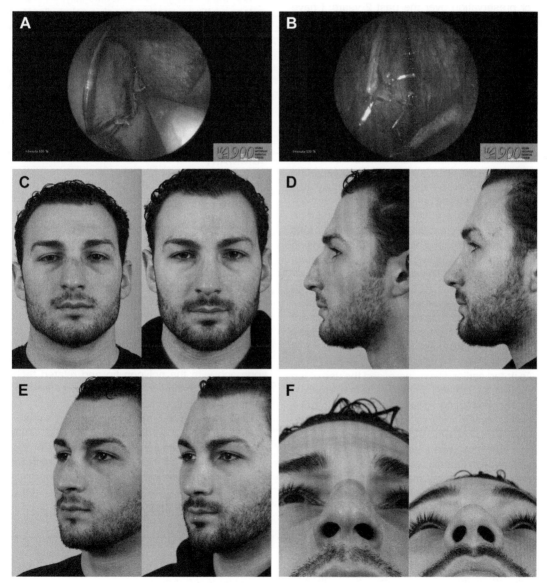

Fig. 20. This patient presented with acute nasal trauma and the deviated nose with a dorsal hump. (*A*) Intraoperative view of the incised Tetris flap. (*B*) Overlapped and sutured Tetris flap to the side opposite the deviation. (*C*) Preoperative frontal view showing the deviated nose (*left*). One year and 3 months postoperative frontal view showing straight nose (*right*). (*D*) Preoperative lateral view showing dorsal hump (*left*). Postoperative lateral view showing straight dorsum (*right*). (*E*) Preoperative oblique view (*left*). Postoperative oblique view (*right*). (*F*) Preoperative base view (*left*). Postoperative base view (*right*).

2. Another major change I have made in structure rhinoplasty is the use of platelet-rich fibrin and fat for dorsal nasal camouflage in patients with thin skin. I use this primarily in revision rhinoplasty cases with thin skin or damaged skin. This technique of platelet rich fibrin (PRF) fat was introduced by Milos Kovacevic.[43] Fat is harvested and chopped into fine pieces and then combined with platelet-rich fibrin to create a sheet of fat that can then be placed over the nasal dorsum for camouflage. I have found this to be very helpful in patients with thin atrophic damaged skin.

For preservation over the past 2 years, I have also made some important changes.

1. I have shifted back to using a 3-mm osteotome to remove the banana-shaped bone strip to execute a "letdown." Initially, I used a push-down, then changed to a letdown, taking out the bone strips using a high and then low cut along the ascending process of the maxilla. I then shifted to using a narrow rongeur to take out the bone strip. Using the rongeur was not as reliable as, in some cases, irregular bone segments were removed. Approximately two years ago, I shifted back to using the 3-mm osteotome to make a high cut, then a low cut on the ascending process of the maxilla to take out a banana-shaped bone strip (**Fig. 19**). Using this technique, I can remove a more consistent segment of bone. This can be a difficult maneuver, so I have also recently developed the banana strip osteotome/gouge(Marina Medical Instruments Inc., Davie, Fla.). This instrument has a left and right-sided version that allows the removal of a bone strip along the ascending process of the maxilla.
2. As noted earlier, I have increased the use of the subdorsal cantilever graft. It is also very effective for reconstructing Asian patients who require the removal of a dorsal implant and immediate reconstruction using a costal cartilage graft.
3. Over the past two years, I have used dorsal preservation techniques for patients presenting with acute nasal trauma and nasal bone fracture. Instead of using an open reduction of the nasal fracture, I am performing a dorsal preservation technique (subdorsal Z-flap, Tetris, or low strip) to correct the deviation and reduce the dorsal hump. I have found this approach to be very effective and provides the patient with an acute nasal fracture with a straight nose with no dorsal hump (**Fig. 20**).
4. I have recently started to use the endonasal approach for select primary rhinoplasty patients.

I use the polygon tip with dorsal preservation with ligament preservation as described by Baris Cakir.[6–8] I have found this technique to have a significant upside in certain primary cases. The primary advantage is the improved control over the supratip with less postoperative supratip swelling due to the preservation of Pitanguy's ligament. With the open structure rhinoplasty approach, I frequently need to inject the supratip with steroids to control the supratip break. With the endonasal polygon tip approach, the supratip position and lateral tip contour are improved with the preservation of Pitanguy's ligament and the scroll ligaments. Additionally, less cartilage grafting is needed as only a columellar strut is used to stabilize the nasal base. In this approach, I do not need a caudal septal extension graft or lateral crural strut grafts. Up to this point in time, I have been very selective in case selection choosing patients with favorable tip orientation (not cephalically positioned), slightly underprojected symmetric tip in need of tip rotation.

SUMMARY

Both structure rhinoplasty and preservation rhinoplasty are very important and effective approaches in rhinoplasty. Structure rhinoplasty is the only viable option for most revision rhinoplasty cases. There are occasional revision cases where dorsal preservation can be used but these are not common.

For primary rhinoplasty, one can use a hybrid approach using dorsal preservation in the upper two-thirds of the nose and structure in the nasal tip (lower third). This hybrid structural preservation rhinoplasty is and will continue to be a powerful option.

I believe the transition to the endonasal approach with the polygon tip and related techniques will continue to increase in popularity as surgeons recognize the benefits.

This is an exciting time in rhinoplasty as a monumental shift is occurring with the preservation movement. As more surgeons take up this philosophy, outcomes will likely improve, and both the patient and surgeon will benefit.

CLINICS CARE POINTS

- Structure rhinoplasty is most appropriate for secondary rhinoplasty.
- Preservation rhinoplasty is most appropriate for primary rhinoplasty patients.

REFERENCES

1. Johnson CM, Toriumi DM. Open structure rhinoplasty. WB: Saunders; 1988.
2. Lothrop OA. An operation for correcting the aquiline nasal deformity. Boston Med Surg J 1914;170: 835–7.
3. Goodale JL. A new method for the operative correction of exaggerated Roman nose. Boston Med Surg J 1989;140:112.
4. Cottle MH, Loring RM. Corrective surgery of the external nasal pyramid and the nasal septum for restoration of nasal physiology. Ill Med J 1946;90: 119–31.
5. Saban Y, Daniel RK, Polselli R, et al. dorsal preservation: the push down technique reassessed. Aesthetic Surg J 2018;38(2):117–31.
6. Cakir B. Aesthetic septorhinoplasty. Heidelberg: Springer; 2016.
7. Cakir B, Oreroglu AR, Daniel R. Surface aesthetics in tip rhinoplasty: a step-by-step guide. Aesthetic Surg J 2014;34(6).
8. Cakir B, Oreroglu AR, Dogan T, et al. A complete subperichondrial dissection technique for rhinoplasty with management of the nasal ligaments. Aesthetic Surg J 2012;32(5):564–74.
9. Daniel RK. The preservation rhinoplasty: A new rhinoplasty revolution. Aesthetic Surg J 2018;38: 228–9.
10. Neves JC, Arancibia-Tagle D. Avoiding aesthetic drawbacks and stigmata in dorsal line preservation rhinoplasty. Facial Plast Surg 2021;37(1):65–75.
11. Rodrigues Dias D, Cardoso L, Santos M, et al. The caucasian hump: radiologic study of the osteocartilaginous vault versus surface anatomy. clinical implications in structured and preservation rhinoplasty. Plast Reconstr Surg 2021;148(3):523–31.
12. Palhazi P, Daniel RK, Kosins AM. The osseocartilaginous vault of the nose: anatomy and surgical observations. Aesthetic Surg J 2015;35(3): 242–51.
13. Saban Y, de Salvador S. Guidelines for dorsum preservation in primary rhinoplasty. Facial Plast Surg 2021;37(1):53–64.
14. Toriumi DM. Caudal septal extension graft for correction of the retracted columella. Op Tech Otol Head Neck Surg 1995;6(4):311–8.
15. Toriumi DM. New concepts in nasal tip contouring. Arch Facial Plast Surg 2006;8(3):156–85.
16. Toriumi DM. Structure rhinoplasty: lessons learned in thirty years. Chicago, IL: DMT Publishing; 2019.
17. Ferraz MBJ, Sella GCP. Indications for preservation rhinoplasty: avoiding complications. Facial Plast Surg 2021;37(1):45–52.
18. Saban Y, Daniel RK, Polselli R, et al. Dorsal preservation: the push down technique reassessed. Aesthetic Surg J 2018;38(2):117–31.

19. Tuncel U, Aydogdu IO, Kurt A. Reducing dorsal hump recurrence following push down-let down rhinoplasty. Aesthetic Surg J 2020. https://doi.org/10.1093/asj/sjaa145.
20. Tuncel U, Aydogdu O. The probable reasons for dorsal hump problems following let-down/push-down rhinoplasty and solution proposals. Plast Reconstr Surg 2019;144(3):378e–85e.
21. Ishida J, Ishida LC, Ishida LH, et al. Treatment of the nasal hump with preservation of the cartilaginous framework. Plast Reconstr Surg 1999;103(6): 1729–33 [discussion 1734-5].
22. Atolini NJ, Lunelli V, Lang GP, et al. Septum pyramidal adjustment and repositioning - a conservative and effective rhinoplasty technique. Braz J Otorhinolaryngol Mar - 2019;85(2):176–82.
23. Kosins AM, Daniel RK. Decision making in preservation rhinoplasty: a 100 case series with one-year follow-up. Aesthetic Surg J 2019;40(1):34–48.
24. Ferreira MG, Santos M, Carmo DOE, et al. Spare roof technique versus component dorsal hump reduction: a randomized prospective study in 250 primary rhinoplasties, aesthetic and functional outcomes. Aesthetic Surg J 2020. https://doi.org/10.1093/asj/sjaa221.
25. Abdelwahab MA, Neves CA, Patel PN, et al. Impact of dorsal preservation rhinoplasty versus dorsal hump resection on the internal nasal valve: a quantitative radiological study. Aesthetic Plast Surg 2020; 44(3):879–87.
26. Patel PN, Kandathil CK, Abdelhamid AS, et al. Matched cohort comparison of dorsal preservation and conventional hump resection rhinoplasty. Aesthetic Plast Surg 2022. https://doi.org/10.1007/s00266-022-03156-3.
27. Alan MA, Kahraman ME, Yuksel F, et al. Comparison of dorsal preservation and dorsal reduction rhinoplasty: analysis of nasal patency and aesthetic outcomes by rhinomanometry, NOSE and SCHNOS Scales. Aesthetic Plast Surg 2022. https://doi.org/10.1007/s00266-022-03151-8.
28. Toriumi DM, Kovacevic M, Kosins A. Structural preservation rhinoplasty. Plast Reconstr Surg 2022; 149(5):1105–20. Epub 2022 Mar 9.
29. Toriumi DM. Subdorsal cantilever graft for elevating the dorsum in ethnic rhinoplasty. Facial Plastic Surgery & Aesthetic Medicine 2022;24(3):143–59.
30. Ozucer B, Cam OH. The effectiveness of asymmetric dorsal preservation for correction of i-shaped crooked nose deformity in comparison to conventional technique. Facial Plast Surg Aesthet Med 2020;22(4):286–93.
31. East C. Preservation rhinoplasty and the crooked nose. Facial Plast Surg Clin North Am 2021;29(1): 123–30.
32. Gola R. Chirurgie maxilla-faciale. Paris: Le François; 1940. p. 1127–33.

33. P S, L D. Correction chirurgicale des difformités congénitales et acquises de la pyramide nasale. Paris: Arnette; 1926. p. 104–5.

34. Cottle MH, Loring RM. Corrective surgery of the external nasal pyramid and the nasal septum for restoration of normal physiology. Ill Med J 1946;90: 119–35.

35. Friedman O, Ulloa FL, Kern EB. Preservation rhinoplasty: the endonasal cottle push-down/let-down approach. Facial Plast Surg Clin North Am 2021; 29(1):67–75.

36. Patel PN, Abdelwahab M, Most SP. A review and modification of dorsal preservation rhinoplasty techniques. Facial Plast Surg Aesthet Med Mar/2020; 22(2):71–9.

37. Patel PN, Abdelwahab M, Most SP. Dorsal preservation rhinoplasty: method and outcomes of the modified subdorsal strip method. Facial Plast Surg Clin North Am 2021;29(1):29–37.

38. Toriumi DM, Kovacevic M. Dorsal preservation rhinoplasty:measures to prevent suboptimal outcomes. Facial Plast Surg Cl N Amer 2020. https://doi.org/ 10.1016/j.fsc.2020.09.009.

39. Neves JC, Arancivia G, Dewes W, et al. The split preservation rhinoplasty: The Vitruvian Man split maneuver. Eur J Plast Surg 2020.

40. Finocchi V, Vellone V, Mattioli RG, et al. A 3-level impaction technique for dorsal reshaping and reduction without dorsal soft tissue envelope dissection. Aesthetic Surg J 2022;42:151–65.

41. Ferreira MG, Ishida LC, Ishida LH, et al. Spare roof technique b. step-by-step guide to preserving the bony cap while dehumping. Plast Reconstr Surg 2022 May 1;149(5):901e–4e. Epub 2022 Apr 26.

42. Tham T, Bhuiya S, Wong A, et al. Clinical outcomes in dorsal preservation rhinoplasty: a meta-analysis. Facial Plast Surg Aesthet Med 2022. https://doi. org/10.1089/fpsam.2021.0312.

43. Kovacevic M, Kosins AM, Göksel A, et al. Optimization of the soft tissue envelope of the nose in rhinoplasty utilizing fat transfer combined with platelet-rich fibrin. Facial Plast Surg 2021 Oct; 37(5):590–8. Epub 2021 Feb 26.

44. Patel PN, Kandathil CK, Buba CM, et al. Global practice patterns of dorsal preservation rhinoplasty. Facial Plast Surg Aesthet Med 2021. https://doi.org/ 10.1089/fpsam.2021.0055.

45. Patel PN, Most SP. Combining open structural and dorsal preservation rhinoplasty. Clin Plast Surg 2022;49(1):97–109.

Reprojecting the Severely Damaged Nose

Grant S. Hamilton III, MD[a],*, Yong Ju Jang, MD[b], Dean M. Toriumi, MD[c]

KEYWORDS

- Rhinoplasty • Saddle nose • Vasculitis • Granulomatosis with polyangiitis • Revision rhinoplasty
- Composite graft • Costal cartilage • Nanofat

KEY POINTS

- Underprojected noses due to trauma, disease, or previous surgery present a challenging constellation of problems that require a breadth of surgical and perioperative techniques.
- Strong central and lateral support is necessary to reproject the contracted nose.
- Techniques continue to evolve for better results in patients with compromised tissues. Three dimensional printing, hyperbaric oxygen therapy, nanofat injections, tissue adhesives, and leukotriene antagonists are some of the technologies that are improving outcomes in these complicated patients.

 Video content accompanies this article at http://www.facialplastic.theclinics.com.

PANEL DISCUSSION

How do you prepare and treat the patient with contracted skin-soft tissue envelope?

How do you manage the contracted inner lining (nasal stenosis)?

What techniques do you use to lengthen the overshortened nose?

What techniques do you use to support the dorsum?

Do you use any special techniques to prevent vestibular stenosis?

How have your techniques in this area changed over the last 2 y?

INTRODUCTION

Treating the patient with a severely damaged nose can pose significant challenges for the rhinoplasty surgeon (Video 1). These patients have sustained traumatic injuries, multiple surgeries, or have catastrophic vasculitic diseases that can make an already challenging operation even more difficult. Scar contracture from damaged skin or underlying disease processes inhibits reprojection of both the dorsum and the tip. Creating a natural nasal contour in these circumstances requires a robust underlying structure and may warrant soft tissue augmentation of either the external soft tissue, nasal lining, or both. In this panel, 3 surgeons, each with decades of experience, will discuss

[a] Division of Facial Plastic and Reconstructive Surgery, Mayo Clinic, 200 First Street Southwest, Rochester, MN 55905, USA; [b] Department of Otolaryngology, Asan Medical Center, University of Ulsan, 88, Olympic-ro 43-gil, Songpa-gu, Seoul 05505, South Korea; [c] Rush University Medical School, 60 East Delaware Place, Suite 1425, Chicago, IL 60611-1495, USA
* Corresponding author. Department of Otorhinolaryngology, Mayo Clinic, 200 First Street Southwest, Rochester, MN 55905.
E-mail address: hamilton.grant@mayo.edu
Twitter: @GrantHamiltonMD (G.S.H.)

Facial Plast Surg Clin N Am 32 (2024) 625–639
https://doi.org/10.1016/j.fsc.2024.06.006
1064-7406/24/© 2024 Elsevier Inc. All rights are reserved, including those for text and data mining, AI training, and similar technologies.

the special considerations and techniques that they use when operating on these challenging patients.

HOW DO YOU PREPARE AND TREAT THE PATIENT WITH CONTRACTED SKIN-SOFT TISSUE ENVELOPE?
Jang

When I encounter patients with a deficient skin-soft tissue envelope (SSTE), I usually recommend skin massage in preparation for surgery. Patients are instructed to pull down the nasal SSTE 5 to 6 times a day for 2 to 5 minutes. This maneuver can release the scar tissue and can lengthen and soften the SSTE before surgery.[1]

Leukotriene antagonists have been reported to have a beneficial effect in preventing capsule contracture related to silicone implant placement—especially in breast augmentation.[2] Based on this, prescription of a leukotriene receptor antagonist to the patients with short noses due to previously inserted silicone nasal implants is becoming a popular practice among many rhinoplasty surgeons in Korea.

In a patient with severely contracted skin, I always discuss with the patient the likelihood of staging the surgery. In the first operation, reconstruction of the septal cartilage framework and dorsal augmentation with glued diced costal cartilage is performed. After this stage, the skin becomes softer and healthier. If the degree of counterrotation or augmentation does not match the esthetic goals of the patient, a second-stage operation can be done to further counter-rotate the tip and augment the nasal dorsum. When approached this way, I often find the SSTE to be more elastic and less contracted making the planned refinement more manageable.

Toriumi

Managing the patient with the underprojected, short nose with contracted skin is one of the most difficult problems to correct. When I first see the patient, I ask them whether they have had a prior infection, prior implant, or skin necrosis. I also ask whether they have had any prior filler injections. Previous infection or alloplastic implant is a key factor in the contracted nose as these criteria can accentuate the degree of contracture. Prior infection can compromise the blood supply to the tissues as well.

During the examination, I assess the tightness of the skin envelope by massaging and pulling on the skin of the tip, columella, and alae. I also assess the blood supply to the tip and columellar skin by pricking the tissues with a 25 gauge needle and monitoring the blood flow from the needle holes. If the blood flow is minimal or sluggish, I will usually pretreat the patient with hyperbaric oxygen (HBO) and possible nanofat injections. The nanofat is harvested from the periumbilical area or inner thighs and processed into nanofat.[3] Then a couple of tenths of a milliliter can be very cautiously injected under the skin using ultrasound guidance. Care must be taken to inject no more than 0.2 to 0.3 cc very slowly and stopping if there is blanching. Then the patient is sent for 5 to 7 consecutive days of HBO treatments at 100% oxygen and 2.2 to 2.6 atm pressure (1 hour sessions). The patient is asked to wait for several weeks to several months to reassess the improvement in the blood supply to the area. In the interim, the patient is asked to perform nasal stretching exercises for 1 minute 20 times a day.[3,4] Once the tissues are relaxed and the blood supply is improved, the patient can then undergo the reconstruction.

For the actual reconstruction, I will consider a range of possible surgical options. In most cases, there is enough relaxation of the tissues for structural grafting in the form of a caudal septal extension graft or caudal septal replacement graft with lateral crural replacement grafts and lateral crural strut grafts. If additional tip projection is needed, a shield tip graft with articulated rim grafts can be added. If the columellar skin closure is too tight to completely close, I will leave a gap in the closure to avoid skin necrosis of the columellar flap. I will place perichondrium over the underlying cartilage under the gap in the columellar closure to encourage healing across the defect (**Fig. 1**A). I will frequently inject some nanofat into the perichondrium to enhance healing. I then apply a thin silicone sheet over the gap in the closure and leave it in place for 4 to 6 weeks to act as a "healing chamber" (**Fig. 1**B and C). The silastic promotes healing and prevents desiccation of the open wound. In most cases, the gap will epithelialize and close the gap in the columellar closure.

In some cases, a composite skin/cartilage graft from the ear will be needed to complete the columellar closure (**Fig. 2**). I use the perichondrial underlay technique to enhance healing of the composite graft (**Fig. 3**).

With larger defects, I will use an interpolated melolabial flap in a 3 stage reconstruction. In this case, the flap can be used to close the columellar defect as well as vestibular skin defects. If the patient does not have a deep nasolabial crease, I will use a paramedian forehead flap to close the columellar defect. I prefer the

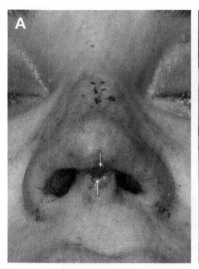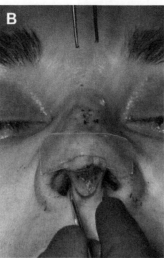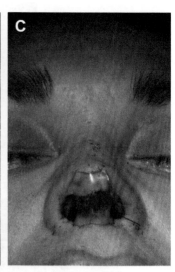

Fig. 1. Gap in columellar closure due to excessive tension. (*A*) Gap in closure indicated by yellow arrows. (*B*) Placing silicone sheeting. (*C*) Silicone sheet "healing chamber" sutured in place.

interpolated melolabial flap because it tends to be less cumbersome to the patient and the scars tend to heal well.

Hamilton

When patients have a contracted and inelastic soft tissue envelope, preparation is the foundation for a successful outcome. This begins with managing expectations. Patients should understand that it is impossible to get their old noses back. Not infrequently, patients will have an unresolved trauma response from their injury, prior surgery, or disease. They may be hoping that the rhinoplasty will undo the psychological trauma of those events. This can be a setup for depression in the immediate postoperative period. When indicated, I recommend that these patients meet with a mental health professional who specializes in trauma therapy before surgery.

Projecting a new structural framework into a compromised skin envelope increases the risk of necrosis and delayed healing. It is an absolute requirement that they must not have smoked for at least several months before surgery. I encourage them to participate in a formal smoking cessation program to increase the likelihood of success. Fortunately, these surgeries are rarely urgent, leaving time for optimization. Similarly, patients with vasculitic diseases should be in remission before surgery. Close coordination with Rheumatology is important when deciding on a patient's suitability for surgery and the timing of surgery relative to his/her medical treatments.

When the skin is deficient or inelastic, I discuss the possibility of a paramedian forehead flap and postoperative HBO therapy. For patients who are coming from out of town, they should also be prepared to stay locally for at least a week in the event that they need HBO treatment.

I have used 3 dimensional (3D) printing of the skull and soft tissue to plan the operation and help with patient education (**Fig. 4**). Having a model of the patient can make it easier to predict whether I will need to harvest 1 rib or 2. In cases after severe craniofacial trauma, a model is an excellent guide to existing reconstruction plates that may need to be incorporated or avoided, depending on the circumstances.

During surgery, local anesthetic and edema can thicken the soft tissue envelope. This thickness comes at the expense of length, making wound closure difficult. Intraoperative tissue massage by gently pushing the edema caudally can be helpful in getting the incision edges to reach. I have had a gap of 5 mm or so be able to be closed by using this technique. When the closure is under some tension, I will use fewer sutures so that I can maximize the blood flow to the skin edges. I also keep an eye on the intraoperative blood pressure. Patients are often relatively hypotensive in surgery and will have better perfusion postoperatively.

HOW DO YOU MANAGE THE CONTRACTED LINING TO REPAIR OR PREVENT NASAL STENOSIS?
Jang

The technique I primarily rely on is grafting the mucosal defect or deficient area with an ear cartilage composite graft. These grafts can be

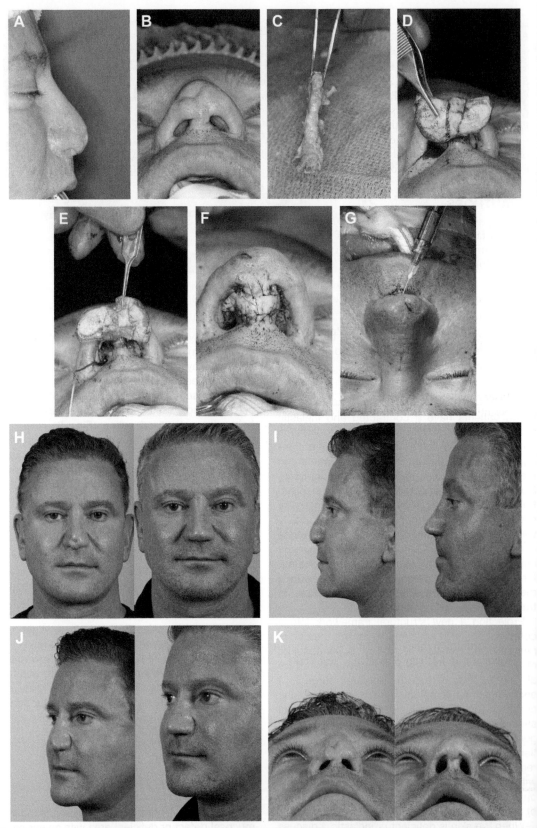

Fig. 2. Patient with underprojected nasal tip due to prior infection. (*A*) Intraoperative lateral view. (*B*) Intraoperative base view. (*C*) Caudal septal replacement graft with native perichondrium attached and wrapped around caudal margin of the graft. (*D*) Entire conchal bowl harvested. (*E*) Skin removed along margin of the graft leaving

harvested in various sizes and from the cymba concha or cavum concha.[5] For larger defects, I take out the graft from the cavum concha. The ear skin defect should be closed with a skin graft taken from the postauricular skin. Relatively small and crescent-shaped defects can be covered with a composite graft harvested from the cymba concha and the donor site can be closed primarily. Septal mucosal defects can be covered with postauricular skin or inferior turbinate mucosal flap.

Toriumi

Internal lining defects must be closed when reconstructing the contracted nose deformity. As the skin envelope is expanded and the nose is lengthened, gaps in the vestibular skin closure may develop and require lining. I usually use composite skin/cartilage grafts from the cymba concha. Most grafts are fusiform in shape and should survive without issues. I use postoperative HBO with patients who undergo composite grafting to the nasal vestibule. In some cases, the columella and vestibular skin defects are closed with an interpolated melolabial flap. I will use interpolated buccal mucosal flaps to close intranasal vestibular skin defects if no harvestable ear is available.

Hamilton

A deficient lining significantly complicates reprojection of the nose. These patients' tips will typically be over-rotated and under-projected. Restoration of the lining is the only way to restore normal proportions. It is first necessary to incise the lining to release it. This determines the size of the defect. Small defects with a vascularized wound bed can be repaired with skin or mucosal grafts. I avoid skin grafts to replace mucosa because this typically leads to crusting. A gingival-labial sulcus flap can be tunneled to the floor of the nose if vascularized tissue is needed. For larger defects, a pericranial flap can be tunneled under the glabella and into the nasal cavity for coverage of cartilage grafts and exposed bone. Pericranium will mucosalize within a couple of weeks if kept moist. Alar retraction from a

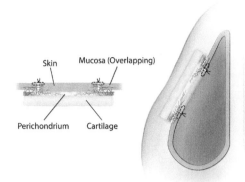

Fig. 3. Illustration demonstrating the perichondrial underlays technique for larger composite grafts. (*Used from* the library of Dean M. Toriumi, MD, with permission; and Image Courtesy: Dean M. Toriumi.)

contracted lining can be fixed with auricular composite grafts.

WHAT TECHNIQUES DO YOU USE TO LENGTHEN THE OVERSHORTENED NOSE?
Jang

Conceptually, I repair the overshortened nose by lengthening both the central compartment and the lateral compartment. The central compartment is evaluated first after elevation of the skin and bilateral septal mucoperichondrial flaps. I typically use autologous costal cartilage to create bilateral extended spreader grafts that are sutured on both sides of the existing L-strut, followed by the placement of end-to-end type 1 caudal extension graft sandwiched between them[6] (**Fig. 5**).

Lateral compartment correction is also necessary to achieve the esthetic goals of the patient. Several techniques are used in lateral compartment correction, including composite conchal cartilage grafts, lateral crural strut grafts, and lateral crural onlay grafts. A critically important aspect in short nose correction is caudally mobilizing the contracted lower lateral cartilages. For the mobilization of the alar cartilage, the junction between the upper lateral and lower lateral cartilages should be dissected and freed from thick,

perichondrium attached to the cartilage. (*F*) Composite graft sutured into columella and closing vestibular defects. (*G*) Injecting nanofat around the composite graft. (*H*) Preoperative frontal view (*left*). One year postoperative frontal view (*right*). (*I*) Preoperative lateral view (*left*). Postoperative lateral view (*right*). (*J*) Preoperative oblique view (*left*). Postoperative oblique view (*right*). (*K*) Preoperative base view (*left*). Postoperative base view (*right*).

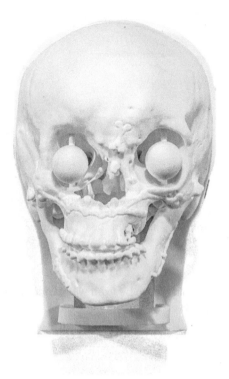

Fig. 4. A 3D printed, 1:1 scale model based on a high-resolution computed tomographic (CT) scan in a patient with a history of significant facial trauma. Note the reconstruction plates and missing bone. In addition to better visualization of these relevant preoperative details, the model makes it possible to make planning measurements before going to the operating room.

fibrous scar tissues. This releasing maneuver is often very difficult. Furthermore, dissection of the scroll area may easily violate the nasal mucosa that should be kept intact to prevent infection. For cases with severe scarring and fibrosis of SSTE in which the lower lateral cartilage cannot reach the new reconstructed caudal septum, a cartilage flap technique is applied.[7] In this maneuver, I dissect the lateral crus of the lower lateral cartilage from the underlying vestibular skin and incise its anterior part to create a medially based cartilage flap, which is later rotated medially to cover the extended spreader graft (**Fig. 6**).

In cases with over-rotation of the tip, counterrotation can be achieved with multilayer tip grafting, shield grafting with or without backstop graft[8] (**Fig. 7**).

Most of the patients with short nose present with concavity of the nasal dorsum that accentuates the overshortened appearance of the nose. Dorsal

augmentation therefore should be done as the final step of correction. My preferred choice of the dorsal augmentation material is glued diced costal cartilage shaped with a mold, which will be detailed later (**Fig. 8**).

Toriumi

To lengthen the short nose, I will use a caudal septal extension graft or caudal septal replacement graft with extended spreader grafts.[3] I will also release the lateral crura and place lateral crural strut grafts to support the lateral compartment of the nose and move the alar margins into proper position. In many Asian patients, I will use a shield tip graft with articulated rim grafts to support the lateral compartment (**Fig. 9**). One of the keys in this technique is to have adequate skin coverage to allow closure of both the columellar closure and any vestibular skin deficiency. Many of these patients will need composite grafts to manage vestibular skin deficiencies (see **Fig. 9**F).

Hamilton

Lengthening the overshortened nose requires strong central support. These patients have a deficient septum that needs to be reinforced or replaced. I exclusively use costal cartilage in these patients—preferably autologous. Even with a deficient septum, there are often remnants caudally and at the keystone that can be used to affix thin but strong costal cartilage grafts. When there is residual dorsal septum, I will use extended spreader grafts overlapping a caudal septal extension/replacement graft. This is a very structurally sound configuration and can effectively counter-rotate the nose. If there is not a caudal septal remnant, it is important to affix the caudal septal replacement graft to the anterior nasal spine. I make a notch either in the graft to accept the spine or in the spine to accept the graft in addition to suturing to make this connection more secure.

Lateral wall support is necessary for both external valve patency and contour. Lateral crural strut grafts or lateral crural replacement grafts of costal cartilage can provide the necessary support.

WHAT TECHNIQUES DO YOU USE TO SUPPORT THE DORSUM?
Jang

Dorsal augmentation is an important part of the correction of short nose as dorsal augmentation eliminates dorsal concavity, thereby creating a

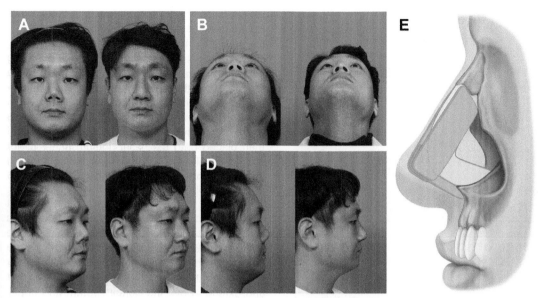

Fig. 5. (*A–E*) This patient presented with a severe short nose deformity. He underwent 2 previous rhinoplasties with silicone augmentation and developed a progressively upturned nose due to capsule contracture. Costal cartilage was used to reinforce and elongate his septum by creating a combination of extended spreader grafts and caudal septal extension graft. His nasal dorsum was augmented with a glued diced costal cartilage graft shaped with a mold. Additional tip grafting was added to further counter-rotate his tip.

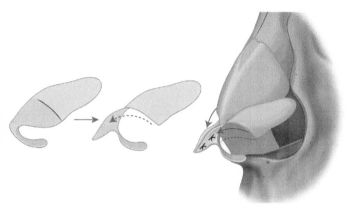

Fig. 6. Cartilage flap technique. This maneuver is a modification of the dome division technique. By using this technique, the lengthened central compartment can be covered, thereby achieving simultaneous elongation of the central and medial compartments of the lower third of the nose.

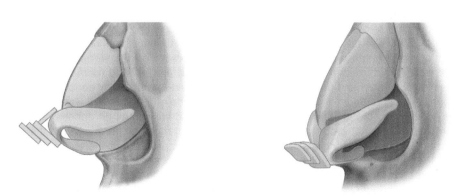

Fig. 7. Multilayer tip grafting technique. Two or 3 layers of cartilage grafts can be placed at the infratip lobule to further elongate the tip. This is often a necessary step for short nose correction.

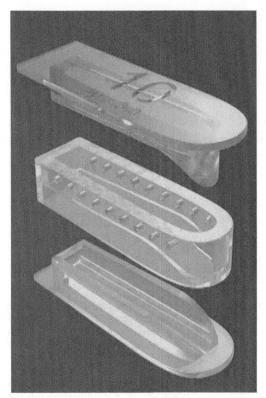

Fig. 8. A set of cartilage mold components to shape the GDCG. This is composed of the base template, guarding frame with holes and compression cap.

second layer of diced cartilage. Finally, the compressor of the mold is applied and pressed together (**Fig. 10**). Through the small holes of the sidewall, excessive glue and fluid around the diced cartilage are removed. The graft is then carefully removed from the mold. It has a convex dorsal surface with or without a soft tissue covering, while the undersurface has a concave shape conforming to the convexity of the nasal dorsum. The graft is then placed onto the nasal dorsum under direct vision—usually in 1 piece but sometimes in segmental manner at the radix and supratip dorsum.

Toriumi

In most revision cases, I will use tall spreader grafts to support the nasal dorsum.[3] These are spreader grafts that have increased vertical height and extend above the dorsal septum and upper lateral cartilages (**Fig. 11**). This will act to augment the dorsum and support the upper two-thirds of the nose. If the dorsum requires more significant augmentation, I will use subdorsal cantilever graft.[10] This graft is placed below the nasal dorsum and allows it to be "pushed up" after the nasal bones and upper lateral cartilages are fully released (**Fig. 12**). I rarely use large dorsal grafts on the dorsum as these other options are more reliable.

Hamilton

If there is a paucity of dorsal septal cartilage causing a saddle nose and precluding fixation of spreader grafts, I will make a structural dorsal graft and build a new framework over the deficient one. There are several key details when using a structural dorsal graft. First, it should be carved from the central part of the rib to minimize the risk of warping. Second, it is important to have a firm attachment to the nasal bones to prevent the graft from sliding into the glabella. I use a few techniques in combination to affix the cephalic end of the graft to the nasal bones. I will reduce the bony dorsum with a step-off that can act as a backstop and provide room for a thicker graft. I also sew a small patch of perichondrium to the undersurface of the cartilage where it will touch the bone that will act as an adhesive to prevent the graft from moving after healing. If the structure is under compression at the end of the case, I will use a Kirschner wire to hold the cephalic end of the graft to the nasal bone. A small cap fits over the exposed end of the wire and I remove the wire in 1 week. Diced cartilage and fibrin glue are useful for camouflaging the edges of the graft.

straighter and longer looking nasal dorsum. For proper dorsal support, the lower two-thirds should be rebuilt with combination of extended spreader grafts and caudal septal extension grafts. Once a stable base is secured, then the desired dorsal contour is created by dorsal onlay grafting using glued diced cartilage graft (GDCG) cartilage shaped with a cartilage mold.[9]

All types of harvested cartilage (septal, conchal, and costal cartilage) are suitable for making of GDCGs. They are diced into less than 0.5 mm fragments using a dermatome blade (Zimmer Surgical Inc., Dover, OH, USA). After taking measurements of the patient's dorsal length and desired thickness, a preformed mold of the desired length and thickness is chosen. When I use costal cartilage, autologous perichondrium is inserted into the mold as covering for the implant. Fascia lata may also be used. One or 2 drops of the fibrin glue are painted onto the covering material, and the frame of the mold was assembled. Then, a thin layer of diced cartilage is placed on top of the fascia or perichondrium, a second layer of glue is painted, an additional layer of diced cartilage is laid on top, and glue was painted over the

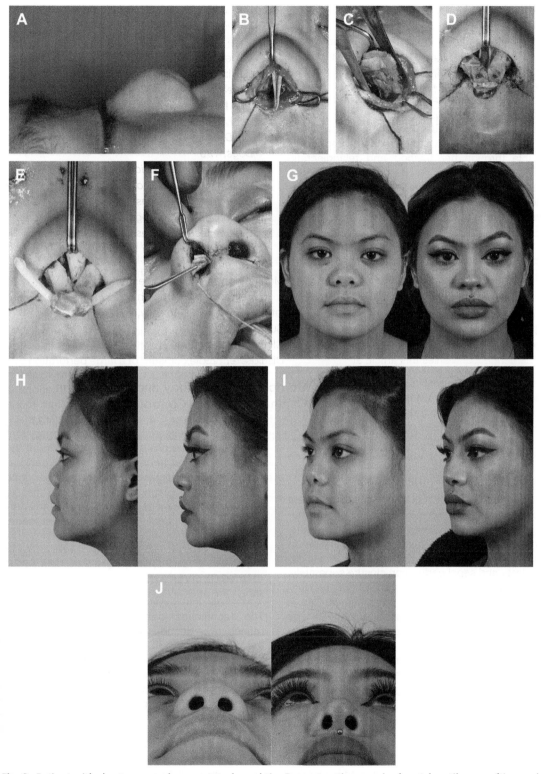

Fig. 9. Patient with short nose and over rotated nasal tip. Reconstruction required costal cartilage grafting and tip grafting. A caudal septal extension graft was stabilized with 2 submucosal spreader grafts to lengthen the nose. (*A*) Intraoperative lateral view showing short nose. (*B*) Placement of 2 submucosal spreader grafts. (*C*) Caudal septal extension graft stabilized with the 2 spreader grafts. (*D*) Shield tip graft with lateral crural grafts

These grafts can be placed either with a cartilage injector or as small patties.

The patient shown in **Fig. 13** had 2 prior rhinoplasties. At the second rhinoplasty, a porous polyethylene implant was placed on the dorsum to correct the saddle nose deformity from the first operation. The implant partially extruded postoperatively and the subsequent scar contracture of her nose was treated with several steroid injections. Preoperatively the remnant implant is visible through her thinned and telangiectatic skin. At her 1 week postoperative visit, she was noted to have a 3 mm area of dehiscence at her incision. With meticulous wound care, her wound was completely closed at 6 weeks. Ten months after surgery, she had a small revision to her scar to correct her retracted columella. She is now 2 years from her last surgery with a stable result.

HOW DO YOU DEAL WITH CONCOMITANT SEPTAL PERFORATIONS?

Jang

In my experience, concomitant rhinoplasty with perforation closure results in a higher postoperative infection rate compared to rhinoplasty alone. The risks are particularly real when the rhinoplasty requires the use of costal cartilage grafting such as extended spreader grafts and caudal septal extension grafts, and the perforation closure is done with an open approach applying advancement flap techniques.[11]

The incisions used for mucosal advancement flap inevitably can serve as a route of contamination from the nasal cavity to the cartilage grafts. Therefore, if the symptoms related to septal perforation are not severe, I recommend performing rhinoplasty and sepal perforation closure separately. However, if the peroration is small where an extensive mucosal elevation and advancement flap is not needed, a simultaneous operation can be considered without much added risk. If it is necessary to close the perforation at the time of the rhinoplasty, an anterior ethmoidal artery septal mucosal flap performed endonasally can be done with little risk of retrograde infection of the cartilage grafts.[12]

Toriumi

I manage septal perforation by raising bilateral bipedicled mucoperichondrial flaps. The flaps are raised from the floor on one side and from above on the opposite side. The flaps take the perforation "out of phase" and each flap compensates for the other sides deficiencies. I place a costal perichondrial graft with injected nanofat between the septal flaps as an interpositional graft.[13] These patients also undergo HBO treatments after surgery to enhance healing.

Hamilton

In most cases, I do not repair the perforation. These patients often have contracted noses due to their large perforations. Attempting to mobilize the lining to close the perforation puts downward tension on the dorsum, working against reprojecting the dorsal height. Pericranium that could provide a vascularized interposition flap in the septum is better used for graft coverage than perforation closure, in my opinion. In patients with vasculitis, I am hesitant to undertake a complex closure of a large perforation due to the substantial risk of recurrence. My conservative approach to large septal perforations is also influenced by my access to custom-made septal prostheses[14] (**Fig. 14**). I will typically place a septal prosthetic in the office after surgery that restores the premorbid nasal airflow without the need for surgery. In cases with smaller perforations, I will elevate and mobilize mucosal flaps with an interposition graft. In some cases, smaller perforations can be treated with an interposition graft and healing by secondary intention.[15]

HOW HAVE YOUR TECHNIQUES IN THIS AREA CHANGED OVER THE LAST 2 YEARS?

Jang

The techniques described here have been refined over decades but have been stable for the last 6 years.[16] Therefore, over the last 2 years, I have consistently used the same techniques adopting cartilaginous dorsum reinforcement with costal cartilage structural grafting and dorsal augmentation with glued diced costal

---

to support the position of the shield graft. (*E*) Camouflaged shield graft with articulated rim grafts to support alar margins. (*F*) Composite grafts placed bilaterally to fill vestibular skin deficiencies. (*G*) Preoperative frontal view showing short nose (*left*). Three year postoperative frontal view showing improved nasal length (*right*). (*H*) Preoperative lateral view showing short nose with over rotated nasal tip (*left*). Postoperative lateral view showing increased nasal length and counterrotation of the nasal tip (*right*). (*I*) Preoperative oblique view (*left*). Postoperative oblique view (*right*). (*J*) Preoperative base view (*left*). Postoperative base view (*right*).

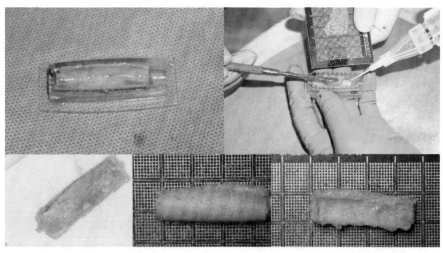

Fig. 10. Making the GDCG with a mold. The convex outer surface is covered with costal perichondrium to reduce the risk of a postoperative dorsal contour irregularity. The inner side has concave surface conforming to the native convexity of the dorsum.

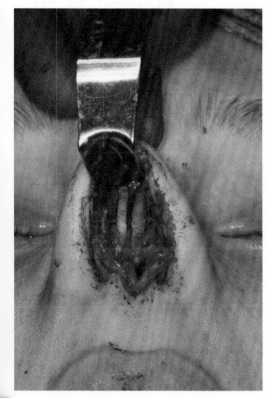

Fig. 11. Tall spreader grafts used to raise the dorsum and reconstruct the middle vault. A thinner graft can be placed between the 2 tall spreader grafts to fill the midline gap. Once the proper height of the dorsum is achieved, the tall spreader grafts are camouflaged with a layer of perichondrium. In patients with thin skin, I will use fat with platelet-rich fibrin as described by Milos Kovacevic.[20]

cartilage. The only recent change in my technique is the occasional use of an additional block of costal cartilage under the glued diced graft (**Fig. 15**). I use this in patients who have severe concavity of the nasal dorsum requiring a substantial degree of augmentation or patients who show a relative deficiency of the cartilaginous dorsum that could not be addressed properly with a single piece of glued diced costal cartilage. Although I do not have long-term results yet, the combination of glued diced cartilage on a cartilage block foundation yielded good cosmetic outcomes with no sign of warping or dorsal contour irregularity.

Toriumi

A major change that I have made is moving away from dorsal onlay grafts to either tall spreader grafts or the subdorsal cantilever graft for dorsal augmentation. I have made these changes over the past 5 years. I have also increased the use of nanofat and HBO to enhance success. There has been an increased incidence of skin necrosis after rhinoplasty, infection, or after simultaneous revision rhinoplasty and upper lip lift. The increase in these problems has necessitated using more flaps for reconstruct complex nasal deformities.

Hamilton

Over the last several years, I have evolved my techniques for using and camouflaging structural dorsal grafts.[17,18] Specifically, I am removing more of the nasal bones in order to accommodate

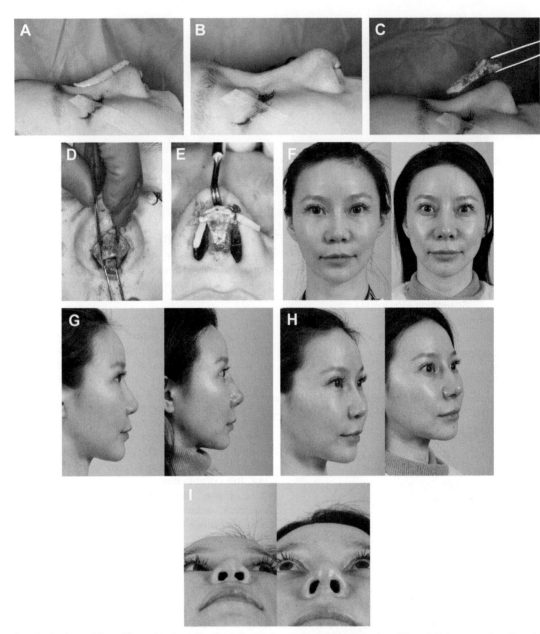

Fig. 12. Patient with a silicone implant that is deformed and required removal and immediate reconstruction. (*A*) Silicone implant removed. (*B*) Low dorsum after implant removed. (*C*) Subdorsal cantilever graft ready to be placed under the dorsum. (*D*) SDCG type B in place and to be fixed to the caudal septal replacement graft. (*E*) Shield tip graft sutured in place with soft tissue and articulated rim grafts. (*F*) Preoperative frontal view (*left*). One and half year postoperative frontal view (*right*). (*G*) Preoperative lateral view (*left*). Postoperative lateral view (*right*). (*H*) Preoperative oblique view (*left*). Postoperative oblique view (*right*). (*I*) Preoperative base view (*left*). Postoperative base view (*right*).

a thicker, stronger graft at its cephalic end without obliterating the natural contour of the radix. Thicker grafts are less prone to fracture or warping. I am also incorporating more nanofat and sub-millimeter diced cartilage for either injection or as patties in combination with fibrin glue. Cartilage scales in fibrin glue are also excellent for camouflage. My threshold for using HBO and medical therapies such as vasodilators and pentoxifylline is also lower.[19]

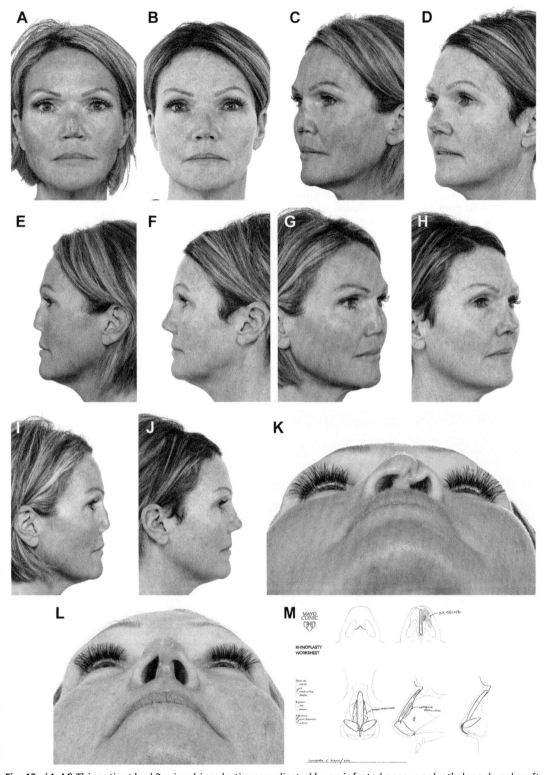

Fig. 13. (*A–M*) This patient had 2 prior rhinoplasties complicated by an infected porous polyethylene dorsal graft. A structural dorsal graft and caudal septal replacement graft were used to provide central support. A lateral crural onlay graft was placed on the right and a lateral crural replacement graft was placed on the left. Diced cartilage was injected alongside the edges of the dorsal graft for camouflage. Perichondrium was used to camouflage the grafts in the nasal tip. Restoring the support and contour of her tip was enough to correct the significant folding in the skin of the infratip lobule.

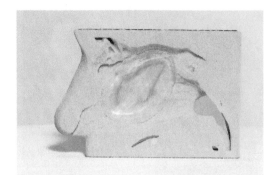

Fig. 14. This is a custom silicone septal prosthesis made from a 3D print of a high-resolution CT scan. These can be placed in the office and are a reliable way to restore a normal physiologic nasal airway in a patient with a large septal perforation.

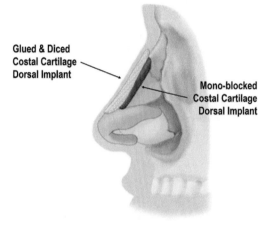

Glued & Diced
Costal Cartilage
Dorsal Implant

Mono-blocked
Costal Cartilage
Dorsal Implant

Fig. 15. When 4 to 6 mm of dorsal augmentation is needed, placement of a block of cartilage under the GDCG can add the necessary dorsal height with minimal risk of warping and contour irregularity.

SUMMARY

Operating on patients with severely damaged and contracted noses can be rewarding for the surgeon and life-changing for the patient. In many cases, these patients have had multiple surgeries, each filled with hope followed by disappointment. A successful operation can help them move past this distressing stage of life. Success depends upon thoughtful planning, preparation, and the restoration of lining, structure and covering. Reinforcement or replacement of the central support of the nose is needed to project the dorsum and counter-rotate and project the nasal tip. This can be accomplished with extended spreader grafts overlapping a caudal extension graft or with a combination of a caudal septal replacement and a structural dorsal graft. Lateral compartment reconstruction is typically accomplished with

lateral crural reinforcement or replacement, sometimes with caudal repositioning. In addition to these surgical techniques, adjunctive medical therapies can improve outcomes in the most challenging cases.

DISCLOSURE

The authors have nothing to disclose.

SUPPLEMENTARY DATA

Supplementary data to this article can be found online at https://doi.org/10.1016/j.fsc.2024.06.006.

REFERENCES

1. Manafi A, Manafi F. Role of Nasal Skin Massage in Optimizing Secondary Rhinoplasty Results. World J Plast Surg 2016;5(1):3–6.
2. Graf R, Ascenco ASK, Freitas RDS, et al. Prevention of Capsular Contracture Using Leukotriene Antagonists. Plast Reconstr Surg 2015;136(5):592e–6e. https://doi.org/10.1097/PRS.0000000000001683.
3. DM T. Lessons Learned in Thirty Years of Structure Rhinoplasty. DMT Solutions 2019.
4. Toriumi DM. Discussion of the Paper Entitled: Autologous Shuffling Lipo-Aspirated Fat Combined Mechanical Stretch in Revision Rhinoplasty for Severe Contractures in Asian Patients. Aesthetic Plast Surg 2023;47(1):292–3. https://doi.org/10.1007/s00266-022-03175-0.
5. Jang YJ, Moon H. Special Consideration in Rhinoplasty for Deformed Nose of East Asians. Facial Plast Surg Clin North Am 2021;29(4):611–24. https://doi.org/10.1016/j.fsc.2021.06.009.
6. Jang YJ, Yoo SH. Dorsal Augmentation in Facial Profiloplasty. Facial Plast Surg 2019;35(5):492–8. https://doi.org/10.1055/s-0039-1695726.
7. Lan MY, Jang YJ. Revision Rhinoplasty for Short Noses in the Asian Population. JAMA Facial Plast Surg Sep-Oct 2015;17(5):325–32. https://doi.org/10.1001/jamafacial.2015.0645.
8. Jang YJ, Kim SH. Tip Grafting for the Asian Nose. Facial Plast Surg Clin North Am 2018;26(3):343–56. https://doi.org/10.1016/j.fsc.2018.03.008.
9. Yoo SH, Kim DH, Jang YJ. Dorsal Augmentation Using a Glued Diced Cartilage Graft Fashioned with a Newly Developed Mold in Asian Rhinoplasty. Plast Reconstr Surg 2022;150(4):757e–66e. https://doi.org/10.1097/PRS.0000000000009568.
10. Toriumi DM. Subdorsal Cantilever Graft for Elevating the Dorsum in Ethnic Rhinoplasty. Facial Plast Surg Aesthet Med May-Jun 2022;24(3):143–59. https://doi.org/10.1089/fpsam.2022.0117.
11. Tran KN, Jang YJ. Incidence and Predisposing Factors of Postoperative Infection after Rhinoplasty: A

Single Surgeon's 16-Year Experience with 2630 Cases in an East Asian Population. Plast Reconstr Surg 2022;150(1):51e–9e. https://doi.org/10.1097/PRS.0000000000009202.

12. Garaycochea O, Santamaria-Gadea A, Alobid I. State-of-the-art: septal perforation repair. Curr Opin Otolaryngol Head Neck Surg 2023;31(1):11–6. https://doi.org/10.1097/MOO.0000000000000857.

13. Toriumi DM, Cappelle QM, Chung V. Use of Costal Perichondrium as an Interpositional Graft for Septal Perforation Closure. JAMA Facial Plast Surg 2017;19(2): 121–7. https://doi.org/10.1001/jamafacial.2016.1367.

14. Onerci Altunay Z, Bly JA, Edwards PK, et al. Three-dimensional printing of large nasal septal perforations for optimal prosthetic closure. Am J Rhinol Allergy 2016;30(4):287–93. https://doi.org/10.2500/ajra.2016.30.4324.

15. Sharma A, Janus J, Diggelmann HR, et al. Healing septal perforations by secondary intention using acellular dermis as a bioscaffold. Ann Otol Rhinol Laryngol 2015;124(6):425–9. https://doi.org/10.1177/0003489414565002.

16. Fung CY, Kim JH, Liao PH, et al. Revision Rhinoplasty Using Glued Diced Costal Cartilage Shaped With Mold for Management of Complicated Silicone Rhinoplasty. Aesthet Surg J 2023;43(11):1237–47. https://doi.org/10.1093/asj/sjad180.

17. Hamilton GS 3rd. Correction of the Saddle Nose Deformity. Facial Plast Surg 2020;36(1):7–17. https://doi.org/10.1055/s-0040-1701644.

18. Hamilton GS. 3rd. Dorsal Failures: From Saddle Deformity to Pollybeak. Facial Plast Surg 2018; 34(3):261–9. https://doi.org/10.1055/s-0038-1653990.

19. Irvine LE, Azizzadeh B, Kerulos JL, et al. Outcomes of a Treatment Protocol for Compromised Nasal Skin in Primary and Revision Open Rhinoplasty. Facial Plast Surg Aesthet Med Mar-Apr 2021;23(2): 118–25. https://doi.org/10.1089/fpsam.2020.0181.

20. Kovacevic M, Kosins AM, Goksel A, et al. Optimization of the Soft Tissue Envelope of the Nose in Rhinoplasty Utilizing Fat Transfer Combined with Platelet-Rich Fibrin. Facial Plast Surg 2021;37(5):590–8. https://doi.org/10.1055/s-0041-1723785.

Appropriate Use of Implants in the Nose

Thomas Romo III, MD[a],*, Alexander E. Graf, MD[b], George Ferzli, MD[c], Sun Hong Kim, MD[d], In-Sang Kim, MD, PhD[e]

KEYWORDS

- Alloplastic implants • Silicone • Meshed implants • Porous implants
- High-density porous polyethylene • Expanded polytetrafluoroethylene • Extrusion
- Marginal incision

KEY POINTS

- Alloplastic implant complication rates in rhinoplasty vary by type of implant used and grafting technique.
- Key properties of implants that vary by implant material type include porous density, pliability, and biological response.
- Using proper techniques, such as, appropriate pocket sizing, appropriate graft carving, and intra-operative antibacterial measures, can minimize complication rates.
- Implants should only be used as columellar strut grafts or as dorsal onlay grafts, both of which anchor the graft to immobile nasal structures and minimize sheering forces placed on the graft.

PANEL DISCUSSION

What is your favorite implant in rhinoplasty and why?

Do you have any special techniques to prevent complications?

In what areas of the nose do you use implants routinely? Are there any areas where you do not use implants?

If you have implant extrusion, how do you manage it?

What are the pros and cons of costal cartilage versus implants in rhinoplasty?

How have your techniques in this area changed over the last 2 years?

WHAT IS YOUR FAVORITE IMPLANT IN RHINOPLASTY AND WHY?
Romo/Graf/Ferzli

While the use of implants in rhinoplasty has been a practice of facial plastic surgery for many years, it remains a subject of great controversy. Which types of implants are best, where in the nose to place implants, and where in the nose to avoid implants are controversial questions. Nasal implants can be broadly categorized by their origin. Autografts are harvested from the same patient. Homografts are harvested from a donor of the same species as the recipient. Xenografts originate from another species, and these are not used in nasal surgery. Alloplasts are manufactured from

[a] Lenox Hill Hospital and Manhattan Eye, Ear & Throat Hospital (MEETH)-Northwell Health Systems, New York, NY, USA; [b] Department of Otolaryngology–Head and Neck Surgery, SUNY Downstate Health Sciences University, Brooklyn, NY, USA; [c] Ferzli Facial Plastic Surgery, New York, NY, USA; [d] Be and Young Aesthetic Surgery Clinic, Seoul, Korea; [e] Department of Otolaryngology and Fascial Plastic Surgery, Labom Plastic Surgery Clinic, Korea
* Corresponding author. Romo Plastic Surgery, 135 East 74th Street, New York, NY 10021.
E-mail address: dr.romo@romoplasticsurgery.com

Facial Plast Surg Clin N Am 32 (2024) 641–652
https://doi.org/10.1016/j.fsc.2024.06.007

synthetic or semisynthetic materials. Autografts are generally considered the gold standard implant and are discussed in detail elsewhere in this issue. For this question, we will focus on alloplast use in rhinoplasty. We will start with a discussion on the accepted use of alloplasts, then review complications, and conclude with a discussion of the 3 most commonly used materials.

Alloplasts are generally accepted for use in 2 categorical scenarios. First, rhinoplasty in the platyrrhine nose, which is a wide and short nose, commonly seen in patients of Asian and African descent. In comparison to Leptorrhine noses, commonly found in Caucasian patients, platyrrhine noses have relatively weak and thin quadrangular cartilage, shortened medial crura, underprojected nasal spine, and a thicker, fattier soft tissue envelope. Platyrrhine noses have comparatively poor tip projection and definition, a wider dorsum, and a more acute nasolabial angle[1–3] (**Fig. 1**). The second scenario is in revision rhinoplasty to restore form and function after loss of structural support and soft tissue volume.[4] A common case that falls into this category is when inexperienced surgeon has over-resected the nasal dorsum, resulting in a narrowed tip and nasal valve collapse. Alloplast implantation in these 2 scenarios is utilized to replace the missing cartilaginous framework for dorsal and/or tip augmentation.

A variety of materials have been used as alloplasts in rhinoplasty. An ideal material would react favorably with the surrounding soft tissues by not causing reactive inflammation and by resisting bacterial growth. An optimal material would be readily available, inexpensive, noncarcinogenic, nontoxic, inert, and sterilizable. Furthermore, it would be pliable and easy to sculpt or mold, but rigid enough to not warp and change shape overtime.[1]

Advantages of alloplast use versus autograft use include reduced operative time, lack of donor-site morbidity, and preservation of shape overtime. Major complications of alloplast use in rhinoplasty include gross infection, visibility, and extrusion, all of which necessitate removal and revision surgery.[5] Minor complications include implant deviation or malpositioning, local tissue inflammation, minor infection resolving with antibiotics, and undesirable esthetic outcome. Complication rates vary by type of alloplast used and by intraoperative maneuver or graft type.[6,7] Moreover, complication rates tend to be higher in revision rhinoplasties compared to primaries.[7,8] To minimize complications when using alloplastic implants in rhinoplasty, certain precautions and surgical principles should always be adhered to. Sterile technique when handling implants is imperative. Implants should only be placed in a precise soft tissue pocket of approximately the same width to minimize migration risk.[2] Excessive skin tension after closure over the implant should always be avoided.[5,9]

Although no perfect alloplastic material exists, many have been used in facial plastic surgery. Today, the most commonly used materials that warrant further discussion are high-density porous polyethylene (HDPPE; Su-Por, Poriferous, GA), silicone, and expanded polytetrafluoroethylene (ePTFE; Gore-Tex, W.L. Gore & Associates, DE). These materials are unique, synthetically manufactured polymers, or repeating units of macromolecules. HDPPE, silicone, and ePTFE each have specific physical properties that dictate variations in their attributes and uses.[10]

High-density porous polyethylene
High-density porous polyethylene implants are well established in facial plastic surgery and have a variety of applications in rhinoplasty. It offers many of the aforementioned properties of an ideal implant. A defining chemical property of HDPPE is that it is 50% porous by volume with an average pore size of 150 μm.[10] This allows for host tissue ingrowth and stabilization, which limits malposition and extrusion risk. While this is a major advantage, extensive host integration can also make removal challenging in cases when it is required.[1] HDPPE is rigid but can be sculpted into the desired shape with warming in hot water. This rigidity allows for true structural support, in contrast to silicone implants. Ready-made HDPPE implants are also

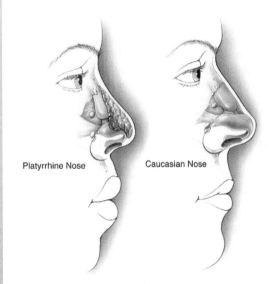

Fig. 1. Anatomy of platyrrhine nose versus Caucasian nose.

Platyrrhine Nose   Caucasian Nose

available for a variety of rhinoplasty grafting techniques. Like silicone, HDPPE carries a risk of infection and extrusion but is commonly accepted as safer than silicone implants.

The complication rate of HDPPE implants varies by grafting technique and anatomic location.[6,7] Davis and colleagues[6] found the highest complication rates when implants were used for extended spreader grafts, caudal septum batten grafts, and caudal septal extension grafts. No complications were seen when implants were used for dorsal onlay grafts or columellar strut grafts.[6] The authors hypothesize that grafts that were used in anatomic locations that are subject to high shearing forces are more likely to have graft failure.[6] Limiting the use of HDPPE alloplasts for spreader grafts, cephalically extended spreader grafts, and dorsal onlay grafts may limit complications.[6] Overall, the removal rate of HDPPE implants is low: a large meta-analysis of 9 studies using Medpor implants found it to be as low as 1.5%.[11]

In those selected rhinoplasty cases that I utilize alloplants for augmentation and structure, I prefer to use HDPPE. I have extensive experience utilizing HDPPE in facial reconstruction. This product was first used by myself for auricular reconstruction in patients with microtia over 30 years ago. Because of late exposures of these auricular implants and the significant difficulty in revision of auricular reconstruction with autologous rib cartilage, I abandoned this product for auricular reconstruction 10 years ago. Very soon after using HDPPE for microtia reconstruction, I instituted using this material for augmentation rhinoplasty in people of color. Alloplasts for augmentation rhinoplasty in Asia had become the standard for many years. Using autologous rib cartilage seemed like an overkill for me in these cases. I had found that HDPPE was easy to carve and customize, provided excellent support in these patients with thick skin, and therefore very reliable over decades with no extrusion or exposures.

Silicone

Silicone implants are another widely used alloplastic material, particularly popular for augmentation in Asian rhinoplasty.[3,5] Alloplasts tend to be more likely used in Asian patients than in Caucasian patients due to greater cultural concern with donor-site morbidity.[3] Silicone meets many of the requirements for an ideal implant: it is inexpensive, inert, easily carved, and resists modification. It is soft and pliable allowing for easy camouflaging in cases of a thin soft tissue envelope. A downside of this property, however, is that it consequently provides limited structural support.[1]

Unlike other commonly used synthetic materials, silicone implants are not porous. A theorized advantage of this is preventing bacterial entry, which may make it less susceptible to infection. However, without pores, the body responds to silicone implants with encapsulation, not soft tissue ingrowth and integration, as seen with porous implants. With time, silicone implants may develop chronic inflammation, malpositioning, and ultimately extrude. A large 2008 meta-analysis found the removal rate of silicone, 6.5%, to be significantly higher than the removal rate of HDPPE and ePTFE, both 3.1%.[12] A more contemporary 2018 meta-analysis found that silicone implants had the highest overall complication rate, 13%, and removal rate, 12%, compared to HDPPE and ePTFE.[11]

I do not use solid silastic implants in the nose because of their tendency to extrude even if they have been in place for many years.

Expanded polytetrafluoroethylene

ePTFE grafts are less frequently used than silicone and HDPPE implants in rhinoplasty today but have great historical significance. For reasons outside of the scope of this study, ePTFE grafts are expensive and not readily available. This alloplast is porous, unlike silicone, but has a smaller average pore size (10–30 μm) than that of HDPPE.[1] This property allows for some advantageous host tissue ingrowth and stabilization, while also allowing for easy explanation, if required. In comparison to silicone implants, malpositioning risk is significantly lower.[13] ePTFE is pliable and sculptable like silicone, which, while advantageous, limits its primary application to soft tissue augmentation, not rigid structural support.

ePTFE is commonly accepted as a very safe implant. A contemporary meta-analysis of 12 studies using ePTFE found that the overall complication rate is 5.3% and the infection rate is 1.2%.[13] A 2018 randomized clinical trial of patients undergoing nasal tip and dorsum augmentation using ePTFE compared outcomes of patients assigned to 2 arms: with or without adjunct conchal cartilage use.[14] During a mean follow-up of 76 patients using ePTFE over 106.9 months, only 3 patients (4%) developed an infection and no patients experienced extrusion.[14]

I do not use ePTFE because of the lack of availability, the expense, and the soft structural nature of the product, which disallows it to be used for structural support.

Kim/Kim

Complications of implants in rhinoplasty are often overrated in the academic community. Implants can be safely used with careful consideration of critical points, as discussed later. Surgeons tend to blame implants easily for complications without exercising appropriate techniques and preventive measures. Experience plays a crucial role in reducing complication rates.[15] My favorite implant in rhinoplasty is silicone. It offers advantages, such as a smooth surface, flexibility, elasticity, various softness, ease of carving, insertion, and removal.[16]

Porous implants like ePTFE and porous polyethylene (Medpor®) are theoretically more prone to bacterial contamination and biofilm formation.[17] Because of tissue ingrowth, these implants adhere to the skin after placement, posing challenges in removal and causing significant skin irregularities upon removal. While initially presenting a smooth appearance without sharp demarcation of the implant margins, adherent skin with tissue ingrowth will make them noticeable overtime, even more than nonporous silicone implants. Additionally, issues regarding collapsibility and deformation arise during extended follow-up periods.

However, complication rates for different implants vary based on surgeons' experience, and some surgeons achieve remarkably low complications with ePTFE. Silicone rubber implants cause fibrous capsule formation, leading to potential long-term contracture, unlike porous implants.[12] However, properly designed, clean, uncontaminated, well-fitted, soft silicone implants create a thin, protective capsule. In contrast, contaminated or poorly fitted stiff implants may result in chronic inflammation and infection and formation of a thick, irregular, contractile capsule, potentially causing a severely contracted nose.[18,19] Apart from rare instances of infection and severe capsular contracture, other issues with silicone implants are generally minor and easily treatable.

DO YOU HAVE ANY SPECIAL TECHNIQUES TO PREVENT COMPLICATIONS?
Romo/Graf/Ferzli

I think of this problem in a sequence of events. First, when possible, use autologous tissue. In my hands, if I am going to use an alloplast in the nose, it is going to be HDPPE. I impregnate the implant with antibiotics. It is then placed in under native skin, not under tension. I do not use under mucosal surfaces and judicially in revision rhinoplasties.

The only problem I have ever had in patients with HDPPE implants is misalignment of the dorsal implant off the midline. This has happened with patients with thick skin. In those rare cases, I

have to dissect out the implant with sharp dull tipped scissors. I have never had difficulty recovering the implant and realigning it in these patients.

Kim/Kim

Preventive measures against infection

1. Before the operation
   - Complete sanitization, shaving of vestibular hair, and scrubbing of the nasal cavity are crucial.
   - Light packing of the posterior nasal cavity with antiseptic-soaked gauzes would be beneficial.
   - Drapes are used, including around the mouth.
2. During the operation

Implant manipulation
   - *Frequent scrubbing* of gloves is strongly recommended, especially right before the manipulation of the implant, and after procedures like graft harvest in different surgical fields.
   - *Careful planning*: Following careful design and carving, the implant is immersed in an antibiotic solution. While repetitive carving may be necessary for optimal adaptation, a desired nose shape, and reduced dead spaces, well-planned surgeries will minimize the implant manipulation.
   - *Cleaning the surgical field and incision wounds*, especially just before implant insertion, can reduce the risk of bacterial contamination of the implant.

Incision and dissection
   - *Marginal incision preferred*: The marginal incision is preferred due to a lower risk of extrusion (**Fig. 2**) and infection compared to the intercartilaginous incision, where the

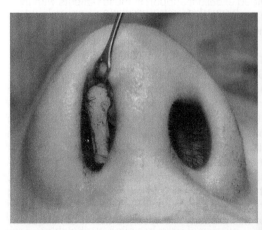

Fig. 2. Silicone extrusion through macerated mucosa.

distal implant margin is in close proximity to the incision.

- *Clean dissection*: Ensure a precise and clean dissection of the surgical plane to minimize tissue damage and bleeding, ensuring tissue viability, preventing hematoma-induced infection, and ascending bacterial infection due to mucosal violation. Water-tight repair is required for any mucosal tear. Osteotomies with minimal mucosal tear are not a contraindication for implant use; however, when the mucosal tear is significant, judicious use of the implant is recommended.

3. After the operation
- In augmentation mammoplasty, post-implant insertion irrigation with triple solution (Bacitracin-Cefazolin-Gentamicin) is known to reduce infection and capsular contracture rates.[20] For augmentation rhinoplasty using implants, concluding procedures with irrigation using antiseptic and antibiotic solutions are recommended.
- Conduct meticulous taping and splinting to deter hematoma, reduce dead space, and immobilize the implant.[21]

Preventive measures against other complications

Appropriate pocket formation
1. As every nose has a degree of asymmetry, augmentation rhinoplasty has the potential to accentuate or exacerbate preexisting asymmetry or deviation. Therefore, a vertical line is drawn upward from the nasal tip to the nasal root and forehead before the surgery in a sitting position. The entire augmentation procedures of the dorsum and tip are executed along the drawn line, ensuring the symmetric creation of the surgical pocket along this reference line.
2. The pocket for the implant should be sized snugly, approximately 10% to 20% wider than the implant width. If the pocket is too wide, the risk of implant deviation arises. If it is too narrow, an implant in an uneasy pocket may deviate or extrude also.

Appropriate design and carving of the implant
1. Implant grade silicones are categorized as soft, medium, and hard in the market according to Shore A hardness scale. Soft silicone implants with 10 to 30 Shore A hardness scale are favored for ease of carving and reduced complications.
2. Each implant is meticulously carved to match the patient's anatomy and desired nose shape. Individualized additional carving is also required intraoperatively for commercially available implants in various shapes and sizes.

3. Novice surgeons tend to oversize implants increasing the potential risks; precise size and length are determined only after implantation into the pocket.
4. Implants are carved to match the patients' radix anatomy, with the proximal end carefully positioned on the mid-pupillary or eyelash line in most Asian patients.

IN WHAT AREAS OF THE NOSE DO YOU USE IMPLANTS ROUTINELY? ARE THERE ANY AREAS WHERE YOU DO NOT USE IMPLANTS?
Romo/Graf/Ferzli

I tend to use implants in augmentation rhinoplasty in the platyrrhine nose. Presently defined by Google as the ethnic nose. For 30 years, I have been utilizing and publishing articles on my techniques for this kind of augmentation rhinoplasty. I use a combination of native septal cartilage and 2 porous polyethylene implants for these cases (**Figs. 3** and **4**). A dorsal tip alloplast always carved smaller and thinner at the tip prior to placement (**Figs. 5** and **6**). The alloplast is used as a columella strut between the medial crura, anterior to the spine and posterior to the domal angles also (**Figs. 7** and **8**). The septal cartilage is used as a plumper graft and infra tip lobule graft. I have had excellent results with these techniques for years (**Figs. 9** and **10**). In revision rhinoplasty, I prefer autologous tissue but have used alloplasts as a columella strut or dorsal graft with good results when patients decline use of their autologous rib cartilage (**Figs. 11** and **12**).

I do not use implants under mucosal surfaces and therefore, I do not use implants for repairing septal perforations or external valve collapse. I

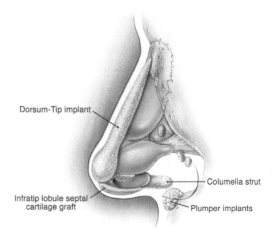

Fig. 3. Preferred alloplastic implant areas, profile view.

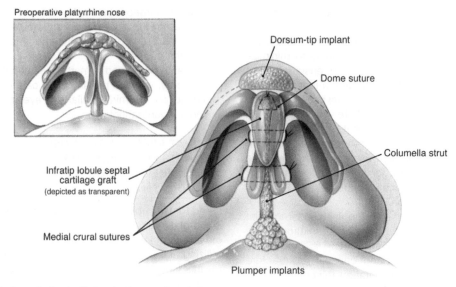

Fig. 4. Preferred alloplastic implant areas, basal view.

do not use implants when there is potential exposure to the internal nose and therefore do not use implants for spreader grafts, extended spreader grafts or caudle extension grafts. I believe the contraindications for using alloplasts in the nose are in patients with septal perforations that can constantly seed the patient's implants with bacteria, patients who smoke or use illicit nasal drugs, those who have overly thin skin, or have a poor blood supply to the skin.

Kim/Kim

I use implants only for the immobile bony and relatively immobile cartilaginous nasal dorsum. For the mobile nasal tip, only autologous materials are used exclusively.

I avoid using implants for the mobile nasal tip not only to prevent potential complications like skin thinning, and extrusion (**Fig. 13**), but also to prevent an unnatural and operated look, which is characterized by a conspicuous, sharp unidome disharmonious with the relatively wide alae of Asian patients, a blunt, thick infratip lobule and a pinched or collapsed appearance of the alar lobules.[3]

However, I recognize that in specific cases, particularly among certain Asian patients with extremely thick skin and weak cartilaginous tip support, using implants for the better tip definition may be required, especially when costal cartilage is not a viable option for various reasons. The L-shaped implant is commonly used in Southeast Asian countries, demonstrating an acceptable complication rate based on the collective experience of patients and surgeons in the region. The L-shaped implant provides medial tip support and a sharper nasal tip appearance, albeit with a variable risk of tip skin problems. To avoid potential tip complications, the tip of the L-shaped implant can be deliberately placed beneath the

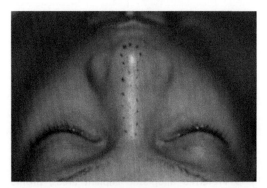

Fig. 5. Dorsal implant skin marking.

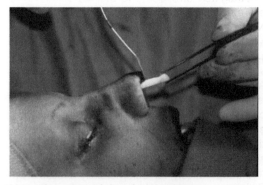

Fig. 6. Placement of dorsal tip implant.

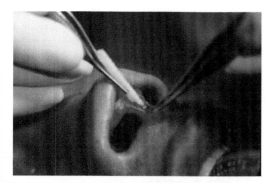

Fig. 7. Placement of columellar strut implant.

lower lateral cartilages as a protective barrier (personal communication with Dr Somyos in Thailand).

Some surgeons utilize an alloplastic implant like porous polyethylene (Medpor®) as a septal extension graft due to the frequently weak and small-sized septal cartilage in Asian patients, especially when a significant amount of tip augmentation is needed. However, porous polyethylene (Medpor®) is susceptible to infection, and it easily extrudes through the membranous septum. Removing the compromised porous implant in membranous septum is particularly demanding due to tissue adhesions and atrophied caudal septum. A technique involving suturing pieces of conchal cartilages on both sides of Medpor® in a sandwich manner for septal extension is believed to have a very low complication rate (personal communication with Dr Le Hanh in Vietnam).

IF YOU HAVE IMPLANT EXTRUSION, HOW DO YOU MANAGE IT?
Romo/Graf/Ferzli

Implant extrusion has not been a problem with this alloplast over the last 30 years. HDPPE is a very inert material. It can be partially exposed and partially integrated under the skin and be in that scenario for years. I have only seen this in auricular

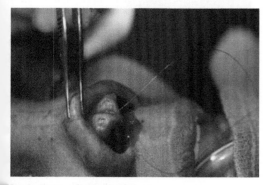

Fig. 8. Suture fixation of dome.

reconstruction. Just as I would do in the nose, I excise the exposed implant. Let the residual structure heal and then re-augment with autologous tissue.

Kim/Kim

Implant extrusion, often associated with infection, requires immediate removal and a course of oral antibiotics for several weeks. Planning a revision operation follows complete infection resolution and normalization of inflamed tissues, typically taking a few months. For near extrusion without overt implant protrusion through the skin or mucosa, salvage attempts can be made for nonporous implants like silicone, with intensive daily irrigation and antibiotic management for a few weeks. However, porous implants like ePTFE have minimal chances of salvage due to ineffective irrigation and antibiotic treatment related to hydrophobic surface pores, necessitating prompt removal. In rare cases of extrusion from chronic implant migration or capsular contracture but without evident infection, the solution involves resecting the extruded implant part and careful wound closure, with a chance of resolving the problem without further complications, while the risk of re-extrusion is discussed with the patient.

WHAT ARE THE PROS AND CONS OF COSTAL CARTILAGE VERSUS IMPLANTS IN RHINOPLASTY?
Romo/Graf/Ferzli

I believe that any completely qualified and trained facial plastic surgeon should know how to perform all techniques of rhinoplasty surgery: aesthetic and reconstructive. If one decides to limit his/her practice to certain types of rhinoplasties, then that is fine as long as he/she is getting good results for his/her patients.

I have a lot of experience with rib cartilage as I have been supervising microtia reconstruction clinics at New York Eye and Ear Infirmary and then Manhattan Eye Ear and Throat Hospital for over 30 years. When using autologous costal cartilage grafts, one downside is the donor-site morbidity. The surface incision site or as patients call it, "The Scar," can become hypertrophic, especially in people of color and not everyone can get one of these grafts out through a 2 cm incision. We recently had one of our most experienced rhinoplasty surgeons present at our Department M&M, a patient with a persistent 1 week pneumothorax post rib graft harvest for revision rhinoplasty. It can happen.

The rib graft then requires carving, slicing, and dicing. This requires a certain level of experience,

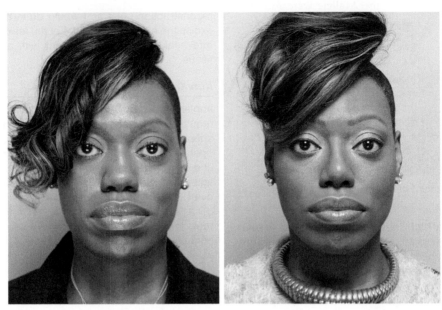

Fig. 9. Platyrrhine nose rhinoplasty with implants, frontal view, preoperative and postoperative photos.

and even with that ability, the graft can twist and warp. Remember, this was such a common consequence that Jack Gunter, M.D. in Dallas, put a k-wire down the length of the graft to prevent it from warping. Also, even as you use a customized rib graft slicer, the amount of grafting material to make these noses, including a caudal extension, extended spreader, dorsal, tip, and columella struts, can make these noses over firm and hard to touch. This is a well-known problem for patients who have experienced this technique.

In order to try and resolve this problem by cubing and dicing of the rib cartilage, then placing this into alloderm or autologous sleeve graft, making a customized sausage has had the problem with sizing being too big or too small. Slicing and placing in fibrin glue, the so-called glue graft has been shown to resorb and cause cobble stoning of the dorsal contour. Even with all these problems, autologous rib cartilage is an invaluable building material for the nose. Like in most ventures, moderation is key.

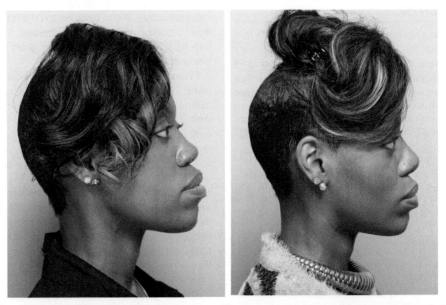

Fig. 10. Platyrrhine nose rhinoplasty with implants, profile view, preoperative and postoperative photos.

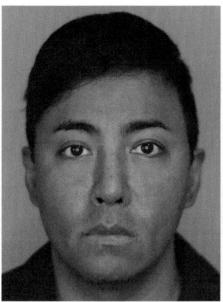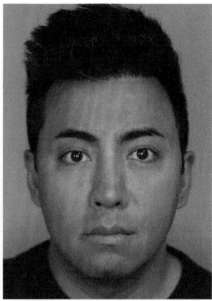

Fig. 11. Revision rhinoplasty with implants, frontal view, preoperative and postoperative photos.

Implants in the nose have a long and varied history of success. Silastic silicone implants cause the body to form a capsule around the implant and are prone to extrusion after trauma, even after many years in place; on the other hand, these implants are used by the thousands in Asia. I never use these implants for nasal reconstruction.

ePTFE or Gore-Tex was and is still widely used for nasal augmentation. Because it is relatively soft and flexible material, it is usually only used for dorsal augmentation in a stacked or rolled manner. W.L. Gore pulled out of the Facial Plastic Surgery market 20 years ago, finding a better market in vascular replacement grafts. HDPPE as an augmentation material for facial reconstruction has had its highs and lows over the last 30 years. One of the renaissances it is having now is its utilization in microtia reconstruction. I have 20 years of experience with this technique and have abandoned it because I have had several patients develop exposures and I ultimately had to remove the alloplastic framework and replace it with an autologous rib graft. This implant should be used judiciously in the nose. There must be good skin

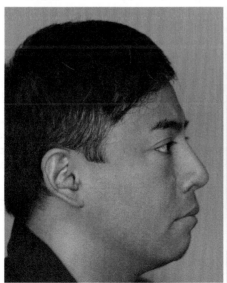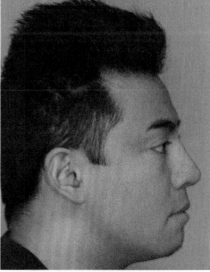

Fig. 12. Revision rhinoplasty with implants, profile view, preoperative and postoperative photos.

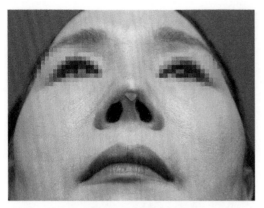

Fig. 13. Silicone extrusion through tip skin.

coverage with a sufficient blood supply to the skin. It should not be used under mucosal surfaces and not placed into tensioned skin tunnels.

Kim/Kim

Pros of costal cartilage
Autologous costal cartilage offers abundant volume and displays resistance to infection.

Cons of costal cartilage
Various complications are associated with the use of costal cartilage, including warping of carved cartilage, the presence of a chest scar, the risk of pneumothorax, and the occurrence of resorption.[22] When rib cartilage is utilized in the nasal tip, it may result in a hard, immobile nasal tip, causing discomfort for the patient. Severely calcified ribs render the cartilage practically unusable. Even mildly or moderately calcified ribs pose challenges, potentially exhibiting significant resorption after implantation. Unfortunately, clinically significant calcification of the rib is not uncommon and is observed in up to 15% of patients.[23]

Costal cartilage, whether diced or carved, is not entirely free from infection, although it is rare. In case of infection, the consequence can be severe:

1. Infected ribs resist standard treatments like irrigation, graft debridement, and antibiotics, with common organisms including Methicillin-resistant Staphylococcus Aureus, Vancomycin-resistant Staphylococcus Aureus, pseudomonas, and anaerobes.
2. Inflammation in costal cartilage can impact nearby nasal cartilages and soft tissue, leading to serious sequelae even after infection resolution. Removing an infected costal cartilage graft for infection control may result in severe nasal contraction, necessitating additional painful reconstructive surgery using another rib cartilage graft.

3. Even after the removal of infected rib cartilage, infection may persist, and tissue contracture may progress further.

Diced rib cartilages, whether glued or wrapped in fascia, are commonly used by many rhinoplasty surgeons; however, they come with disadvantages:

1. Difficulty in carving makes it difficult to accommodate various nasal shapes and to meet diverse esthetic needs.
2. Common issues with diced ribs include visible or palpable irregularities due to graft resorption, difficult tight molding, and surgical implantation.
3. Revision surgery becomes extremely difficult for diced ribs, as fine modifications and partial or complete removal are challenging. Additional augmentation or touch-up procedures may require another rib harvest, unless remnants are stored following various protocols by surgeons.

Pros of implants
From a pure esthetic standpoint, implants hold advantages over rib cartilages. They exhibit no absorption, deformation, scarring, or complications related to graft harvest. Implants are readily available in various sizes and shapes, without limitation in supply volume. Carving them into the desired shape is easy, and unlike rib cartilage, they offer softness and elasticity.

Implants are easy to insert and remove, simplifying revision surgery compared to rib cartilage grafts. Except for severe but rare complications like infection and contracture, most mild complications can be easily treated.

Cons of implants
Implants may be prone to infection and extrusion if not used cautiously, but the problems are preventable. While other issues like encapsulation and calcification are inherent and unavoidable, but they can be reduced through precise surgical techniques.

HOW HAVE YOUR TECHNIQUES IN THIS AREA CHANGED OVER THE LAST 2 YEARS?
Romo/Graf/Ferzli

None, but alloplasts in nasal reconstructive surgery will become passee when 3 dimensional-printed autologous cartilage grafts become available.

Kim/Kim

No significant but only minor changes in my basic implant techniques over the past 2 years.

1. Endonasal approach:
   The author now favors the endonasal approach more for augmentation rhinoplasty, finding it faster, less aggressive,

and less prone to bacterial contamination compared to the open approach. Symmetric pocket dissection can be achieved effectively through a marginal incision on one side by ensuring midline dissection without diagonal direction, preventing implant deviation.

2. Implant softness:

Softer implants offer advantages in preventing complications related to mechanical properties, while stiffer implants are preferred for achieving the desired nasal profile. The authors have used very soft implants with about 10 Shore A hardness scale and now prefer to use slightly stiffer implants about 15 Shore A hardness scale in recent years, finding it is easier to produce and maintain a desired nasal shape with them, while fair softness, flexibility, and carvability are maintained.

SUMMARY

In the right clinical scenarios, alloplastic implants can be used in rhinoplasty with great success. Complication rates tend to be overstated in the literature and can be minimized with surgeon experience, appropriate implant usage, and proper intraoperative techniques. Severe complications, extrusion and infection, are rare. Alloplastic materials can be used in concert with autologous grafting materials. Surgeons should select the implant material, which have varying physical properties and characteristics, that they are most comfortable with and are best suited to their patients.

CLINICS CARE POINTS

- Preoperative evaluation and careful patient selection when deciding whether to use alloplastic materials versus autologous materials are crucial.

- Select the implant material that you are most comfortable with, have had success using, and meet your patient's needs.

- Use implants only to graft immobile bony and/or relatively immobile cartilaginous structures, specifically the nasal dorsum or as a columellar strut.

- For the mobile nasal tip, only autologous grafting materials should be employed.

- Implants should be placed in appropriately sized tissues pockets, never under mucosal surfaces, and never closed under skin tension.

- Sterile technique and intraoperative antiseptic washings are imperative to limit complications.

DISCLOSURES

No disclosures.

REFERENCES

1. Romo T 3rd, Pearson JM. Nasal implants. Facial Plast Surg Clin North Am 2008;16(1):123–32.
2. Peng GL, Nassif PS. Rhinoplasty in the african american patient: anatomic considerations and technical pearls. Clin Plast Surg 2016;43(1):255–64.
3. Kim IS. Augmentation rhinoplasty using silicone implants. Facial Plast Surg Clin North Am 2018;26(3):285–93.
4. Romo T 3rd, Kwak ES. Nasal grafts and implants in revision rhinoplasty. Facial Plast Surg Clin North Am 2006;14(4):373–87.
5. Wei J, Dai C, Li S. Revision rhinoplasty in asians. Clin Plast Surg 2023;50(1):141–9.
6. Davis SJ, Landeen KC, Sowder JC, et al. Complications associated with use of porous high-density polyethylene in rhinoplasty. Facial Plast Surg Aesthet Med 2022;24(5):337–43.
7. Winkler AA, Soler ZM, Leong PL, et al. Complications associated with alloplastic implants in rhinoplasty. Arch Facial Plast Surg 2012;14(6):437–41.
8. Yap EC, Abubakar SS, Olveda MB. Expanded polytetrafluoroethylene as dorsal augmentation material in rhinoplasty on Southeast Asian noses: three-year experience. Arch Facial Plast Surg 2011;13(4):234–8.
9. Dong L, Hongyu X, Gao Z. Augmentation rhinoplasty with expanded polytetrafluoroethylene and prevention of complications. Arch Facial Plast Surg 2010;12(4):246–51.
10. Sclafani AP, Romo T. Alloplasts for nasal augmentation: clinical experience and scientific rationale. Facial Plast Surg Clin North Am 1999;7(1):43–54.
11. Liang X, Wang K, Malay S, et al. A systematic review and meta-analysis of comparison between autologous costal cartilage and alloplastic materials in rhinoplasty. J Plast Reconstr Aesthet Surg 2018;71(8):1164–73.
12. Peled ZM, Warren AG, Johnston P, et al. The use of alloplastic materials in rhinoplasty surgery: a meta-analysis. Plast Reconstr Surg 2008;121(3):85e–92e.
13. Hoang HLT, Januszyk M, Boyd JB. A systematic review of complications associated with nasal augmentation implants: expanded polytetrafluoroethylene (Gore-Tex) versus silicone. J Cosmet Med 2018;2(1):27–31.
14. Gu Y, Yu W, Jin Y, et al. Safety and efficacy of cosmetic augmentation of the nasal tip and nasal dorsum with expanded polytetrafluoroethylene: a

randomized clinical trial. JAMA Facial Plast Surg 2018;20(4):277–83.

15. McCurdy JA Jr. Considerations in Asian cosmetic surgery. Facial Plast Surg Clin North Am 2007; 15(3):387–397, vii.

16. Genther DJ, Papel ID. Surgical nasal implants: indications and risks. Facial Plast Surg 2016;32(5): 488–99.

17. Perez-Kohler B, Bayon Y, Bellon JM. Mesh infection and hernia repair: a review. Surg Infect 2016;17(2): 124–37.

18. Pajkos A, Deva AK, Vickery K, et al. Detection of subclinical infection in significant breast implant capsules. Plast Reconstr Surg 2003;111(5):1605–11.

19. Jirawatnotai S, Mahachitsattaya B. Analysis of subclinical infections and biofilm formation in cases of capsular contracture after silicone augmentation rhinoplasty: Prevalence and microbiological study. Arch Plast Surg 2019;46(2):160–6.

20. Ajdic D, Zoghbi Y, Gerth D, et al. The relationship of bacterial biofilms and capsular contracture in breast implants. Aesthet Surg J 2016;36(3):297–309.

21. Ozucer B, Yildirim YS, Veyseller B, et al. Effect of postrhinoplasty taping on postoperative edema and nasal draping: a randomized clinical trial. JAMA Facial Plast Surg 2016;18(3):157–63.

22. Wee JH, Park MH, Oh S, et al. Complications associated with autologous rib cartilage use in rhinoplasty: a meta-analysis. JAMA Facial Plast Surg 2015;17(1):49–55.

23. Sunwoo WS, Choi HG, Kim DW, et al. Characteristics of rib cartilage calcification in Asian patients. JAMA Facial Plast Surg 2014;16(2):102–6.

Safety in Rhinoplasty
Avoidance and Management of Complications

Parsa P. Salehi, MD, MHS[a,b,*], Anna Frants, MD[b,c], Oren Friedman, MD[d],
Jonathan Sykes, MD[e,f], Paul Nassif, MD[b,g]

KEYWORDS

• Rhinoplasty • Nasal surgery • Septoplasty • Complications • Outcomes

KEY POINTS

• Frequent postoperative checks can allow for early detection of rhinoplasty complications. This early detection allows for early intervention and may ultimately save the patients' rhinoplasty result.
• Patient dissatisfaction can be minimized with appropriate preoperative counseling, which includes comprehensive informed consent and setting expectations during the preoperative appointment.
• Postoperative skin compromise may be treated with topical nitroglycerin, hyperbaric oxygen treatment, a variety of medications, and leech therapy; patients should be monitored closely until resolution is achieved.

PANEL DISCUSSION

Infections? How to diagnose and treat them?

What is your most common complication?

What patients and what procedures are at greater risk? Is the length of surgery a risk factor?

Do you use additional treatments like hyperbaric chamber, nasal soaks, or other treatments?

What does your consent form include regarding complications?

How have your techniques in this area changed over the last 2 years?

INTRODUCTION

The nose is central to identity, and nasal appearance is critical in determining body image and personality development.[1,2] Studies have shown that both nasal cosmesis and function play a role in social interactions, self-confidence, quality of life, and daily function.[1,3,4] As such, rhinoplasty has become one of the most popular operations in the world.[5]

Despite its popularity, rhinoplasty carries inherent risks, and complications can occur during or after surgery. Patient dissatisfaction can stem from a broad range of underlying issues both

[a] SalehiMD Plastic Surgery, Newport Beach, CA, USA; [b] NassifMD Plastic Surgery, 120 South Spalding Drive #301, Beverly Hills, CA 90212, USA; [c] Specialty Aesthetic Surgery, New York, NY, USA; [d] Facial Plastic Surgery, Otorhinolaryngology Head and Neck Surgery, University of Pennsylvania Perelman School of Medicine, Philadelphia, PA, USA; [e] Facial Plastic Surgery, University of California, Davis Medical Center, Davis, CA, USA; [f] Sykes Fascial Plastic Surgery, Beverly Hills, CA, USA; [g] Department of Otolaryngology–Head and Neck Surgery, University of Southern California, Keck School of Medicine, Los Angeles, CA, USA
* Corresponding author.
E-mail address: DrParsaSalehiResearch@gmail.com
Twitter: @DrParsaSalehi (P.P.S.); @Dr.AnnaFrants (A.F.); @DrPaulNassif (P.N.)

Facial Plast Surg Clin N Am 32 (2024) 653–668
https://doi.org/10.1016/j.fsc.2024.06.008

subjective and objective in nature; complications of rhinoplasty include scar, asymmetries, irregularities, imperfections, nasal airway obstruction, skin ischemia or necrosis, nasal collapse, nasal deformity, and overcorrection or undercorrection of a perceived nasal irregularity. Understanding these potential complications, along with strategies for their avoidance and management, is essential for ensuring patient safety and optimizing surgical outcomes.

Complications may arise before, during, or after surgery, necessitating careful consideration, assessment, counseling, and management by plastic surgeons. This article aims to provide a comprehensive overview of complications in rhinoplasty, along with strategies for prevention and intervention.

Question 1: Infections? How to Diagnose and Treat Them?

Salehi/Frants/Nassif

The risk of infection is inherent in any surgical procedure, including rhinoplasty. The risk of infection is significantly higher in revision rhinoplasty cases since the blood supply is not as good as in primary rhinoplasty, and there may be more cartilaginous grafts present with revision rhinoplasty that increase the chance for infection.[6–14]

To minimize the risk of infection, both primary and revision rhinoplasty patients are given a structured regimen of oral, topical, and intranasal antibiotic treatments. These are summarized in **Tables 1** and **2**.

In primary rhinoplasty, patients are instructed to use hypochlorous acid sprays and mupirocin ointment beginning 5 days before surgery. Beginning on postoperative day 1, patients are instructed to continue the aforementioned regimen, while also maintaining excellent wound care and beginning a 5 day course of oral antibiotics. Mupirocin ointment is applied to bilateral nostrils preoperatively and postoperatively to minimize the chance of methicillin-resistant *Staphylococcus aureus* (MRSA) infection.

In revision rhinoplasty patients are instructed to add ciprofloxacin soaks (**Fig. 1**) beginning 5 days before surgery. Beginning on postoperative day 1, patients are instructed to continue the aforementioned regimen with the addition of a second 5 day course of oral antibiotics.

The senior author has incorporated ciprofloxacin antibiotic soaks as part of routine preoperative and postoperative care for revision rhinoplasty patients. The ciprofloxacin soak protocol consists of crushing two 500 mg ciprofloxacin tablets and mixing the powder with 1000 mL of normal saline.

A 5.08 cm x 5.08 cm gauze is saturated with the resulting solution and placed carefully in each nostril using a cotton-tipped applicator (see **Fig. 1**).

Any postoperative worsening erythema, foul odor perception, or obvious purulent drainage from any of the incisions is concerning for infection. The patient should be evaluated immediately and cultured. Mupirocin ointment is continued. If an organism is identified, antibiotic treatment should be started promptly. In cases in which clinical suspicion for infection is high, oral antibiotic therapy may be started prior to culture results, and updated as needed.

Friedman

Infections following rhinoplasty are relatively rare events, with reported estimates ranging from 0% to 4%.[15] Rhinoplasty is considered to be a "clean contaminated" operation—organisms living as part of the normal biome, either inside the nose or as skin flora outside of the nose, are also within the surgical field and are, therefore, the most likely potential sources of infection.[16] Recognizing infections early allows for prompt treatment, thereby avoiding long-term irreversible and potentially devastating sequelae. Anecdotally, we have found patients with a history of smoking, radiation therapy, intranasal drug use, chronic pseudomonal or staphylococcal carrier state, or systemic vasculitis to have a higher rate of infection. Among this patient population, we are on higher alert and will see them back in the office more frequently following surgery. The famous and wise Philadelphian Benjamin Franklin advised, "An ounce of prevention is worth a pound of cure," and being that I practice in Philadelphia, I heed his advice vigorously. Specifically, our high-risk patients may at times be asked to swab their nose with betadine solution, irrigate hydrogen-peroxide, or wash with chlorhexidine preoperatively to help reduce risks of postop infections. Intraoperatively, prior to the first surgical incision, we have also at times "prepped" the nose with hydrogen-peroxide irrigations. Among revision rhinoplasty patients who have had prior postnasal surgery infections, or among patients who are chronically colonized with *Staphylococcus* or *Pseudomonas* or other potentially pathologic organisms, preoperative nasal swab culture-directed prophylactic antibiotics[17,18] may be considered. *S aureus* is responsible for most infections after rhinoplasty; however, methicillin-resistant forms and even gram-positive coliforms should be suspected in at-risk patients.[17]

Infections following rhinoplasty may present as cellulitis, vestibulitis, incisional wound breakdown, cartilage graft necrosis, prolonged crusting,

Table 1
Medication protocol for primary rhinoplasty

Begin 5 Days before Surgery	
Hypochlorous acid spray	Spray in nose and mouth 2× daily for 5 d. Start 5 d before surgery
Mupirocin ointment/antibiotic	Apply inside of nostrils 2× daily for 5 d. Start 5 d before surgery
The Night before Surgery	
Famotidine 20 mg	Take one tablet the night before surgery to reduce throat irritation postoperatively
Take the Morning of Surgery	
Aprepitant	1 tablet with a small sip of water upon arrival at the surgery center
Gabapentin	Given in preoperative holding area, weight based per anesthesiologist
Begin the Evening of Surgery—These Are Optional	
Pain control	Alternating acetaminophen and ibuprofen, age-appropriate, maximum dose, every 4 h If needed for severe pain: tramadol: 1 tab every 6 h as needed for pain (take with food)
Benzodiazepine	Half to 1 tab every 6 h as needed for anxiety
Ondansetron	1 tab every 12 h as needed for nausea
Promethazine	Half to 1 tab every 8 h as needed for nausea
Probiotics (Optional)	Follow package instructions as directed
Colace	Take twice a day for 7 d
Begin the Day after Surgery	
Hydrogen peroxide and distilled water	Clean all incisions with three-fourths distilled water and one-fourth hydrogen peroxide twice a day (to clear any crusting/scabbing)
Arnica tablets/gel	Take 1 tablet twice a day for 7 d. Gel as needed for bruising
Sinus irrigation	Do sinus irrigations at least twice a day for 7 d. Can continue as needed after 1 wk
Mupirocin ointment	Apply to incisions and inside nostrils twice a day for 7 d
Cefadroxil	Take 1 capsule twice a day for 5 d
Medrol dose pack	Follow package instructions as directed
Antihistamine	Take as needed for congestion (Please avoid decongestants, general antihistamine recommended instead)
Begin at 1 wk Postop	
Nasal saline spray	As needed for nasal dryness for 2–3 mo
Aquaphor ointment	Apply to all incisions twice daily, begin after sutures are removed
Begin at 2 wk Postop or When Incision Lines Heals	
Silicone-based scar gel	Start 2 wk after surgery. Use for 2–3 mo; use on incision lines

septal abscess, suture abscess, septal perforation, external nasal abscess, and more advanced regional infections including intracranial infections transmitted through vascular channels from the nose to the intracranial cavity. Although rare, central nervous system extension of nasal infection may present a life-threatening complication.[19] Most minor infectious complications encountered are either self-limited or they may be successfully managed with simple measures. Postoperative nasal hygiene is advocated among all patients to prevent infections—saline irrigations, topical

Table 2
Antibiotic protocol for revision rhinoplasty

Begin 5 Days before Surgery	
Hypochlorous acid spray	Spray in nose and mouth 2× daily for 5 d. Start 5 d before surgery
Cipro soaks	(2-Cipro 500 mg tablets dissolved in 1000 mL sodium chloride solution) Twice a day for 5 d prior to surgery. See Cipro soaks attachment for instructions
Mupirocin ointment	Apply inside of nostrils 2× daily for 5 d. Start 5 d before surgery
The Night before Surgery	
Famotidine 20 mg	Take one PEPCID tablet the night before surgery to reduce throat irritation postoperatively
Take the Morning of Surgery	
Aprepitant	1 tablet with a small sip of water upon arrival at the surgery center
Gabapentin	Given in preoperative holding area, weight based per anesthesiologist
Begin the Evening of Surgery—These Are Optional	
Pain control	Alternating acetaminophen and ibuprofen, age-appropriate, maximum dose, every 4 h As needed for severe pain: tramadol: 1 tab every 6 h as needed for pain (take with food)—(we strongly discourage narcotic use)
Benzodiazepine	Half to 1 tab every 6 h as needed for anxiety
Ondansetron	1 tab every 12 h as needed for nausea
Promethazine	Half to 1 tab every 8 h as needed for nausea
Probiotics (optional)	Follow package instructions as directed
Colace	Take twice a day for 7 d
Begin the Day after Surgery	
Hydrogen peroxide and distilled water	Clean all incisions with three-fourths distilled water and one-fourth hydrogen peroxide twice a day (to clear any crusting/scabbing)
Cipro soaks/antibiotic soak	(2-Cipro 500 mg tablets dissolved in 1000 mL sodium chloride solution) Twice a day for 10 d after surgery
Arnica tablets/gel	Take 1 tablet twice a day for 7 d. Gel as needed for bruising
Nasal sinus irrigation	Do sinus irrigations at least twice a day for 7 d. Can continue after 7 d as needed
Mupirocin ointment/antibiotic	Apply to incisions and inside nostrils twice a day for 7 d
Ciprofloxacin	1 tablet twice a day for 5 d
Cefadroxil	Take 1 capsule twice a day for 5 d
Medrol dose pack	Follow package instructions as directed
Antihistamine	Take as needed for congestion (Please avoid decongestants, general antihistamine recommended instead)
Begin at 1 Wk Postop	
Nasal saline spray	As needed for nasal dryness for 2–3 mo
Aquaphor ointment	Apply to all incisions twice daily, begin after sutures are removed
Begin at 2 Wk Postop or When Incision Lines Heals	
Silicone-based scar gel	Start 2 wk after surgery. Use for 2–3 mo; use on incision lines

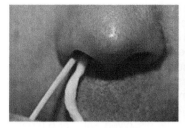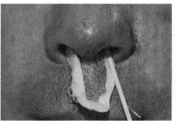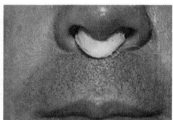

Fig. 1. Ciprofloxacin soaks.

antibiotic ointment, and cleaning the incisions and surgical areas. The most important advice for diagnosing and treating infectious complications following surgery is to be aware of, and open to, their possible occurrence. The slightest sign of infection such as the most minimal amount of erythema or tenderness in a particular area may indicate a looming infection which, if managed early, may resolve without any consequence. Conversely, if the surgeon is not aware of, concerned about, or worse—is dismissive of—early signs and symptoms of infection, significant long-term problems may ensue.

Cellulitis may be identified as redness, warmth, pain, and tenderness in a particular region of the nose. This may involve the skin externally, which is easily visible to the patient and clinician and, therefore, relatively easy to identify and treat promptly. Cellulitis involving the internal nasal skin, or vestibulitis inside of the nostril, may be more difficult to see and, therefore, to identify promptly. We should remain vigilant and search for signs of infection if patients are complaining of associated symptoms. Once identified, cellulitis and vestibulitis may be easily treated—if it involves an intact area of skin and not an incision-line, these infections may be managed with oral antibiotics. Ideally, culture-directed antibiotics would be employed, but most often when infections are identified early and treated early, there is improvement or resolution before the culture and sensitivities return from the laboratory. Generally, for otherwise healthy and nonimmunocompromised patients, we use empiric antibiotic therapy with amoxicillin–clavulanic acid or a first-generation cephalosporin such as cephalexin (or clindamycin, if β-lactam allergy). If the area infected involves a suture line or sutured area as in the septum, treatment begins with the removal of any irritating or inciting contributors such as suture material that may serve as a nidus of infection or crusts that may be providing cover for underlying bacterial growth. For these open wounds or suture-line or suture-related infections, topical soap and water or topical hydrogen peroxide scrubs to the affected region are very helpful. Additionally, topical antibiotic ointment

such as mupirocin or povidone-iodine may be used. More advanced infections such as nasal or septal abscesses may require incision and drainage along with topical therapies and likely systemic antibiotics and potentially hospitalization.

Sykes

Postoperative rhinoplasty infections are uncommon. The vast vascular supply and lymphatic drainage of the nose likely account for the low infection incidence, despite operating in a field that is exposed to nasal and sinus flora and is considered clean contaminated.

The exception to this rare infection rate occurs when a foreign body, such as an alloplast implant, is used during the nasal reconstruction. Alloplasts, such as high-density polyethylene (Medpor–Porous polyethylene, Stryker, Kalamazoo, MI) or gore-Tex (expanded-polytetrafluoroethylene) can be colonized with bacteria during their implantation. This will often result in chronic inflammation or even infection. Infection in rhinoplasty with the use of alloplasts can occur at any time after surgery. Although infections can occur in the early postoperative period, chronic inflammation or infection can happen many years after the surgery and this chronic inflammatory condition is common.

Diagnosis of postrhinoplasty infections requires a careful examination and a high clinical suspicion. A common source of inflammation or infection is from intraoperative suture placement. Mini suture abscesses from transcolumellar sutures are common. These can be treated with suture removal and wound care (topical antibiotic ointment). If the suture abscess is from nasal tip sutures, access to these is more difficult, and removal of the offending suture(s) requires anesthesia of the area and an incision (endonasal or open approach) to expose the area and remove the contaminating suture.

Question 2: What Is Your Most Common Complication?

Salehi/Frants/Nassif

The most common complication in both primary and revision rhinoplasty is unsatisfactory esthetic outcome. This complication is difficult to measure or objectify, as it is defined by patients' perceptions of what their ideal outcome should be from a functional and cosmetic standpoint. As such, quantifying the success and goals of rhinoplasty surgery is quite difficult. Successful outcomes are contingent on both the surgeon's execution (optimizing both cosmetics and function) and the patient's *perception* of these outcomes. In many cases, the patient may be bothered by an outcome the surgeon finds acceptable (or even optimal).

As such, the best way to minimize complications is astute clinical examination skills and decision-making and exhaustive preoperative and postoperative counseling of realistic expectations and healing timeline. For instance, we routinely tell patients that they will require a full 3 years to heal after rhinoplasty, especially revision cases. Prior to the 3 year healing window, we often do not entertain further revision surgeries unless there is an obvious functional deficit or cosmetic deformity.

Clinicians should always monitor for body dysmorphia and/or unrealistic expectations, as these patients often are unhappy with their outcomes, regardless of surgeon's skill. Notably, there has been a rise of addictive social media use in recent years; this rise has negatively impacted the mental wellness and body image distortion in certain patients.[20] Further, social media use has coincided with a notable rise in misinformation surrounding plastic surgery.[20] Now more than ever, plastic surgeons have a duty to assess and counsel patients thoroughly; in the end, the surgeon that carefully selects patients will minimize unsatisfactory esthetic outcomes.

Friedman

Overall rhinoplasty complications are best divided into 2 categories: early complications and longer term complications. In addition, it is worth highlighting that I can comment from personal experience on the most common early and longer term complications I see among my own patients, but it is more difficult to comment on the very long-term complications I may not be aware of among my surgical patients who may have sought revision surgery elsewhere. I can, however, also comment on the most common reasons patients might seek my opinion for revision rhinoplasty after surgery performed elsewhere.

1. My early complications: The most common complication I see in the early weeks after surgeries that I perform relate to suture-related irritation and low-grade infection. In my earlier years of practice, I noticed problems with irritation from polyester poly (p-dioxanone) (PDS) suture material placed under the septal flaps. Patients experience slight tenderness in the region of the suture and knot, they may develop microabscesses that become visible under the septal mucosa, and often there may be extrusion of the suture material—before the suture material ever dissolved—at 3 or 6 months or longer after surgery. As a result, I moved away from using any slow-dissolving or permanent suture materials submucosally in the septum and only used that suture material when there is a more robust and highly vascular soft tissue coverage available to help bury the suture material more deeply and to help dissolve the material more quickly and without overlying superficial signs of irritation or infection (I continue to use PDS and permanent suture for lower lateral and upper lateral cartilage fixation as this is buried under the thickness of the well-vascularized and cushioned nasal skin). I now use mostly absorbable chromic suture and plain gut suture, placed in an extramucosal location, for nearly all septal work including fixation of cartilage grafts as needed. These sutures generally dissolve quickly, may easily be removed if they are causing irritation and infection and crusting, and are sufficient to provide the necessary strength and support for securing tissues in position until permanent scar tissue associated with proper wound healing fixes them more permanently.

2. My longer term complications: The most common complication I find in the longer term is persistent edema. Common belief led many surgeons to covey to their patients that the permanent result of their surgery would be visible at 12 months postoperatively. Over time, it has become clear that I do not see the expected surgical result at 12 months, and I find that the patients are swollen for much longer than that. As a result, I counsel my patients that they will continue to see resolution of swelling and settling of tissues for a period of 18 to 24 months before the "final result" takes shape. And even after that, I know there will continue to be changes to the skin envelope that will alter the appearance of the nose. A highly satisfactory rhinoplasty outcome is certainly visible in the early postoperative period, within 6 weeks of surgery, both from the patient's perspective and from my perspective, but I know that the nasal appearance will only continue to improve over time as the swelling resolves more fully. Despite this

knowledge and communication of such to the patient preoperatively and again postoperatively, delays in visualizing the ultimate surgery outcome are a source of anxiety and, at times, frustration for the patient and for our team.

There are a number of factors that have been shown to predispose patients to increased and prolonged edema including skin thickness,[21,22] external rhinoplasty approaches,[23,24] osteotomies,[25] and extent of nasal tip dissection.[26] Patient compliance with postoperative rhinoplasty care instructions may also determine the degree of edema, including maintaining the nasal splint and tape, icing the eyes and nose, elevating the head of bed, mobilizing early after surgery, minimizing sun exposure, and others.

In our quest for optimal results and rapid recovery, surgeons have sought ways of improving edema following rhinoplasty. Osteotomy technique has been studied, and periosteal preservation[27] and piezoelectric osteotomy[28–30] have been shown to be helpful in reducing postoperative edema. A 2021 meta-analysis failed to show the external approach to lateral osteotomy beneficial for postoperative swelling and bruising.[25] In conjunction with the anesthesia team, we often employ intraoperative systemic steroids to reduce postoperative nausea and vomiting, but this practice has also been shown effective in reducing the degree of edema seen on postoperative day 1 compared to placebo.[31,32] A single perioperative systemic steroid dose has proven useful, with additional benefit obtained from an additional short postoperative course of steroids.[31] In a meta-analysis of 18 randomized controlled trials, no significant difference was found between the type of steroid used among dexamethasone, methylprednisolone, or betamethasone.[32]

While nasal taping and external splinting after rhinoplasty are the standard practice, there is little evidence to support the practice. At times, surgeons may use tissue glue to seal the "deadspace" between the skin-soft-tissue-envelope and the underlying bony-cartilage skeleton in hopes of reducing edema. Additional recommendations to help control edema include the use of *Arnica montana* and bromide as supplements to help with swelling and bruising. A recent randomized controlled trial using 3 dimensional-printed rhinoplasty splints found superior results for long-term edema reduction of the nose at 6 months and 1 year compared to control (taping; $P \le .05$), as well as consistent reductions in the tip and dorsum, specifically (1 year, $P \le .1, .01$, respectively).[33] A commonly accepted practice for the reduction of edema in the early postoperative months following rhinoplasty, which we also incorporate into our practice as needed, includes the injection of triamcinolone into the subcutaneous tissue, especially in the supratip region. Care should be taken in avoiding too superficial an injection or too much injected steroid as skin atrophy and scar may complicate the injection.

3. Complications requiring revision surgery: The most common reasons patients present to me for corrective revision rhinoplasty following primary surgery that was performed elsewhere include nasal obstruction, crooked nose deformities, and dorsal irregularities. The details of my approach to these problems are beyond the scope of this publication, but are mentioned for completeness.

Sykes

The 2 most common infectious complications after rhinoplasty include reaction/infection related to intraoperative suture placement and endonasal infection from postobstructive sinus cavity contaminants. In that the normal draining sinus ostia are often obstructed from postoperative edema or inspissated blood and mucous, it is prudent to use perioperative oral antibiotics as prophylaxis to prevent these infections. Intranasal sinus infections from postobstructive (intranasal packing/stents or intranasal edema) are usually limited by perioperative oral antibiotics and do not typically require intravenous antibiotics or surgical drainage. In most cases, perioperative sinus infections are well treated with a combination of oral antibiotics, nasal saline irrigation, and intranasal decongestant sprays.

Question 3: What Patients and What Procedures Are at Greater Risk? Is the Length of Surgery a Risk Factor?

Salehi/Frants/Nassif

The patients most at risk for complications are revision rhinoplasty patients (with a greater risk with each subsequent surgery), thick-skinned patients, thin-skinned patients, patients suffering from body dysmorphia, patients with unrealistic expectations, prior filler injections to the nose, foreign body injection/implant in the nose, and patients with underlying medical comorbidity.

For instance, patients with underlying autoimmune disease, such as granulomatosis with polyangiitis (GP), are at greater risk for complications. Patients with GP have up to a 20% complication rate,[34] 50% disease recurrence rate,[34,35] and 25% graft resorption rate.[36] Patients with GP are at greater risk for postoperative graft necrosis and infection.[34] In GP nasal reconstructions, autologous tissue is preferred, with either costal cartilage or calvarial bone grafts.[34] Some advocate for calvarial bone grafts over costal cartilage given GP's tendency to destroy cartilage; though this has not been our experience.[34,37]

Excluding complications of general anesthesia (which we rarely experience), we have not found that the length of surgery has an impact on the surgical risks or outcomes. Often times, more challenging cases may take longer, but that does not necessarily negatively impact the outcomes. In fact, we advocate that in challenging cases the surgeon proceeds with caution and attention to detail to maximize postoperative outcomes.

Friedman

Complications following rhinoplasty are reported with variable incident rates in different studies. In general, surgery performed for patients with poor blood supply as may occur in smokers, patients who have undergone radiation therapy, and patients with vascular insufficiency or vasculitis is of higher risk and prone to complications. Revision surgery, due to scar tissue, altered circulation, need for more aggressive maneuvers, need for cartilage grafts taken from secondary sites, requirements for more comprehensive reconstruction with a greater number and larger incisions and wider areas of soft tissue disruption and dissection are also higher risk situations that require greater care and awareness. A review of the American College of Surgeons' National Surgical Quality Improvement Program database[38] found that the incidence of all complications was 5.4%. Some of the commonly cited surgical complications, and those specifically listed on the American Society of Plastic Surgery's "Consent for Rhinoplasty," were systematically reviewed by Sharif-Askary and colleagues[15] and I will comment on various factors that may contribute to higher risks for some of the listed complications.

Nasal septal perforation Nasal septal perforation is said to occur in under 3% of patients undergoing rhinoplasty. Certain factors may contribute to septal perforation following nasal surgery including surgeon unfamiliar with septoplasty techniques, patients with particularly thin mucosa, patients with nasal crusts and ulcerations who undergo surgery when crusts and ulcers are present, severe septal deviations, revision nasal surgery where septal cartilage and bone has been previously resected, and others. If there is a postoperative infection, or suture irritation or infection, this may trigger septal perforation. In a study specifically looking at patients undergoing repair of septal perforation, we found that among 81 repair

procedures, the rate of infection was 3.7% and those patients with infection following surgery were predisposed to a failure of perforation repair.[39] I find that approximating torn septal mucosal flaps if present, excellent postoperative nasal hygiene, and the application of silicone splints during the healing process help prevent the occurrence of septal perforation.

Infection Infection is reported to occur in less than 4% of rhinoplasty patients. Strategies for prevention, identification, and management of infections have been discussed earlier in this publication and the reader is referred to the earlier sections for review or surgical and patient factors associated with this complication. In general, the American Academy of Otolaryngology-Head and Neck Surgery (AAOHNS) Clinical Practice Guidelines do not recommend prophylactic antibiotics for a period greater than 24 hours.[40] There remains variability in surgeon practice.[3,41,42] Among patients undergoing revision rhinoplasty, the use of antibiotic "soaks" or "irrigations" have been shown to be beneficial.[43] An additional study revealed that women undergoing revision rhinoplasty with rib cartilage had a higher rate of postoperative infection.[44]

Bleeding In most patients, rhinoplasty is achieved without complications of postoperative bleeding that requires packing after surgery, and with the extremely rare occurrence of septal hematoma. Conversely, ecchymosis following rhinoplasty is common. Light-skinned and light-eyed patients with thinner skin seem to be more prone to severe ecchymosis, and I generally quote to patients a 33% occurrence of ecchymosis based on anecdotal experience. Patients are instructed to use ice packs on their eyes for 72 hours after surgery, 20 minutes on and 20 minutes off. Among patients who bruise easily by history, I recommend A montana, bromide,[45] early and aggressive mobilization, elevated head of bed, and at times oral systemic steroid taper.

Nasal airway obstruction Historically, nasal airway obstruction has been one of the most common long-term complications following rhinoplasty.[46] This is especially true following a purely reductive cosmetic rhinoplasty.[47] During standard "Joseph" dorsal reduction cosmetic rhinoplasty, failure to address septal deviation and/or reconstruct a weak nasal valve results in an increased risk of postoperative nasal airway obstruction. In rhinoplasty education today, facial plastic surgeons continue to appropriately emphasize the confluence of form and function in the nasal organ and recognize the extreme importance and value in addressing both aspects of the nose among our patients.[48] A variety of surgical techniques have been developed and employed to manage functional aspects of the nose[49] and may often be used in conjunction with rhinoplasty techniques to improve patient quality of life.[50] Given the significant impact nasal obstruction has on a patient's sleep quality and life quality, when performing cosmetic rhinoplasty, surgeons should also aim to improve nasal breathing function.

Sykes

Patients that have preoperative colonization with large amounts of bacteria that are not part of typical respiratory flora are at greater risk of developing postoperative intranasal infections. The most common of these bacterium is MRSA. If the patient is a known carrier of MRSA, preoperative treatment with oral antibiotics known to kill MRSA and topical antibiotic ointment mupirocin for at least 7 days is advised.

Several patient types and conditions increase the incidence of perioperative rhinoplasty infections. These include patients undergoing revision rhinoplasty, especially in those cases in which the skin-soft tissue envelope has been compromised and the vascularity to the skin is compromised or is in question. Additionally, chronic nicotine use and or diabetes mellitus changes the skin vascularity. In patients with these conditions, the infection rate may be increased.

In patients with potentially compromised vascularity to the skin-soft tissue envelope, perioperative treatments with hyperbaric oxygen is indicated.

Question 4: Do You Use Additional Treatments Like Hyperbaric Chamber, Nasal Soaks, or Other Treatments?

Salehi/Frants/Nassif

In addition to the protocols discussed in **Tables 1** and **2**, we do advocate for hyperbaric chamber therapy in patients. Ideally, all patients would undergo hyperbaric oxygen therapy immediately before and for 3 to 5 days after surgery. In revision rhinoplasty patients, especially in the case of multiple revisions, we may require patients to undergo hyperbaric oxygen therapy as a condition for surgery. In cases where postoperative venous congestion is noted, we again send patients for hyperbaric oxygen therapy. Depending on the severity of postoperative concern, our typical protocol is at least five 1 hour treatment sessions at 2.0 atmosphere absolute (ATA) or ten 1 hour treatment sessions at 2.0 ATA.

In addition to daily hyperbaric oxygen treatments, our protocol for venous nasal skin congestion postoperatively includes a multifaceted

treatment protocol, with close follow-up until symptoms resolve. We utilize a combination of topical nitroglycerin 2% ointment and *Hirudo medicinalis* therapy (with antibiotic prophylaxis) in the immediate postoperative period, oral aspirin 81 mg daily, and, in severe cases, oral pentoxifylline. Other considerations include avoiding postoperative dressings/splints/tape to avoid pressure and improve postoperative wound monitoring. In patients with underlying autoimmune disease history, providers may consider rheumatologic testing to assess disease reactivation. As with any complication, consistent communication and regular follow-up are critical.

Friedman

I routinely insist that patients stop smoking prior to proceeding with nasal surgery. For routine postrhinoplasty care, I instruct patients to avoid strenuous activities and heavy weight lifting for 10 days, to use ointment in the nose at least 4 times daily, to use saline nasal spray 6 sprays each nostril 6 times a day, to apply saline irrigations to the nose 2 to 3 times daily, and to try to wash any suture lines with soap and water 1 to 2 times daily. Among healthy patients undergoing primary rhinoplasty, the listed instructions form the extent of our basic routine. I generally see patients in follow-up within the first 10 days after surgery, then again a week or two later depending on how things are looking, then again at 1 month after surgery and then at 3 months, 6 months, and 12 months after surgery, and I am always looking vigilantly for any signs of healing problems or developing complications. Among patients undergoing major revision rhinoplasty with rib grafts, recent former smokers, after head and neck radiation therapy, former drug users, patients with vascular issues, and patients with history of chronic bacterial colonization or high risk of this as with patients who are health care workers, I am more vigilant and add more cautionary instructions and follow up. I will routinely have these patients use topical povidone-iodine ointment, chlorhexidine, and/or hydrogen peroxide preoperatively and at times postoperatively if they are at high risk of infection. At the very first sign of suture irritation or infection or cellulitis, I will remove the affected suture and perform a thorough cleaning in the office. The patient will be instructed to more frequently perform soap and water cleansing of the affected area at home, and in addition to the mupirocin antibiotic ointment, I may start the patient on an antibiotic irrigation (ie, gentamicin or other) as well as a possible topical steroid. If there appears to be exposed cartilage or threat of exposed cartilage, I will often place the patient on oral antibiotics and possibly oral steroid if there is significant inflammation in the region. A culture is taken, and the patient may be started on very strong broad-spectrum antibiotics if the threat of wound breakdown or cartilage loss is significant, for example, levofloxacin and clindamycin. Patients are instructed to be aware of, and seek medical attention immediately, if they develop gastrointestinal issues or loose stools because of any of these treatments. Very rarely have I instituted hyperbaric oxygen therapy for a routine primary or revision rhinoplasty, but in a patient with the risk factors mentioned, this would be considered as clinically indicated.

A recent study of over 3000 patients published by Toriumi and colleagues[43] showed reduced infections when antibiotic soaks or irrigations were used in rhinoplasty as compared with control patients ($P = .0053$). The effect reported was most evident among revision rhinoplasty patients. Chien and colleagues[39] reported on 81 septal perforation repairs among whom the rate of infection was 3.7%, but they noted a significantly lower chance of success of perforation repair among patients who developed infections as compared with the patients who did not develop infection.

Sykes

If the patient has a history of chronic nasal drainage (especially if the drainage is purulent), preoperative nasal cultures are indicated. Treatment should be individualized and directed by culture results.

In patients with potentially compromised vascularity to the skin-soft tissue envelope, perioperative treatments with hyperbaric oxygen are indicated. Also, if the patient develops a postoperative infection, which includes possible vascular compromise or skin ischemia, postoperative hyperbaric oxygen chamber treatments may be indicated. Use of a hyperbaric chamber of at least 4 ATA is advisable. Daily treatments for 7 to 10 days (3 preoperative and 7 postoperative) are indicated.

Question 5: What Does Your Consent Form Include Regarding Complications?

Salehi/Frants/Nassif

Our consent includes all the standard risks of surgery including bleeding, infection, damage to surrounding structures, need for future surgery, cosmetic dissatisfaction, and death. Notably, several topics are discussed (as applicable) at the time of consultation and again at the preoperative visit (**Table 3**). A thorough discussion of these factors is essential in managing expectations with patients.

Friedman

Consent form includes bleeding, infection, nasal obstruction, vision loss, cosmetic dissatisfaction, septal perforation, need for revision surgery, cerebrospinal fluid leak, pain, loss of smell, and risks associated with anesthesia including death.

Sykes

All preoperative informed choice consents should include generalized information regarding the risk of postoperative infection. If prior nasal infection is known, discussion and documentation of an increased risk of perioperative infection should be performed.

A specific discussion relating to the risk of skin compromise, scarring, and the possibility that the infection will affect the final esthetic or functional outcome. This discussion is most important for revision rhinoplasty cases and for the patients with preoperative conditions that may negatively affect healing (smoking, diabetes mellitus, collagen vascular disorders, and so forth).

Question 6: How Have Your Techniques in This Area Changed over the Last 2 Years?

Salehi/Frants/Nassif

We continue to use the diced cartilage glue graft (DCGG) and refine the various grafts that may be created from it.[51–56] DCGG is an excellent tool, as it allows for precise shaping of cartilage grafts and nasal refinement, while providing a layer of camouflage to mask sharp edges. We have found that by mincing the cartilage finely (finer than minced garlic) and applying a thin layer of fibrin glue, we minimize the amount of resorption and unpredictability.

The most significant change to our practice in the past 2 years has been the greater emphasis on dorsal preservation rhinoplasty approaches.[57,58] The dorsal preservation approach allows for optimal dorsal hump reduction while preserving a patient's natural dorsal anatomy.[57] Patient selection and training in dorsal preservation is key to performing these surgeries.

Recently, we have moved toward more endonasal rhinoplasty approaches. The impetus for this change was primarily to minimize postoperative swelling. One of the most frequent complaints of patients after rhinoplasty are postoperative swelling, and it has been our experience that with the endonasal approach patients are less swollen and have a shorter course of postoperative edema. As with any surgery, patient selection is critical in pursuing closed approach rhinoplasty.

Friedman

Throughout my career, I have performed both endonasal and external rhinoplasty, and at different

Table 3
Specific complications discussed at every preoperative visit

Complication	Discussed Material
Expectations	Our goal is improvement, but not perfection. We made this clear to the patient
Morphed images	We showed the patient computer morphs that are not guaranteed surgical results but to help guide surgical discussion. We reminded the patient that the morphs are realistic, but the results are not exact and are not a guarantee. We made clear that even with the morphs, we cannot promise an exact result or promise to over deliver. We showed her the disclaimer on the morphing program that "Simulation—actual results will differ"
Fibrin glue use	We also need to use fibrin glue for the patient. Fibrin glue is made of pooled blood products that has been used safely in surgery for decades. We combine the glue with very finely diced cartilage to create soft moldable grafts to refine the nose, similar to spackling
Asymmetries	We showed pre-existing asymmetries of the face. We want the patient to be aware of the inherent asymmetries of the facial skeleton that will not be changed by this surgery but may affect how the nose looks as it sits on the face. We specifically discussed that we are unable to change the location of the nostril attachment to the face
Rib	Taking cartilage from the rib involves a small incision in the breast crease or pectoral groove that hides well. The cartilage is harvested from the right side, unless there is a medical and/or surgical contraindication. We discussed the risk of pneumothorax. A pneumothorax would require a postoperative chest tube, further procedures, and possibly hospital admission
Cartilage grafts	We discussed that with placement of cartilage there are always several risks, namely rejection of cartilage, warping of cartilage, chondritis, infection of cartilage, and graft rejection
General risks	We discussed the risks of rhinoplasty including asymmetric healing, scarring, bleeding, septal hematoma, septal perforation, saddle nose, infection, damage to surrounding structures, need for future surgeries, need for revision, unsatisfactory results, cosmetic changes, and unsatisfactory cosmetic results
Counseling	In our counseling, we reviewed that the goal with surgery is an improvement and not perfection. We answered the patient's questions regarding healing, including that the patient may have some ecchymosis and mild pain in the immediate postoperative period. All preoperative questions were answered, and a thorough discussion took place about the postoperative course, realistic expectations, and that much time is taken for the nose and face to heal following surgery, which may take up to 3 y. The patient realized the impossibility of creating perfection and realized asymmetries were inevitable because of natural nasal contour irregularities and because the nose is 3-dimensional. The national average need for a revision due to healing, scarring, or other factors is about

(continued on next page)

Table 3
(continued)

Complication	Discussed Material
	22%. We discussed that *no* nose heals perfectly, and there is nothing we can do to control this. We told the patient that we will only do what is safe and natural. The patient understands
Revision policy	Patient understands revision policy. If a revision is necessary and/or desired, there will be additional fees and charges to be paid by the patient. The patient has read and understands this
Thick skin	The patient does have thick skin, so this may be a limiting factor for her in terms of how small we can get the nose
Nasal tip	We discussed that patient's tip will drop after surgery. We discussed that since we expect a slight drop after surgery, we will overrotate the nasal tip during surgery to account for this. We made clear that this is an unpredictable process, and the tip may remain overrotated, or in some cases drop lower. Our goal will be to optimize rotation, so that once the patient is healed, the tip will be where the patient desires
Pinched nose	We specifically discussed with the patient that we will not attempt any maneuvers that may jeopardize patient's airway and/or breathing. We also discussed that the "pinched" or "defined" look is not normal anatomy. We specifically emphasized to the patient that we will not do any maneuvers that will pinch his tip. We made this clear to the patient multiple times. We emphasized to the patient the impossibility of creating perfection and that asymmetries are inevitable because of natural nasal contour irregularities and because the nose is 3-dimensional. We made clear multiple times that we will not make the tip more "pinched." In fact, we discussed that we will likely widen the tip to improve the airway
Dorsal profile	Esthetically, patient desires a very refined, pointed nose with a steep slope—"ski slope." We discussed that we need to balance a natural look with a safe surgery that will not worsen her breathing. We discussed that aggressive hump reduction has the potential for an increased nasal obstruction and cosmetic deformities (eg, inverted-V deformity). We will do our best to balance a natural esthetic with optimal function. Patient understands this
Alar base modification	We specifically discussed the risk of scarring and hyperpigmentation with this maneuver. We discussed the risk of asymmetries
PDS plate	We discussed the risks of PDS plate including scarring, extrusion, need for removal, implant rejection, and nasal obstruction
Auricular cartilage	We discussed that there is a small possibility we may need to use ear cartilage to achieve the desired surgical goals. This may incur additional surgical time and cost. This involves a postauricular incision. We will use cartilage from the bowl of the ear. Healing will involve a cotton bolster ball in the ear. Taking cartilage from here may result in the ear becoming less prominent, which is why we use the more prominent ear for grafting.

(continued on next page)

Table 3
(continued)

Complication	Discussed Material
Latera implant	Risks, benefits, and indications discussed. Risks include abscess, implant protrusion, facial pain/discomfort, and failure to absorb. Treatment of these complications include antibiotics, steroid injections, and even removal of implant
Rhinoplasty video	Patient did review Dr Nassif's video on rhinoplasty complications, expected postoperative healing/course, and need for 3 y for full healing

times, the balance has shifted between which technique predominates. I have always been enamored with the simplicity and minimal invasiveness of endonasal rhinoplasty, as I think there are fewer risks of various healing complications—and I subscribe to Bobby Simons' thinking that it should be termed "endonasal rhinoplasty" rather than "closed rhinoplasty," since the word "closed" connotes a lack of visibility, and the reality is that with endonasal rhinoplasty, the surgeon is afforded excellent visualization of the important structures. On the other hand, I have also always been enamored with the precision, beauty, and outstanding results that so many external rhinoplasty teachers and leaders promoted and demonstrated. I have tried to emulate surgery from the masters of both endonasal and external rhinoplasty schools and have found that in the right patient, and with the right technical maneuvers, both surgical approaches allow for outstanding results. Over the past 2+ years, I have continued to favor endonasal approaches to rhinoplasty, and I incorporate the many lessons of external structural rhinoplasty to the endonasal approach.[59] The "Cottle rhinoplasty technique," which in the most recent 5 years has been categorized as a "preservation rhinoplasty" technique, is originally an endonasal operation that combines the most important aspects of functional rhinological surgery with modifications to nasal shape. I continue to perform this operation through the endonasal approach primarily, and I predict that over the next 5 to 10 years, there will be a significant shift toward more frequent use of endonasal rhinoplasty and likely also more Cottle and other preservation techniques. It seems to me that the minimally invasive nature of the operation, and the application of fundamental rhinological and structural grafting principles, allows for reduced complications and faster healing.

Sykes

As surgeons gain more experience, their clinical recognition of and suspicion for possible complications increase. If conditions exist preoperatively that increase the risk of perioperative infection postrhinoplasty, a protocol should exist to minimize the incidence of infection and/or skin compromise. This may consist of the following interventions:

- Perioperative oral antibiotics
- Perioperative topical antibiotics (ointment)
- Perioperative hyperbaric oxygen treatments
- Intraoperative antibiotic irrigations

SUMMARY

The following descriptions summarize common rhinoplasty complications.

Asymmetries and Irregularities

It is critical to perform careful preoperative nasal analysis to note and discuss existing baseline asymmetries and irregularities. Patients are often hypercritical in analyzing their noses postoperatively, so they may notice and be bothered by a pre-existing asymmetry that they had not previously noted. The surgeon should have a very detailed discussion with their patient about which of these imperfections can and will be modified intraoperatively and which cannot be altered. Examples include hemifacial microsomia and differences in alar base height, midface projection, and eyebrow position and height. Additionally, there may be inherent differences in the underlying bony and cartilaginous framework. For example, nasal bones may be oblique or vertical, there may be asymmetric prominence or configuration of cartilages. The baseline imperfections are often more extreme with revision rhinoplasty. We always counsel our patients that asymmetries, contour irregularities, and imperfections will persist postoperatively.

To minimize the appearance of any contour irregularities, we take care intraoperatively to smooth out apparent irregularities of the underlying bony and cartilaginous framework. Unless a patient has extremely thick nasal skin, most irregularities that are visible in the framework will also be visible percutaneously once the nasal skin envelope swelling subsides. We routinely use DCGGs to create smooth contours and to decrease the chance of visible irregularities.

Overcorrection and Undercorrection

The preoperative consultation is key in defining the esthetic goals of surgery. The authors routinely create simulations of patient photos while their patients are present to show the proposed changes are. The authors also create a nasal diagram that specifies surgical maneuvers and highlights exact location of planned cartilaginous grafts that is reviewed with each patient preoperatively. These steps provide patients with an opportunity to evaluate proposed changes and to work together with the surgeon so that the final goals and vision of reconstruction are aligned. A PowerPoint slideshow is created for each patient, which includes preoperative photos of the nose from all views and the computer-morphed images; the slideshow is displayed on a screen intraoperatively. On the operative bed, photos are then taken prior to incision and at the conclusion of the case (before extubating). The on-the-table result is carefully analyzed by the surgeon to confirm that the desired result was achieved. If any modification is made, a new set of photos is taken and again critically analyzed prior to the conclusion of the surgery. The authors note that these additional steps have decreased the rate of revision surgery and has led to increased patient satisfaction.

Bleeding

Bleeding is a common complication during rhinoplasty. Excessive bleeding particularly from osteotomy sites or along the maxillary crest can lead to septal hematoma, pollybeak deformity, and excessive ecchymosis of the soft tissues. Preoperative administration of tranexemic acid is safe and may decrease bleeding, edema, and ecchymosis in patients undergoing rhinoplasty.[1] Meticulous hemostasis intraoperatively is important to minimize the chance of hematoma formation. If a small perforation is not created accidentally while elevating the mucoperichodrial flaps during the septoplasty, then it is recommended to create a small opening in one of the flaps to ensure there is a path of egress for any blood that may be accumulated between the flaps. Also, temporary application of manual pressure over the osteotomy sites may prevent significant ecchymosis and edema at the osteotomy sites.

Infection

See "Question 1: Infections? How to Diagnose and Treat Them?" section.

Poor Wound Healing and Skin Compromise or Necrosis

Poor wound healing may result due to pre-existing conditions, technical error, and/or complications that arise during surgery. Control of comorbidities preoperatively can significantly decrease the likelihood of skin compromise after rhinoplasty. Patients with a history of nicotine use should be counseled on the additional risk this carries for wound breakdown and skin necrosis. Smokers are instructed to avoid all nicotine-containing products (including gum and patches) at least 6 weeks prior to surgery and continue to abstain perioperatively and postoperatively. The authors routinely perform urine nicotine testing preoperatively to confirm patient adherence to protocol. Diabetic patients should optimize their blood glucose prior to proceeding with rhinoplasty, as elevated blood glucose levels can increase the chance of poor wound healing and infection.

Care must be taken to carefully reapproximate tissue during closure to minimize the chance of widened scar or dehiscence. Dehiscence along suture lines may increase the chance of postoperative infection. Patients with a history of multiple prior nasal surgeries or previous dermal filler injections to the nose should be counseled regarding potential for postoperative complications. Preoperative hyperbaric oxygen therapy should be considered in smokers and those with a history of prior skin compromise.

The risk of skin compromise or, in extreme cases, skin necrosis is significantly higher in revision rhinoplasty surgery. This is due to decreased blood supply to the nasal tip, potential prior defatting of the skin envelope, possible prior infections, and scar tissue.

Nasal Airway Obstruction

Every patient should be evaluated for nasal airway obstruction preoperatively. If present, it is important to assess and understand the contributing factors including external nasal valve collapse, internal nasal valve collapse, and nasal septal deviation. As part of the preoperative discussion with patients, we often highlight the general principle that aggressive reduction rhinoplasty (in an effort to create a smaller nose) may destabilize major and minor tip support structures. Aggressive reduction rhinoplasty often leads to nasal airway obstruction in the postoperative period, sometimes progressing years after the surgery. As such, we maintain structural rhinoplasty principles.

CLINICS CARE POINTS

- Aside from meticulous surgical technique and planning, the best way to prevent complications is to counsel patients on pre-operative and post-operative expectations.

- When compliations arise, frequent follow up is recommended.

DISCLOSURE

The authors declare that there is no relevant conflict of interest. The authors declare that there is no funding support.

REFERENCES

1. Bulut OC, Wallner F, Oladokun D, et al. Long-term quality of life changes after primary septorhinoplasty. Qual Life Res 2018;27(4):987–91.
2. Naraghi M, Atari M. Development and validation of the expectations of aesthetic rhinoplasty scale. Arch Plast Surg 2016;43(4):365–70.
3. Talmadge J, High R, Heckman WW. Comparative outcomes in functional rhinoplasty with open vs endonasal spreader graft placement. Ann Plast Surg 2018;80(5):468–71.
4. East C, Badia L, Marsh D, et al. Measuring patient-reported outcomes in rhinoplasty using the FACE-Q: a single site study. Facial Plast Surg 2017;33(5):461–9.
5. Plastic Surgery Statistics Report. 2020. Available at: https://www.plasticsurgery.org/documents/News/Statistics/2020/plastic-surgery-statistics-full-report-2020.pdf.
6. Irvine LE, Azizzadeh B, Kerulos JL, et al. Outcomes of a treatment protocol for compromised nasal skin in primary and revision open rhinoplasty. Facial Plast Surg Aesthet Med 2021;23(2):118–25.
7. Kerolus JL, Nassif PS. Correcting bad results in facial plastic surgery. Facial Plast Surg Clin North Am 2019;27(4):xv.
8. Kerolus JL, Nassif PS. Treatment protocol for compromised nasal skin. Facial Plast Surg Clin North Am 2019;27(4):505–11.
9. Nassif PS. Male revision rhinoplasty: pearls and surgical techniques. Facial Plast Surg 2005;21(4):250–70.
10. Nassif PS, Lee KJ. Asian rhinoplasty. Facial Plast Surg Clin North Am 2010;18(1):153–71.
11. Peng GL, Nassif PS. Rhinoplasty in the African American patient: anatomic considerations and technical pearls. Clin Plast Surg 2016;43(1):255–64.
12. Shtraks JP, Peng GL, Nassif PS. Utilization of leech therapy after rhinoplasty. Plast Reconstr Surg 2022;149(6):1090e–5e.
13. Wilkins SG, Sheth AH, Kayastha D, et al. Adverse events associated with bioabsorbable nasal implants: A MAUDE database analysis. Otolaryngol Head Neck Surg 2023;168(5):1253–7.
14. Yoo DB, Peng GL, Azizzadeh B, et al. Microbiology and antibiotic prophylaxis in rhinoplasty: a review of 363 consecutive cases. JAMA Facial Plast Surg 2015;17(1):23–7.
15. Sharif-Askary B, Carlson AR, Van Noord MG, et al. Incidence of postoperative adverse events after rhinoplasty: a systematic review. Plast Reconstr Surg 2020;145(3):669–84.
16. Kim SH, Tan KL, Lee SY, et al. Effect of chlorhexidine pretreatment on bacterial contamination at rhinoplasty field. SpringerPlus 2016;5(1):2116.
17. Yoo DB, Peng GL, Azizzadeh B, et al. Microbiology and antibiotic prophylaxis in rhinoplasty: a review of 363 consecutive cases. JAMA Facial Plast Surg 2015;17(1):23–7.
18. Moon KC, Jung JE, Dhong ES, et al. Preoperative nasal swab culture: is it beneficial in preventing postoperative infection in complicated septorhinoplasty? Plast Reconstr Surg 2020;146(1):27e–34e.
19. Lawson W, Kessler S, Biller HF. Unusual and fatal complications of rhinoplasty. Arch Otolaryngol Chic Ill 1960 1983;109(3):164–9.
20. Salehi PP, Suhail-Sindhu T, Salehi P. Re: "Analysis of online videos on facial feminization surgery: what are patients watching on tiktok and youtube?" by ziltzer et al: concerns regarding proliferation of social media (especially tiktok) as a source of facial feminization surgery information. Facial Plast Surg Aesthet Med 2023;25(6):530.
21. Ozucer B, Yildirim YS, Veyseller B, et al. Effect of postrhinoplasty taping on postoperative edema and nasal draping: a randomized clinical trial. JAMA Facial Plast Surg 2016;18(3):157–63.
22. Vahidi N, Wang L, Peng GL, et al. Rhinoplasty for thick-skinned noses: a systematic review. Aesthetic Plast Surg 2023;47(5):2011–22.
23. Sakallioğlu Ö, Cingi C, Polat C, et al. Open versus closed septorhinoplasty approaches for postoperative edema and ecchymosis. J Craniofac Surg 2015;26(4):1334–7.
24. Kiliç C, Tuncel Ü, Cömert E, et al. Effect of the rhinoplasty technique and lateral osteotomy on periorbital edema and ecchymosis. J Craniofac Surg 2015;26(5):e430–3.
25. Kim JS, Kim SH, Hwang SH. Method of lateral osteotomy to reduce eyelid edema and ecchymosis after rhinoplasty: a meta-analysis. Laryngoscope 2021;131(1):54–8.
26. Gupta R, John J, Ranganathan N, et al. Outcomes of closed versus open rhinoplasty: a systematic review. Arch Plast Surg 2022;49(5):569–79.
27. Kim JS, Kim SH, Lee H, et al. Effects of periosteal elevation before lateral osteotomy in rhinoplasty: a meta-analysis of randomized controlled trials. Clin Exp Otorhinolaryngol 2020;13(3):268–73.
28. Mirza AA, Alandejani TA, Al-Sayed AA. Piezosurgery versus conventional osteotomy in rhinoplasty: A systematic review and meta-analysis. Laryngoscope 2020;130(5):1158–65.

29. Khajuria A, Krzak AM, Reddy RK, et al. Piezoelectric osteotomy versus conventional osteotomy in rhinoplasty: a systematic review and meta-analysis. Plast Reconstr Surg Glob Open 2022;10(11):e4673.

30. Kisel J, Khatib M, Cavale N. A comparison between piezosurgery and conventional osteotomies in rhinoplasty on post-operative oedema and ecchymosis: a systematic review. Aesthetic Plast Surg 2023;47(3):1144–54.

31. Hwang SH, Lee JH, Kim BG, et al. The efficacy of steroids for edema and ecchymosis after rhinoplasty: a meta-analysis. Laryngoscope 2015;125(1):92–8.

32. Wu TJ, Huang YL, Kang YN, et al. Comparing the efficacy of different steroids for rhinoplasty: A systematic review and network meta-analysis of randomized controlled trials. J Plast Reconstr Aesthetic Surg JPRAS 2023;84:121–31.

33. Patel A, Townsend AN, Gordon AR, et al. Comparing postoperative taping vs customized 3d splints for managing nasal edema after rhinoplasty. Plast Reconstr Surg Glob Open 2023;11(9):e5285.

34. Ezzat WH, Compton RA, Basa KC, et al. Reconstructive techniques for the saddle nose deformity in granulomatosis with polyangiitis: a systematic review. JAMA Otolaryngol Head Neck Surg 2017;143(5):507–12.

35. Congdon D, Sherris DA, Specks U, et al. Long-term follow-up of repair of external nasal deformities in patients with Wegener's granulomatosis. Laryngoscope 2002;112(4):731–7.

36. Lasso JM, La Cruz ED. Reconstruction of wegener granulomatosis nose deformity using fascia lata graft. J Craniofac Surg 2018;29(8):2179–81.

37. Salehi PP, Salehi P, Shtraks J, et al. Facial rejuvenation in a patient with granulomatosis with polyangiitistreatment protocol for compromised skin flap. J Craniofac Surg 2023;34(8):2453–4.

38. Knoedler S, Knoedler L, Wu M, et al. Incidence and risk factors of postoperative complications after rhinoplasty: a multi-institutional ACS-NSQIP analysis. J Craniofac Surg 2023;34(6):1722–6.

39. Chien L, Yver CM, Shohat S, et al. Predictors of success of endonasal septal perforation repair: a 10-year experience. Facial Plast Surg Aesthetic Med 2024;26(2):117–23.

40. Ishii LE, Tollefson TT, Basura GJ, et al. Clinical practice guideline: improving nasal form and function after rhinoplasty. Otolaryngol–Head Neck Surg 2017;156(2_suppl):S1–30.

41. Olds C, Spataro E, Li K, et al. Postoperative antibiotic use among patients undergoing functional facial plastic and reconstructive surgery. JAMA Facial Plast Surg 2019;21(6):491–7.

42. Kullar R, Frisenda J, Nassif PS. The more the merrier? should antibiotics be used for rhinoplasty and septorhinoplasty?-a review. Plast Reconstr Surg Glob Open 2018;6(10):e1972.

43. Toriumi DM, Kowalczyk DM, Cristel RT, et al. Evaluation of postoperative infection rates in 3084 rhinoplasty cases using antibiotic soaks and/or irrigations. Facial Plast Surg Aesthetic Med 2021;23(5):368–74.

44. Tran KN, Jang YJ. Incidence and predisposing factors of postoperative infection after rhinoplasty: A Single Surgeon's 16-Year Experience with 2630 Cases in an East Asian Population. Plast Reconstr Surg 2022;150(1):51e–9e.

45. Knackstedt R, Gatherwright J. Perioperative homeopathic arnica and bromelain: current results and future directions. Ann Plast Surg 2020;84(3):e10–5.

46. Courtiss EH, Goldwyn RM. The effects of nasal surgery on airflow. Plast Reconstr Surg 1983;72(1):9–21.

47. Luu NN, Friedman O. Septal deviation after septorhinoplsty: causes and surgical management. Facial Plast Surg 2020;36(1):72–7.

48. Friedman O, Cook TA. Conchal cartilage butterfly graft in primary functional rhinoplasty. Laryngoscope 2009;119(2):255–62.

49. Go BC, Frost A, Friedman O. Addressing the nasal valves: the endonasal approach. Facial Plast Surg 2022;38(1):57–65.

50. Saleh AM, Younes A, Friedman O. Cosmetics and function: quality-of-life changes after rhinoplasty surgery. Laryngoscope 2012;122(2):254–9.

51. Codazzi D, Ortelli L, Robotti E. Diced cartilage combined with warm blood glue for nasal dorsum enhancement. Aesthetic Plast Surg 2014;38(4):822–3.

52. Dong J, Luo X, Dong W. Crushed septal cartilage-covered diced cartilage glue (CCDG) graft: a hybrid technique of crushed septal cartilage. Aesthetic Plast Surg 2022;46(5):2623–4.

53. Swaroop GS, Reddy JS, Mangal MC, et al. Autogenous control augmentation system - A refinement in diced cartilage glue graft for augmentation of dorsum of nose. Indian J Plast Surg 2018;51(2):202–7.

54. Tasman AJ, Suárez GA. The diced cartilage glue graft for radix augmentation in rhinoplasty. JAMA Facial Plast Surg 2015;17(4):303–4.

55. Tasman AJ. Dorsal augmentation-diced cartilage techniques: the diced cartilage glue graft. Facial Plast Surg 2017;33(2):179–88.

56. Tasman AJ. Replacement of the nasal dorsum with a diced cartilage glue graft. Facial Plast Surg 2019;35(1):53–7.

57. Ferreira MG, Toriumi DM, Stubenitsky B, et al. Advanced preservation rhinoplasty in the era of osteoplasty and chondroplasty: how have we moved beyond the cottle technique? Aesthet Surg J 2023;43(12):1441–53.

58. Toriumi DM. My first twenty rhinoplasties using dorsal preservation techniques. Facial Plast Surg Clin North Am 2023;31(1):73–106.

59. Go BC, Frost AC, Friedman O. The use of endonasal spreader grafts in preservation rhinolplasty. Plast Reconstr Surg 2023;151(3):398e–401e.

UNITED STATES POSTAL SERVICE ®

Statement of Ownership, Management, and Circulation
(All Periodicals Publications Except Requester Publications)

1. Publication Title: FACIAL PLASTIC SURGERY CLINICS OF NORTH AMERICA

2. Publication Number: 013 – 122

3. Filing Date: 9/18/2024

4. Issue Frequency: FEB, MAY, AUG, NOV

5. Number of Issues Published Annually: 4

6. Annual Subscription Price: $432.00

7. Complete Mailing Address of Known Office of Publication (Not printer) (Street, city, county, state, and ZIP+4®)
ELSEVIER INC.
230 Park Avenue, Suite 800
New York, NY 10169

Contact Person: Malathi SAmayan
Telephone (include area code): 91-44-4299-4507

8. Complete Mailing Address of Headquarters or General Business Office of Publisher (Not printer)
ELSEVIER INC.
230 Park Avenue, Suite 800
New York, NY 10169

9. Full Names and Complete Mailing Addresses of Publisher, Editor, and Managing Editor (Do not leave blank)

Publisher (Name and complete mailing address)
Dolores Meloni, ELSEVIER INC.
1600 JOHN F KENNEDY BLVD. SUITE 1600
PHILADELPHIA, PA 19103-2899

Editor (Name and complete mailing address)
Stacy Eastman ELSEVIER INC.
1600 JOHN F KENNEDY BLVD. SUITE 1600
PHILADELPHIA, PA 19103-2899

Managing Editor (Name and complete mailing address)
PATRICK MANLEY, ELSEVIER INC.
1600 JOHN F KENNEDY BLVD. SUITE 1600
PHILADELPHIA, PA 19103-2899

10. Owner (Do not leave blank. If the publication is owned by a corporation, give the name and address of the corporation immediately followed by the names and addresses of all stockholders owning or holding 1 percent or more of the total amount of stock. If not owned by a corporation, give the names and addresses of the individual owners. If owned by a partnership or other unincorporated firm, give its name and address as well as those of each individual owner. If the publication is published by a nonprofit organization, give its name and address.)

Full Name	Complete Mailing Address
WHOLLY OWNED SUBSIDIARY OF REED/ELSEVIER, US HOLDINGS	1600 JOHN F KENNEDY BLVD. SUITE 1600 PHILADELPHIA, PA 19103-2899

11. Known Bondholders, Mortgagees, and Other Security Holders Owning or Holding 1 Percent or More of Total Amount of Bonds, Mortgages or Other Securities. If none, check box ☑ None

Full Name	Complete Mailing Address
N/A	

12. Tax Status (For completion by nonprofit organizations authorized to mail at nonprofit rates) (Check one)
The purpose, function, and nonprofit status of this organization and the exempt status for federal income tax purposes:
☒ Has Not Changed During Preceding 12 Months
☐ Has Changed During Preceding 12 Months (Publisher must submit explanation of change with this statement)

PS Form 3526, July 2014 [Page 1 of 4 (see instructions page 4)] PSN: 7530-01-000-9931 PRIVACY NOTICE: See our privacy policy on www.usps.com.

---

13. Publication Title: FACIAL PLASTIC SURGERY CLINICS OF NORTH AMERICA

14. Issue Date for Circulation Data Below: AUGUST 2024

15. Extent and Nature of Circulation

		Average No. Copies Each Issue During Preceding 12 Months	No. Copies of Single Issue Published Nearest to Filing Date
a. Total Number of Copies (Net press run)		172	141
b. Paid Circulation (By Mail and Outside the Mail)	(1) Mailed Outside-County Paid Subscriptions Stated on PS Form 3541 (Include paid distribution above nominal rate, advertiser's proof copies, and exchange copies)	129	92
	(2) Mailed In-County Paid Subscriptions Stated on PS Form 3541 (Include paid distribution above nominal rate, advertiser's proof copies, and exchange copies)	0	0
	(3) Paid Distribution Outside the Mails Including Sales Through Dealers and Carriers, Street Vendors, Counter Sales, and Other Paid Distribution Outside USPS®	19	18
	(4) Paid Distribution by Other Classes of Mail Through the USPS (e.g., First-Class Mail®)	7	10
c. Total Paid Distribution [Sum of 15b (1), (2), (3), and (4)]		155	120
d. Free or Nominal Rate Distribution (By Mail and Outside the Mail)	(1) Free or Nominal Rate Outside-County Copies included on PS Form 3541	16	20
	(2) Free or Nominal Rate In-County Copies included on PS Form 3541	0	0
	(3) Free or Nominal Rate Copies Mailed at Other Classes Through the USPS (e.g., First-Class Mail)	0	0
	(4) Free or Nominal Rate Distribution Outside the Mail (Carriers or other means)	1	1
e. Total Free or Nominal Rate Distribution (Sum of 15d (1), (2), (3) and (4))		17	21
f. Total Distribution (Sum of 15c and 15e)		172	141
g. Copies not Distributed (See Instructions to Publishers #4 (page #3))		0	0
h. Total (Sum of 15f and g)		172	141
i. Percent Paid (15c divided by 15f times 100)		90.1%	85.11%

* If you are claiming electronic copies, go to line 16 on page 3. If you are not claiming electronic copies, skip to line 17 on page 3.

16. Electronic Copy Circulation

	Average No. Copies Each Issue During Preceding 12 Months	No. Copies of Single Issue Published Nearest to Filing Date
a. Paid Electronic Copies		
b. Total Paid Print Copies (Line 15c) + Paid Electronic Copies (Line 16a)		
c. Total Print Distribution (Line 15f) + Paid Electronic Copies (Line 16a)		
d. Percent Paid (Both Print & Electronic Copies) (16b divided by 16c × 100)		

☒ I certify that 50% of all my distributed copies (electronic and print) are paid above a nominal price.

17. Publication of Statement of Ownership
☒ If the publication is a general publication, publication of this statement is required. Will be printed
in the __NOVEMBER 2024__ issue of this publication.
☐ Publication not required.

18. Signature and Title of Editor, Publisher, Business Manager, or Owner

Malathi Samayan

Malathi Samayan - Distribution Controller

Date: 9/18/2024

I certify that all information furnished on this form is true and complete. I understand that anyone who furnishes false or misleading information on this form or who omits material or information requested on the form may be subject to criminal sanctions (including fines and imprisonment) and/or civil sanctions (including civil penalties).

PS Form 3526, July 2014 (Page 3 of 4) PRIVACY NOTICE: See our privacy policy on www.usps.com